D1253741

HAND AND WRIST

ORTHOPAEDIC SURGERY ESSENTIALS

HAND AND WRIST

ORTHOPAEDIC SURGERY ESSENTIALS

Adult Reconstruction
Daniel J. Berry, MD
Scott P. Steinmann, MD

Foot and Ankle
David B. Thordarson, MD

Hand and Wrist
James R. Doyle, MD

Oncology and Basic Science
Timothy A. Damron, MD
Carol D. Morris, MD

Pediatrics
Kathryn E. Cramer, MD
Susan A. Scherl, MD

Spine
Christopher M. Bono, MD
Steven R. Garfin, MD

Sports Medicine
Anthony A. Schepsis, MD
Brian D. Busconi, MD

Trauma
Charles Court-Brown, MD
Margaret McQueen, MD
Paul Tornetta III, MD

ORTHOPAEDIC SURGERY ESSENTIALS

HAND AND WRIST

Series Editors

PAUL TORNETTA III, MD
Professor
Department of Orthopaedic Surgery
Boston University School of Medicine;
Director of Orthopaedic Trauma
Boston University Medical Center
Boston, Massachusetts

THOMAS A. EINHORN, MD
Professor and Chairman
Department of Orthopaedic Surgery
Boston University School of Medicine
Boston, Massachusetts

Author

JAMES R. DOYLE, MD
Emeritus Professor of Surgery (Orthopaedics)
John A. Burns School of Medicine
University of Hawaii
Honolulu, Hawaii

DREXEL UNIVERSITY
HEALTH SCIENCES LIBRARIES
HAHNEMANN LIBRARY

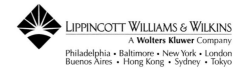
LIPPINCOTT WILLIAMS & WILKINS
A **Wolters Kluwer** Company
Philadelphia • Baltimore • New York • London
Buenos Aires • Hong Kong • Sydney • Tokyo

Acquisitions Editor: Bob Hurley
Developmental Editor: Grace Caputo, Dovetail Content Solutions
Managing Editor: Michelle LaPlante
Project Manager: Nicole Walz
Senior Manufacturing Manager: Ben Rivera
Marketing Director: Sharon Zinner
Design Coordinator: Holly Reid McLaughlin
Cover Designer: Andrew Gatto
Compositor: TechBooks
Printer: Edwards Brothers

WE
39
H235
2006

© 2006 by LIPPINCOTT WILLIAMS & WILKINS
530 Walnut Street
Philadelphia, PA 19106 USA
LWW.com

All rights reserved. This book is protected by copyright. No part of this book may be reproduced in any form or by any means, including photocopying, or utilized by any information storage and retrieval system without written permission from the copyright owner, except for brief quotations embodied in critical articles and reviews. Materials appearing in this book prepared by individuals as part of their official duties as U.S. government employees are not covered by the above-mentioned copyright.

Printed in the USA.

Library of Congress Cataloging-in-Publication Data
Hand and wrist / book editor, James R. Doyle.
     p. ; cm.—(Orthopaedic surgery essentials)
   Includes bibliographical references and index.
   ISBN 0-7817-5146-2 (case)
   1. Hand–Surgery. 2. Wrist–Surgery. 3. Orthopedic surgery.   I. Doyle, James R. II. Series.
      [DNLM: 1. Hand–surgery–Handbooks. 2. Hand Injuries–surgery–Handbooks. 3. Wrist–surgery–Handbooks. 4. Wrist Injuries–surgery–Handbooks. WE 39 H235 2005] RD559.H35725
   2005 617.5′75–dc22

2005016072

Care has been taken to confirm the accuracy of the information presented and to describe generally accepted practices. However, the authors, editors, and publisher are not responsible for errors or omissions or for any consequences from application of the information in this book and make no warranty, expressed or implied, with respect to the currency, completeness, or accuracy of the contents of the publication. Application of this information in a particular situation remains the professional responsibility of the practitioner.

The authors, editors, and publisher have exerted every effort to ensure that drug selection and dosage set forth in this text are in accordance with current recommendations and practice at the time of publication. However, in view of ongoing research, changes in government regulations, and the constant flow of information relating to drug therapy and drug reactions, the reader is urged to check the package insert for each drug for any change in indications and dosage and for added warnings and precautions. This is particularly important when the recommended agent is a new or infrequently employed drug.

Some drugs and medical devices presented in this publication have Food and Drug Administration (FDA) clearance for limited use in restricted research settings. It is the responsibility of the health care provider to ascertain the FDA status of each drug or device planned for use in their clinical practice.

To purchase additional copies of this book, call our customer service department at (800) 638-3030 or fax orders to (301) 824-7390. International customers should call (301) 714-2324.

Visit Lippincott Williams & Wilkins on the Internet: http://www.LWW.com. Lippincott Williams & Wilkins customer service representatives are available from 8:30 am to 6:00 pm, EST.

10 9 8 7 6 5 4 3 2 1

This textbook is dedicated to the orthopaedic teaching staff of the John A. Burns School of Medicine at the University of Hawaii. It is dedicated to the memory of the illustrious past chairs of the Division of Orthopaedics, Ivar Larson and Allen Richardson, as well as a living emeritus chair, friend, and mentor, Lawrence Gordon.

It is dedicated to the memory of those outstanding teachers, Eugene Lance and Alan Pavel, who taught all of us the value of scholarship and excellence in surgery.

It is dedicated to those who continue the tradition of excellence in teaching, Robert Atkinson, Daniel Singer, John Smith, and all those who continue to give their time and energy to the advancement of the orthopaedic residency training program at the University of Hawaii.

It is dedicated to those who made the paths to excellence straight and level in so many ways, including Albert Chun Hoon, Tom Whelan, Ruth Ono, Sue Arakaki Harada and Tori Marciel.

It is dedicated to my residents—they taught me more than they will ever know.

CONTENTS

SECTION I: BASIC ANATOMY

SECTION II: OUTPATIENT CLINIC

SECTION III: EMERGENCY DEPARTMENT

CONTRIBUTING AUTHORS

Kevin Cunningham, MD
Attending Anesthesiologist
McGuire Veterans Administration Hospital
Richmond, Virginia

Charles L. McDowell, MD
Clinical Professor of Orthopaedic
  and Plastic (Hand) Surgery
Medical College of Virginia
Chief of Hand Surgery Service
McGuire Veterans Administration Hospital
Richmond, Virginia

SERIES PREFACE

Most of the available resources in orthopaedic surgery are very good, but they either present information exhaustively—so the reader has to wade through too many details to find what he or she seeks—or they assume too much knowledge, making the information difficult to understand. Moreover, as residency training has advanced, it has become more focused on the individual subspecialties. Our goal was to create a series at the basic level that residents could read completely during a subspecialty rotation to obtain the essential information necessary for a general understanding of the field. Once they have survived those trials, we hope that the *Orthopaedic Surgery Essentials* books will serve as a touchstone for future learning and review.

Each volume is to be a manageable size that can be read during a resident's tour. As a series, they will have a consistent style and template, with the authors' voices heard throughout. Content will be presented more visually than in most books on orthopaedic surgery, with a liberal use of tables, boxes, bulleted lists, and algorithms to aid in quick review. Each topic will be covered by one or more authorities, and each volume will be edited by experts in the broader field.

But most importantly, each volume—*Pediatrics, Spine, Sports Medicine*, and so on—will focus on the requisite knowledge in orthopaedics. Having the essential information presented in one user-friendly source will provide the reader with easy access to the basic knowledge needed in the field; mastering this content will give him or her an excellent foundation for additional information from comprehensive references, atlases, journals, and online resources.

We would like to thank the editors and contributors who have generously shared their knowledge. We hope that the reader will tell us what works and does not work.

—Paul Tornetta III, MD
—Thomas A. Einhorn, MD

PREFACE

This volume is part of a series of focused and concise textbook reviews designed to facilitate the learning process for orthopaedic residents as they rotate through various subspecialty services in their training. I hope it will serve as a tool that will facilitate the rapid acquisition of knowledge so that the time spent on an upper extremity service will be as productive as possible. The concise information in this text may also be useful to residents in plastic surgery and general surgery as well as other disciplines that may be involved in care of the hand and wrist.

My aim was to cover basic core concepts and facts that will act as building blocks or starting points for the development of the reader's own knowledge base of hand and wrist care. Please note that this text is not designed to be a comprehensive work on the hand and wrist but rather an illustrated guide and outline that will give the reader an overview of the field.

Much of the content reflects the work of friends and mentors, colleagues, authors, professional organizations, and publishers that have generously shared their knowledge of both published and unpublished work. References are not cited in the text, and the Suggested Reading list may give only a hint of the sources of the material utilized or presented by the writer. These lists are at the end of each chapter, and are intended to expand on the basic information presented in the chapter but are not intended to represent a comprehensive bibliography.

I made every effort to ensure that all these contributions (either reproduced or modified) have been recognized. I owe a great debt to my past and present mentors and colleagues for my own knowledge base and hope that any failure to source appropriated concepts or facts will be considered an unintentional oversight.

Textbooks require a joint effort. I thus am indebted to Executive Editor Robert Hurley at Lippincott Williams & Wilkins for his dedication to excellence and patient and professional guidance, and to Grace Caputo, of Dovetail Content Solutions, who saw me through this process in such a delightful and professional manner. I am also indebted to my long-time friend and colleague, Charles McDowell, who wrote the chapter on anesthesia techniques. It was Dr. McDowell who suggested that a text such as this would be useful for residents. I greatly appreciate his support and encouragement before and during the writing of this textbook. Last, but certainly not least, I wish to express my gratitude to Elizabeth Roselius for her skillful interpretations of my many sketches and for her excellent depictions of important points of anatomy and technique.

Finally, I would like a parting word with the residents who are the most likely readers of this text. Your residency years may be akin to the classic words that Charles Dickens wrote in the opening of his book about the French Revolution, *A Tale of Two Cities:* "It was the best of times. It was the worst of times." After your passage through this experience you will—as most have done— look back on it as the best time or experience of your life. Find joy and meaning in your passage. Remember that your learning process is based on the gift of knowledge given to you by colleagues who have gone before you. Appreciate and respect that knowledge, use it wisely, challenge it when needed, and add to it at every opportunity.

—James R. Doyle, MD

HAND AND WRIST

ANATOMY

1.1 SURFACE ANATOMY

The most appropriate starting point is the hand's surface anatomy. Much can be learned about the deeper structures in the hand by correlating external landmarks such as skin creases and eminences to underlying anatomic structures.

PALMAR HAND

External Landmarks

The landmarks of the palmar side of the hand are depicted in Figure 1.1-1. These landmarks are identified by inspection of the skin creases and eminences, and by palpation for the bony landmarks of the pisiform and the hook process of the hamate bone.

Flexion Creases

The wrist, thenar, palmar, and digital flexion creases are skin flexion lines seen near synovial joints. These creases provide "folding points" in the skin, similar to the creases in a road map. Two creases are present over the proximal interphalangeal (PIP) joints, which account for the increased angles of flexion at these joints. By comparison, only one crease is found adjacent to the metacarpophalangeal (MCP) and distal interphalangeal (DIP) joints. Flexion creases are usually at right angles to the long axis of the metacarpals and phalanges, and parallel to the flexion-extension joint axis of motion. The pronounced obliquity of the thenar crease reflects the opposing movement of the thumb. It must be noted, however, that only one of the 17 creases (the thumb MCP joint) lies directly over the joint. Look at your own hand and note that the MCP flexion crease lies at the midpoint between the MCP and PIP joints.

Figure 1.1-2 depicts the relationship between these various skin creases and the underlying joints, and will allow you to locate the underlying joint structures with a high degree of confidence.

Thenar and Hypothenar Eminences

The thenar eminence is formed by the abductor pollicis brevis (APB), the most superficial of the thenar group, and the flexor pollicis brevis (FPB). Both overlie the deeper opponens pollicis (OP). The ulnar-sided counterpart of the thenar eminence is the hypothenar eminence, which is formed by the abductor and flexor digiti minimi (ADM, FDM) and the opponens digiti minimi (ODM).

Bony Landmarks

Pisiform Bone
This relatively superficial and easily palpated carpal bone is located on the ulnar side of the base of the hand, and it aids in the identification of the flexor carpi ulnaris (FCU) tendon, the underlying ulnar neurovascular bundle, and the more distal and radial hook process of the hamate bone.

Hook Process of the Hamate Bone
This process of the hamate may be palpated approximately 2 cm distal and 1 cm radial to the more prominent pisiform. It marks the beginning of the oblique course of the motor branch of the ulnar nerve.

Relationship of the Superficial Landmarks and the Deeper Structures

A unique system of lines may be drawn on the hand that will permit the examiner to accurately locate the underlying deeper structures. These lines and the underlying structures are depicted in Figure 1.1-3.

DORSAL HAND

External Landmarks

The external landmarks on the dorsum of the hand are illustrated in Figure 1.1-4.

1

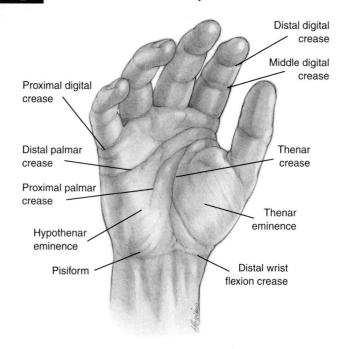

Figure 1.1-1   Landmarks of the palmar hand.

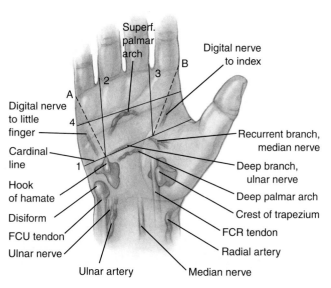

Figure 1.1-3   Kaplan described a unique system of lines that may be drawn on the palmar side of the hand and that coincide with the underlying structures.

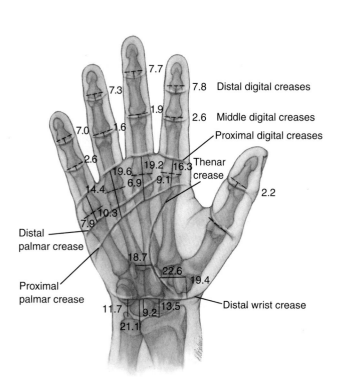

Figure 1.1-2   Wrist, thenar, palmar, and digital skin flexion creases and their relationship to the underlying joints and bones.

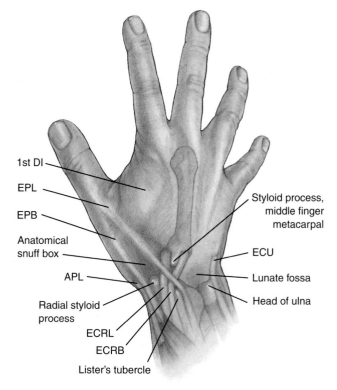

Figure 1.1-4   Landmarks on the dorsal hand.

Bony Landmarks

Lister's Tubercle

This bony landmark is located about 0.5 cm proximal to the dorsal articular margin of the distal radius, in line with the cleft between the index and middle finger metacarpals. It is easily palpated and marks the fulcrum, or turning point, for the extensor pollicis longus (EPL) tendon on its way to the terminal phalanx of the thumb. It lies in a groove just ulnar to Lister's tubercle. The extensor carpi radial brevis (ECRB) tendon is just radial to Lister's tubercle in a similar groove on the distal aspect of the radius.

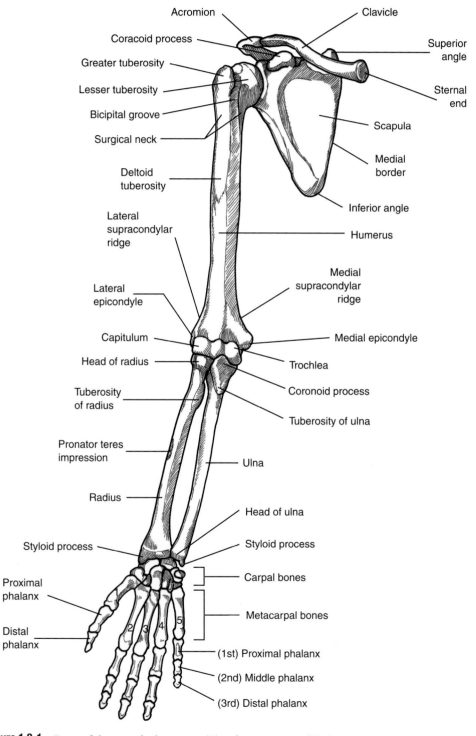

Figure 1.2-1   Bones of the upper limb: anterior (**A**) and posterior view (**B**). *Figure continues.*

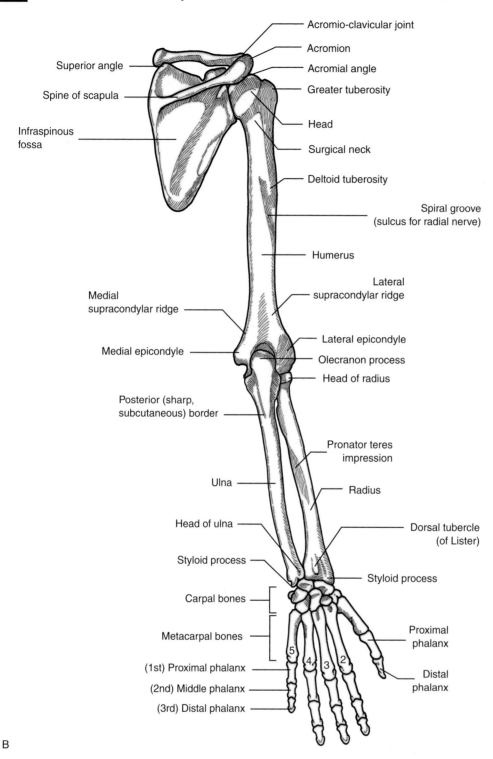

Acromio-clavicular joint
Acromion
Acromial angle
Greater tuberosity
Head
Surgical neck
Deltoid tuberosity
Spiral groove
(sulcus for radial nerve)
Superior angle
Spine of scapula
Infraspinous
fossa
Humerus
Lateral
supracondylar ridge
Medial
supracondylar ridge
Medial epicondyle
Lateral epicondyle
Olecranon process
Head of radius
Posterior (sharp,
subcutaneous) border
Pronator teres
impression
Ulna
Radius
Head of ulna
Dorsal tubercle
(of Lister)
Styloid process
Styloid process
Carpal bones
Metacarpal bones
Proximal
phalanx
Distal
phalanx
(1st) Proximal phalanx
(2nd) Middle phalanx
(3rd) Distal phalanx

B

Figure 1.2-1 (*continued*)

Styloid Process of the Middle Finger Metacarpal

The styloid process of the middle finger metacarpal is located on the metacarpal's dorsal and radial base. It points to the articular interface between the capitate and the trapezoid, and is just proximal to the point of insertion of the ECRB tendon.

Radial Styloid

This distal projection of the radial side of the radius forms a visible and easily examined landmark that is palpable both palmar and dorsal to the abductor pollicis longus (APL) and extensor pollicis brevis (EPB) tendons that run across its apex.

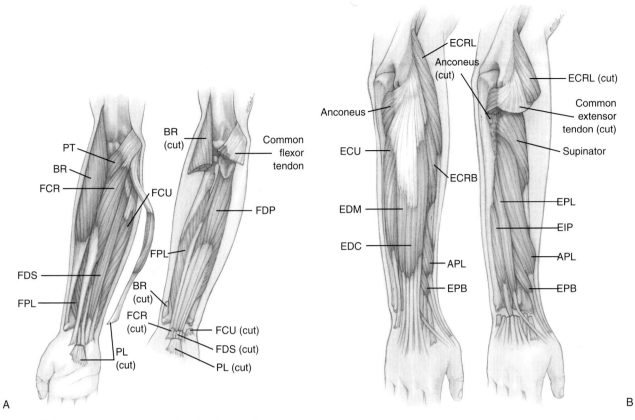

Figure 1.2-2 (**A**) Flexor forearm muscles. (**B**) Extensor forearm muscles.

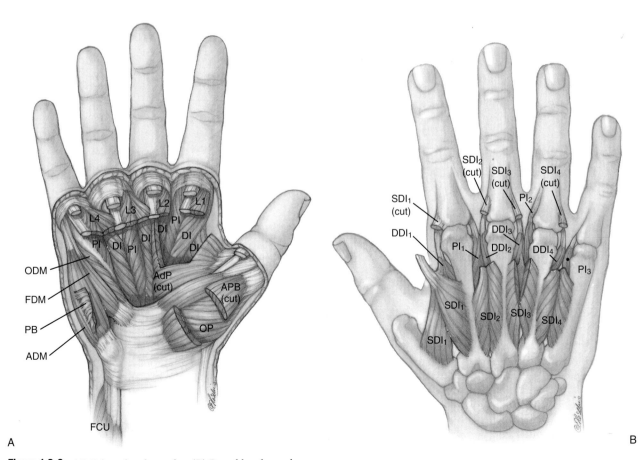

Figure 1.2-3 (**A**) Palmar hand muscles. (**B**) Dorsal hand muscles.

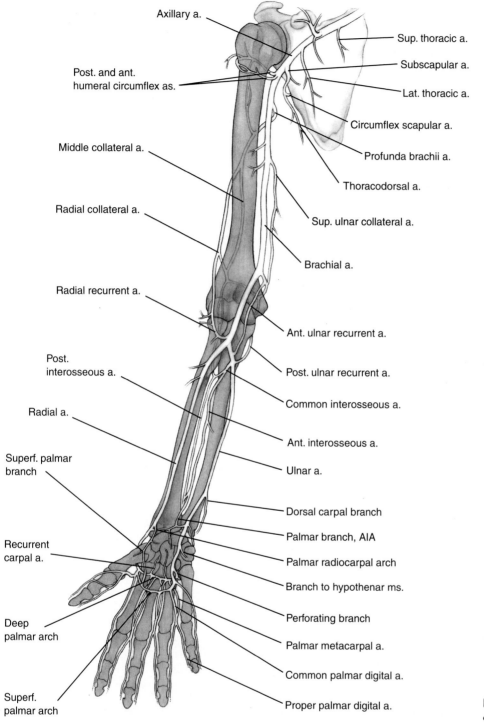

Axillary a.

Sup. thoracic a.

Subscapular a.

Post. and ant.
humeral circumflex as.

Lat. thoracic a.

Circumflex scapular a.

Middle collateral a.

Profunda brachii a.

Thoracodorsal a.

Radial collateral a.

Sup. ulnar collateral a.

Brachial a.

Radial recurrent a.

Ant. ulnar recurrent a.

Post.
interosseous a.

Post. ulnar recurrent a.

Common interosseous a.

Radial a.

Ant. interosseous a.

Superf. palmar
branch

Ulnar a.

Dorsal carpal branch

Palmar branch, AIA

Recurrent
carpal a.

Palmar radiocarpal arch

Branch to hypothenar ms.

Perforating branch

Deep
palmar arch

Palmar metacarpal a.

Common palmar digital a.

Superf.
palmar arch

Proper palmar digital a.

Figure 1.2-4   Arteries of the upper
extremity.

Distal Head of the Ulna

The distal aspect of the ulna is slightly expanded and contains a head and a comparatively small styloid process. The head is most noticeable and prominent when the forearm is pronated. The short styloid process is a rounded dorsoulnar projection from the ulnar head that is most palpable in supination, and is about 1 cm proximal to the plane of the radial styloid. The apex of the triangular fibrocartilage attaches to the palmar-radial base of the styloid process. The

extensor carpi ulnaris (ECU) tendon runs in a groove along the dorsal aspect of the ulnar head.

Other Dorsal Landmarks

Anatomic Snuff Box

This depression on the radial side of the wrist is a narrow triangle with its apex distal that is bordered dorsoulnarly by the EPL, radially by the abductor pollicis longus (APL),

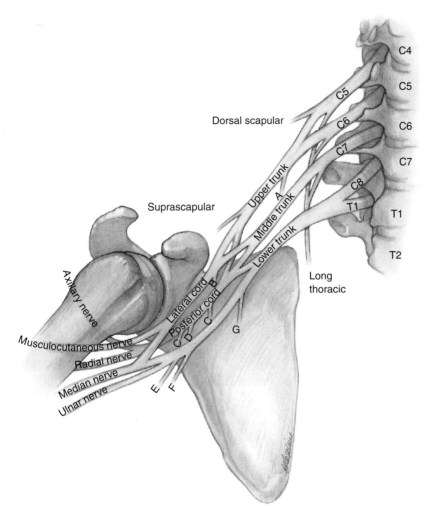

Figure 1.2-5   Schematic illustration of the brachial plexus, associated major branches, peripheral branches and muscles they innervate. A, nerve to subclavius; B, lateral pectoral nerve; C, subscapular nerve; D, thoracodorsal nerve; E, medial antebrachial cutaneous nerve; F, medial brachial cutaneous nerve; G, medial pectoral nerve.

and extensor pollicis brevis (EPB) tendons, and proximally by the distal margin of the extensor retinaculum. It contains the dorsal branch of the radial artery; in its dorsoulnar corner, the tendon of the extensor carpi radialis longus (ECRL); and superficially, one or more branches of the superficial branch of the radial nerve. The carpal scaphoid bone lies beneath this fossa and tenderness in this area following trauma may indicate an injury of this bone.

Lunate Fossa
The lunate fossa is a palpable central depression located on the dorsum of the wrist, in line with the longitudinal axis of the third metacarpal just ulnar and distal to Lister's tubercle, and beginning immediately distal to the dorsal margin of the radius. It is, on average, approximately the size of the pulp of your thumb, and it marks the location of the carpal lunate in the proximal carpal row.

1.2 SYSTEMS ANATOMY

The following figures and discussion represent and are designed to provide an overall perspective on the deeper anatomy—the skeletal, muscular, vascular, and neural anatomy—of the upper extremity. The perspective spans from the shoulder and neck for discussions of the skeletal, neural, and vascular anatomy, and from the elbow for the muscular system.

SKELETAL ANATOMY

The osseous structures of the upper limb include the humerus, the radius and ulna, eight carpal bones, five metacarpals, and 14 phalanges. The upper extremity skeleton is depicted in Figure 1.2-1.

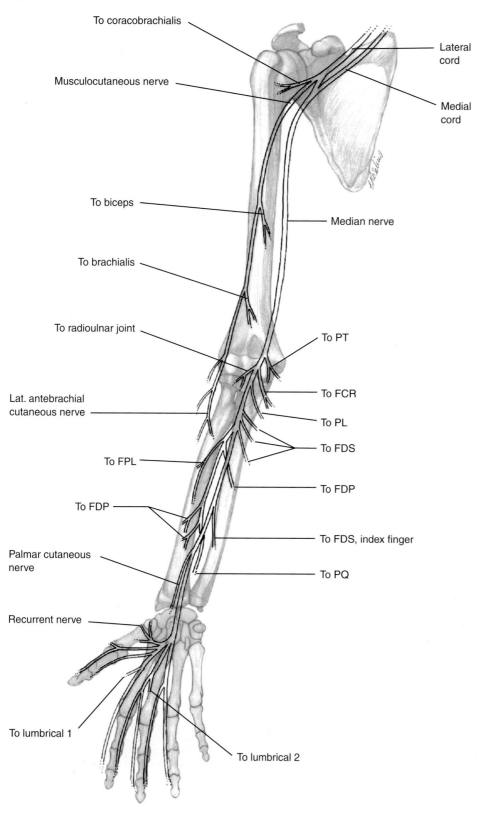

To coracobrachialis

Musculocutaneous nerve

Lateral cord

Medial cord

To biceps

Median nerve

To brachialis

To radioulnar joint

To PT

To FCR

Lat. antebrachial cutaneous nerve

To PL

To FDS

To FPL

To FDP

To FDP

To FDS, index finger

Palmar cutaneous nerve

To PQ

Recurrent nerve

To lumbrical 1

To lumbrical 2

Figure 1.2-5 (*continued*)

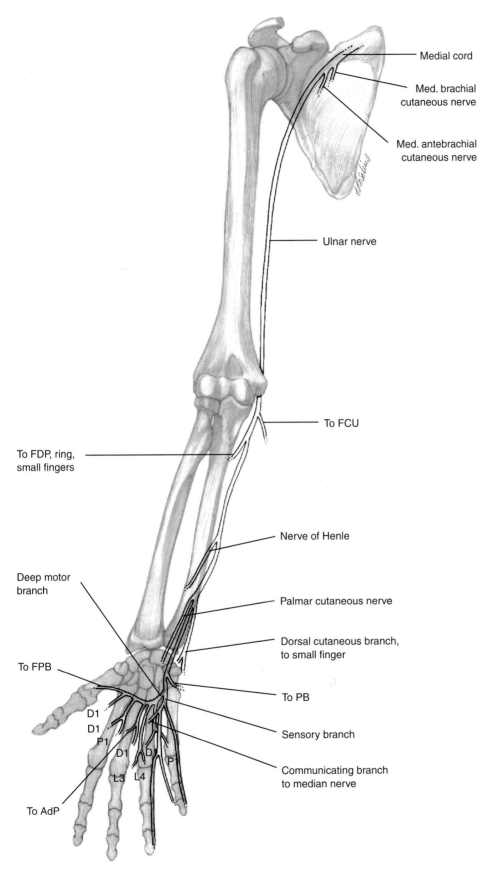

Medial cord

Med. brachial
cutaneous nerve

Med. antebrachial
cutaneous nerve

Ulnar nerve

To FCU

To FDP, ring,
small fingers

Nerve of Henle

Deep motor
branch

Palmar cutaneous nerve

Dorsal cutaneous branch,
to small finger

To FPB

To PB

D1
D1
P1

Sensory branch

D1   D
L3   L4
P1

Communicating branch
to median nerve

To AdP

Figure 1.2-5 (*continued*)

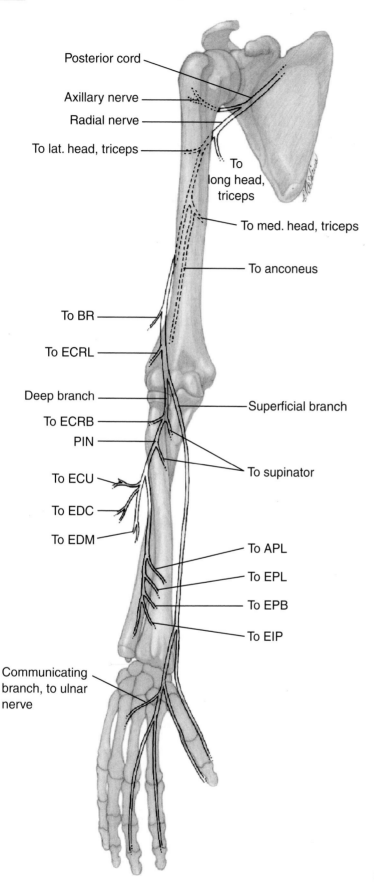

Posterior cord

Axillary nerve

Radial nerve

To lat. head, triceps

To long head, triceps

To med. head, triceps

To anconeus

To BR

To ECRL

Deep branch

Superficial branch

To ECRB

PIN

To supinator

To ECU

To EDC

To EDM

To APL

To EPL

To EPB

To EIP

Communicating branch, to ulnar nerve

Figure 1.2-5 (*continued*)

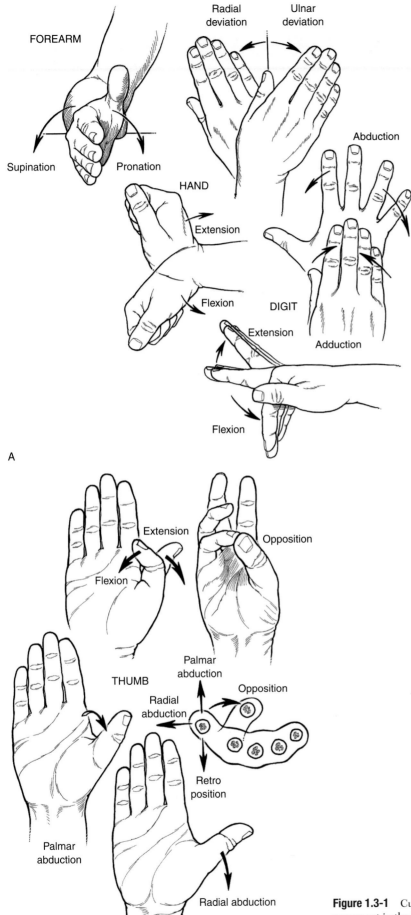

Figure 1.3-1 Currently accepted terminology and depiction of movement in the forearm, wrist, fingers: wrist, forearm (**A**), thumb (**B**).

TABLE 1.3-1 ANATOMIC BASIS FOR MOVEMENT IN THE UPPER EXTREMITY

Joint/Motion	Muscle	Nerve	Root
Elbow			
Flexion	Brachialis	Musculocutaneous	C5+C6+C7
	Biceps	Musculocutaneous	C5+C6
Extension	Triceps	Radial	C6+C7+C8
Forearm			
Supination	Biceps	Musculocutaneous	C5+C6
	Supinator	Radial	C7+C8
Pronation	Pronator teres	Median	C6+C7
	Pronator quadratus	Anterior interosseous branch of median	C7+C8
Wrist			
Flexion	Flexor carpi radialis	Median	C6+C7
	Flexor carpi ulnaris	Ulnar	C7+C8+T1
Extension	Extensor carpi radialis longus	Radial	C6+C7
	Extensor carpi radialis brevis	Radial	C7+C8
	Extensor carpi ulnaris	Radial	C7+C8
Finger MCP			
Flexion	Medial two lumbricals	Ulnar	C8+T1
	Lateral two lumbricals	Median	C8+T1
Extension	Extensor digitorum communis, extensor indicis, extensor digiti minimi	Posterior interosseous of radial	C7+C8
Abduction	Dorsal interossei*	Ulnar	C8+T1
	Abductor digiti minimi	Ulnar	C8+T1
Adduction	Palmar interossei*	Ulnar	C8+T1
Finger PIP			
Flexion	Flexor digitorum superficialis	Median	C8+T1
Extension	Extensor digitorum communis, extensor indicis, extensor digiti minimi	Posterior interosseous of radial	C7+C8
Finger DIP			
Flexion	Flexor digitorum profundus	Ulnar; anterior interosseous of median	C8+T1
Extension	Extensor digitorum communis, extensor indicis, extensor digiti minimi	Posterior interosseous of radial	C7+C8
Thumb			
Palmar abduction	Abductor pollicis longus	Radial	C7+C8
	Abductor pollicis brevis	Median	C8+T1
Dorsal adduction	Adductor pollicis	Ulnar	C8+T1
Thumb MCP			
Flexion	Flexor pollicis brevis deep head	Ulnar	C8+T1
	Flexor pollicis brevis superficial head	Median	C8+T1
Extension	Extensor pollicis brevis	Radial	C7+C8
Thumb IP			
Flexion	Flexor pollicis longus	Median	C7+C8
Extension	Extensor pollicis longus	Radial	C7+C8

DIP, distal interphalangeal; IP, interphalangeal; MCP, metacarpophalangeal; PIP, proximal interphalangeal.
*The dorsal and palmar interossei are abductors and adductors, respectively, of the fingers. They also flex the MCP joints and extend the PIP and DIP joints. These so-called intrinsic muscles are the balancing and mediating forces between the powerful *extrinsic* flexors and extensors of the fingers. Loss of the intrinsic muscles results in significant deformity in the hand and the reader is referred to the Doyle/Botte reference in Suggested Reading, pages 581–595 and chapter 13 of this text for a comprehensive discussion of the anatomy and function of these muscles.

MUSCULAR ANATOMY

The muscles of the forearm are depicted in Figure 1.2-2 and the hand in Figure 1.2-3.

VASCULAR ANATOMY

The vascular anatomy from the axillary artery to the hand is depicted in Figure 1.2-4.

NEURAL ANATOMY

The brachial plexus, median, ulnar, and radial nerves and the muscles they innervate are depicted in Figure 1.2-5.

1.3 TERMINOLOGY OF MOVEMENT

It is important to learn the language of movement as it relates to forearm, wrist, fingers, and thumb functions. Figure 1.3-1 depicts the accepted terminology used to describe the various movements seen and tested in the hand, wrist, and forearm. Consistent use of these terms will allow all health care providers to easily communicate their findings to each other. Health workers might also develop a reasonable diagnosis and treatment plan if they note the absence of a specific movement. Table 1.3-1 provides the anatomic basis for movement in the upper extremity; learning it will aid in making a diagnosis and help to establish the site and level of an injury.

Table 1.3-2 covers the grading of muscle strength, which helps to document the degree of disability as a baseline. It is a useful tool in monitoring the presence or absence of recovery.

SUGGESTED READING

Bugbee WD, Botte MJ. Surface anatomy of the hand. Clin Orthop 1993;296:122–126.
Doyle JR, Botte MJ. Surgical anatomy of the hand and upper extremity. Philadelphia: Lippincott Williams & Wilkins, 2002.
Kaplan EB. Functional and surgical anatomy of the hand. 2nd Ed. Philadelphia: JB Lippincott, 1965:265–270.

TABLE 1.3-2 GRADING OF MUSCLE STRENGTH

Grade	Strength	Description
5	Normal	Complete ROM against gravity with full resistance
4	Good	Complete ROM against gravity with some resistance
3	Fair	Complete ROM against gravity
2	Poor	Complete ROM with gravity eliminated
1	Trace	Evidence of slight contraction; no joint motion
0	Zero	No evidence of contraction

ROM, range of motion.

PEARLS

- Knowledge of anatomy is the key to diagnosis, treatment, and surgery in the hand and wrist.
- Continually review the anatomy of the hand, wrist, and forearm; use the landmarks on your own hand and wrist to visualize the deeper structures.
- Remember that anatomy is three dimensional.
- Dissect in the anatomy laboratory with your resident colleagues.
- Learn by repetition.

CONGENITAL DEFORMITIES

Orthopaedics is both science and art. The art of orthopaedics includes the surgeon's demeanor, which has often been called "bedside manner." The evaluation and treatment of congenital deformities requires the appropriate application of both science and art in order to effectively deal with an infant or child with a congenital deformity, or with his or her parents and extended family. We live in a society where physical perfection is highly valued, so the words of Robert E. Carroll in 1989 bear repeating:

> "Two body regions are constantly under scrutiny: the face and the hands. These areas are rarely covered, and are perceived as symbolic of the individual. Furthermore, they are very sensitive areas used for communication. Since there is constant awareness of these two body areas, what can be more important than the functional and esthetic restoration of the upper extremities? The management of these complex problems carries with it both great responsibility and rewards."

A congenital deformity may carry with it disappointment, frustration, fear, and rejection. The initial doctor visit or evaluation is often associated with anxiety or even guilt, which can alter what might be considered normal responses in other medical situations. Upper limb deformities are very noticeable and are difficult to conceal. This often worsens the deformity's social or emotional impact on the patient and family.

The role of the upper extremity surgeon is to provide support and information. Positive comments about other physical attributes of the child are helpful to the parents and to the patient. Your projection of a caring and accepting caregiver will do much to help the parents along their difficult path of acceptance of the deformity. Information about support groups will be helpful to the family. Upper extremity surgeons will need to offer more than technical expertise; they will need to become part of a team of thoughtful and experienced professionals including pediatricians, geneticists, and social workers. Finally, the use of inappropriate descriptive and potentially offensive terms such as lobster claw hand or club hand should be abandoned. A suitable and internationally accepted system of classification and nomenclature has been developed and is best used to write and speak about these deformities. Some have proposed that "congenital differences" is a more appropriate descriptive phrase than "congenital deformities."

CLASSIFICATION

Being able to classify congenital deformities of the upper limb is necessary to exchange ideas and concepts for diagnosing and treating them. The currently accepted classification system is given in Box 2-1. It is based on embryonic failure during development and relies on clinical diagnosis for placement of the various and most prominent anomalies. This system has been revised and adopted by the Congenital Anomalies Committee of the International Federation of Societies for Surgery of the Hand (IFSSH). Although no classification system is perfect, the current system is the best that exists at this time and is used worldwide. It has also been observed that research on embryogenesis has rendered some of the information outdated regarding pathogenesis of limb malformations used in this classification. Although many investigators have expressed difficulties in classifying specific anomalies in this system, it has provided a framework for discussion. Central deficiencies (cleft hand) and brachysyndactyly, along with ulnar deficiencies in particular, have provided areas of controversy since the original classification system was adopted, but it is beyond the scope of this text to further define them. Defects in human limb formation have been connected to gene mutations that may encode signaling proteins, transcription factors, and receptor proteins. Some limb defects have been mapped to a specific chromosomal segment and molecular defect. Table 2-1 provides a currently available genetic classification.

NORMAL UPPER LIMB DEVELOPMENT[1]

Embryonic growth begins with fertilization of the egg followed by attachment of the fertilized egg to the uterine

---

[1] This section has been adapted with permission from Light TR. Development of the hand. In: Green DP, Hotckiss RN, Pederson WC, eds. Green's operative hand surgery. 4th Ed. New York: Churchill Livingstone, 1993.

BOX 2-1 EMBRYOLOGIC CLASSIFICATION OF CONGENITAL DEFORMITIES OF THE UPPER EXTREMITY

I. Failure of formation of parts (arrest of development)
   A. Transverse arrest
      1. Shoulder
      2. Arm
      3. Elbow
      4. Forearm
      5. Wrist
      6. Carpal
      7. Metacarpal
      8. Phalanx
   B. Longitudinal arrest
      1. Radial ray deficiency
      2. Ulnar ray deficiency
      3. Central ray deficiency
      4. Intersegmental deficiency (phocomelia)
II. Failure of differentiation of parts
   A. Soft-tissue involvement
      1. Disseminated
         a. Arthrogryposis
      2. Shoulder
      3. Elbow and forearm
      4. Wrist and hand
         a. Cutaneous syndactyly
         b. Camptodactyly
         c. Thumb-in-palm deformity
         d. Deviated/deformed digits
   B. Skeletal involvement
      1. Shoulder
      2. Elbow
         a. Elbow synostosis
      3. Forearm
         a. Proximal radioulnar synostosis
         b. Distal radioulnar synostosis
      4. Wrist and hand
         a. Osseous syndactyly
         b. Synostosis of carpal bones
         c. Symphalangia
         d. Clinodactyly

C. Congenital tumorous conditions
      1. Hemangiotic
      2. Lymphatic
      3. Neurogenic
      4. Connective tissue
      5. Skeletal
III. Duplication
      1. Whole limb
      2. Humeral segment
      3. Radial segment
      4. Ulnar segment
         a. Mirror hand
      5. Digit
         a. Polydactyly
            1. Radial (preaxial)
            2. Central
            3. Ulnar (postaxial)
IV. Overgrowth
      1. Whole limb
      2. Partial limb
      3. Digit
         a. Macrodactyly
            1. With fibrolipoma of nerve
            2. No fibrolipoma of nerve
V. Undergrowth
      1. Whole limb
      2. Whole hand
      3. Metacarpal
      4. Digit
         a. Brachysyndactyly
         b. Brachydactyly
VI. Congenital constriction band syndrome
VII. Generalized skeletal abnormalities
   A. Chromosomal
      1. Madelung's deformity

Taken from Kozin, S. Congenital anomalies. In: Trumble T, ed. Hand surgery update 3, hand, elbow and shoulder. Rosemont, IL: American Society for Surgery of the Hand, 2003:603–604.

wall. The transition from embryo to fetus occurs at about 8 weeks, and is hallmarked by the appearance of the primary ossification center in the proximal humerus. Embryogenesis is characterized by the appearance of new organ systems and the fetal period by differentiation, maturation, and enlargement of existing organs. The changes in the early limb bud into the mature arm, forearm, and hand rely on four interdependent developmental processes: *morphogenesis* (the process by which a part assumes a particular shape); *cell differentiation* (the process by which individual cells, under genetic control, become specialized for carrying out specific functions); *pattern formation* (the process by which cellular differentiation is spatially organized); and *growth* (the enlargement of the structure reflecting both cell proliferation and matrix elaboration).

Embryogenesis

Streeter identified 23 stages of embryonic development based on his histological study of sectioned embryos (Table 2-2). The upper limb develops from the arm bud, which is an outgrowth from the ventrolateral body wall located opposite the fifth through seventh cervical somites. The arm bud first appears at approximately 26 to 27 days of gestation (3 to 5 mm crown-rump length; Table 2-2 and Fig. 2-1). Development in the arm bud occurs from proximal to distal and is composed of a mass of somatic mesoderm-derived mesenchyme covered by ectoderm. As the arm bud grows, it assumes a flipper-like shape. At day 33, blood circulation is established to the paddle-like arm bud.

At days 33 to 36 (7 to 9 mm crown-rump length), the hand plates are evident as a flattened structure. Vessels

TABLE 2-1 GENETIC CLASSIFICATION OF LIMB DEFECTS

Molecular Defect	Syndrome	Limb Defect	Gene	Chromosome
Transcription factor	Holt-Oram	Radial deficiency	TBX5	12q24.1
	Synpolydactyly	Syndactyly, polydactyly, brachydactyly	HOXD13	2q31-q32
	Townes-Brocks	Polydactyly	SALL1	16q12
	Waardenburg types I and III	Syndactyly	PAX3	2q35
	Hand-foot-genital	Brachydactyly	HOXA13	7p15-p14.2
	Saethre-Chotzen	Brachydactyly, syndactyly	TWIST	7p21
	Ulnar mammary	Deficiency and duplication	TBX3	12q24.1
	Pallister-Hall	Polydactyly	GL13	7p13
	Creig cephalopoly syndactyly	Syndactyly, polydactyly	GL13	7p13
Signaling protein	Grebe	Severe brachydactyly	CDMP1	20q11.2
	Hunter-Thompson	Brachydactyly	CDMP1	20q11.2
	Aarskog	Brachydactyly	FGD1	Xp11.2
Receptor protein	Apert	Syndactyly	FGFR2	10q26
	Pfeiffer	Brachydactyly, syndactyly	FGFR1	8p11.2-p11.1
			FGFR2	8p11.2-p11.1
	Jackson-Weiss	Syndactyly, brachydactyly	FGFR2	10q26
Unknown	Split-hand-foot	Syndactyly, fusion		7q21, Xq26, 10q24
	Tarsal-carpal coalition	Brachydactyly, fusions		17q
	Nager Syndrome	Posterior limb deficiency		9q32

Taken from Kozin, S. Congenital anomalies. In: Trumble T, ed. Hand surgery update 3, hand, elbow and shoulder. Rosemont, IL: American Society for Surgery of the Hand, 2003:601.

TABLE 2-2 STREETER STAGES OF HUMAN EMBRYONIC DEVELOPMENT

Stage	Age (days)	Crown-Rump Length	Events
1			Fertilization
2			Zygote divides
3			Early blastocyte
4	6		Implantation begins
5	9–10		Complete blastocyte implantation
6	11–15		Primary villi
7	16–20		Notochord appears
8	20–21		Neural plate develops
9	21–22		Neural groove develops
10	23	2.0–3.5 mm	Embryo straight; heart begins to beat
11	24–25	2.5–4.5 mm	Embryo curved
12	26–27	3.0–5.0 mm	Arm buds appear
13	28–31	4.0–6.0 mm	Arm buds are flipper-like
14	32	5.0–7.0 mm	Forelimbs are paddle-shaped
15	33–36	7.0–9.0 mm	Hand plates formed
16	37–40	8.0–11.0 mm	Foot plates form
17	41–43	1.1–1.4 cm	Finger rays appear
18	44–46	1.3–1.7 cm	Notches between finger rays
19	47–48	1.6–1.8 cm	Fingers begin to separate
20	49–51	1.8–2.2 cm	Fingers separate and elongate
21	52–53	2.2–2.4 cm	
22	54–55	2.3–2.8 cm	Toes separate and elongate
23	56	2.7–3.1 cm	Head rounded

Taken from Light TR. Development of the hand. In Green DP, Hotckiss RN, Pederson WC, eds. Green's operative hand surgery.4th Ed. New York: Churchill Livingstone,1993:333–338.

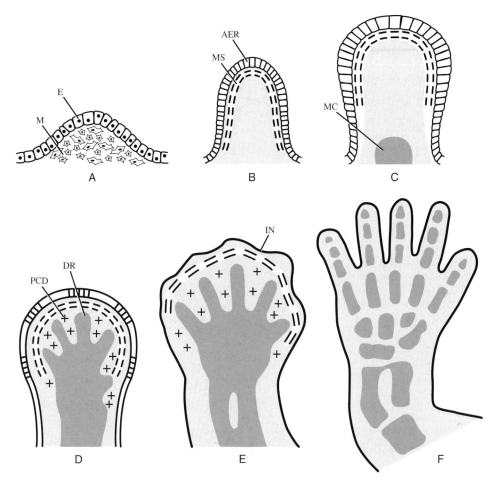

Figure 2-1 Normal limb bud development. (**A**) At 28 days. (**B**) At 34 days. (**C**) At 36 days. (**D**) At 40 days with programmed cell death of mesenchymal tissue between digital ray mesenchymal condensations. (**E**) At 42 days. (**F**) At 50 days showing individual digits and well-defined web spaces. AER, apical ectodermal ridge; DR digital ray; E, ectoderm; IN, interdigital notch; M, mesoderm; MC, mesenchymal condensation; MS, marginal sinus; PCD, physiologic cell death. (Taken from Yasuda M. Pathogenesis of preaxial polydactyly of the hand in human embryos. J Embryo Exp Morph 33:745–756, 1975.)

grow into the limb from proximal to distal. At 5 weeks, a constriction demarcates the arm from the forearm. A more proximal depression will become the axillary fossa. At 41 to 43 days (11 to 14 mm crown-rump length), the finger rays appear. At 50 days, individual digital metacarpal and phalangeal mesenchymal condensations are histologically visible. At day 52 or 53 (22 to 24 mm crown-rump length), the fingers are entirely separate. In the seventh week, the upper limb rotates 90 degrees on its longitudinal axis, so that the elbow points dorsally. Embryogenesis ends during the eighth week.

Limb Formation

Three interactions help guide limb formation. The first is between the mesenchyme of the limb bud and the apical ectodermal ridge (AER). This interaction influences and guides proximal to distal axis limb differentiation, and is the process that distinguishes the arm from the forearm and the forearm from the hand. The second set of interactions controls differentiation along the dorsal to palmar axis, the distinction between the dorsum of the finger with a fingernail, and the soft tissue of the pulp. The third set of interactions controls cellular differentiation across the anteroposterior (AP) axis and causes the thumb to assume a morphologic form distinctly different from the little finger.

The three critical regions of the limb bud that signal or control outgrowth and pattern formation are the AER, the dorsal ectoderm, and the zone of polarizing activity (ZPA). The dorsal ectoderm controls palmar to dorsal differentiation, which results in distinctly different flexor and extensor surfaces.

The anteroposterior (AP) interactions are controlled by a cluster of mesenchymal cells along the postaxial border of the limb bud, the zone of polarizing activity (ZPA). The morphogens elaborated within the ZPA diffuse and create a gradient that helps control differentiation in the AP plane. Retinoids are vitamin A-derived substances that may signal digital differentiation from the polarizing region.

The AER is a transient ectodermal thickening at the tip of the limb bud that is present during critical transitions in limb development. The AER induces the differentiation of the underlying mesoderm. The mesoderm elaborates morphogens that maintain the AER. The progress zone is a region of subectodermal mesoderm that defines proximodistal relationships. The theory of positional information suggests that the ultimate role or position of an individual cell is determined by the length of time that a cell spends in the progress zone, and by the number of times the cell undergoes mitosis before exiting from the progress zone. These interactions are critical for coordinating limb pattern formation.

Apoptosis, or programmed cell death, is an integral element of orderly limb embryogenesis. The resorption of tissue between the digital mesenchymal condensations results from the release of lysosomal enzymes from cells. The antichondrogenic effects of the ectoderm and digital cartilage inhibit interdigital mesenchymal cells from forming cartilage. As those interdigital cells migrate toward digital condensations to participate in chondrogenesis, the interdigital zone experiences a decrease in cell density and cell death.

Genetic Control of Limb Differentiation

The four Hox genes (HoxA–D) regulate patterning during the development of the limbs, and help regulate the timing and extent of local growth rates within the embryonic limb. Mutation in the HoxDl3 position has been demonstrated to lead to human synpolydactyly deformities in the hands and feet. Three proteins (Sonic hedgehog [Shh], FGFs, and Wnt-7a) are believed to establish the pattern of Hox gene expression. The Hox code, in conjunction with other gene products, is thought to provide more detailed positional and morphogenic information to competent mesenchymal cells, enabling them to form precartilaginous skeletal cell condensations of appropriate size and at appropriate sites.

Fetal Development

The upper limb is completely formed in miniature during embryogenesis, and limbs grow rapidly during fetal development. Areas of cartilage are replaced by expanding primary ossification centers, and joints move in utero in response to muscle contraction.

Postnatal Development

After birth, the hand begins to explore its environment. Initial behaviors are shaped by subcortical reflexes. By the end of the first year of life, the child begins to purposefully manipulate objects, using his or her hands in a coordinated fashion. Hand preference or dominance is evident by 3 or 4 years of age.

ABNORMAL UPPER LIMB DEVELOPMENT

Abnormal limb development may be secondary to *malformation* (poor formation of tissue that initiates a chain of additional abnormalities), *deformation* (from mechanical forces applied to a normally formed embryo or fetus), *disruption* (destructive forces or problems such as infection that affect normal embryos or fetuses), or *dysplasia* (conditions that arise from the abnormal arrangement of cells into tissues).

Causes of Common Congenital Deformities

Syndactyly

Digital ray separation is the result of the interactions between the AER and the underlying mesoderm. Syndactyly

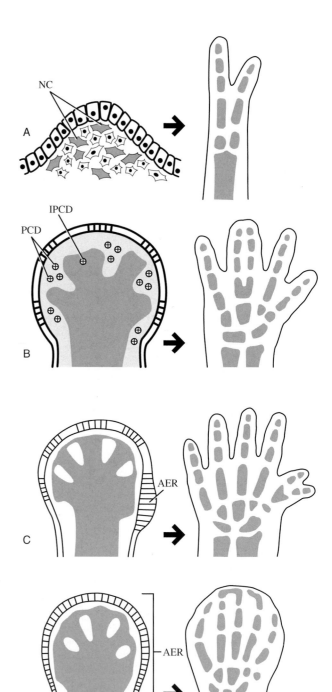

Figure 2-2 Pathogenesis of limb deformities. (**A**) Mesenchymal cell death leads to a reduction deformity of the hand. (**B**) Failure of cell death results in syndactyly of adjacent digits. (**C**) Polydactyly results from hyperplasia of the apical ectodermal ridge (AER). (**D**) Disrupted ridge metabolism that results in failure of breakdown of the AER may result in complete complex syndactyly. AER, apical ectodermal ridge; IPCD, inhibited physiologic cell death; NC, necrotic cells; PCD, physiologic cell death.

represents the failure of the normal separation of the digital rays from one another. When there is a failure of the normal interdigital programmed cell death, interdigital webbing will persist as syndactyly (Fig. 2-2).

Polydactyly

Polydactyly represents an inappropriate definition of digital rays, reflecting an abnormality in the interaction between limb bud ectoderm and mesoderm. Thumb polydactyly may be related to prolonged ectodermal cells in the tip of the limb bud that induce an abnormal notch in the radial mesenchymal tissue. Studies have shown that implantation on the anterior side of the limb bud of FGF-soaked beads or of portions of the ZPA will result in a mirror duplication of the limb. In some instances, an inappropriate number of digital condensations are formed. In other instances of polydactyly, one of the five digital condensations becomes partially split longitudinally. Digital definition occurs as the process of interdigital apoptosis defines separate rays. If this process occurs in an abnormal location, further splitting of the hand plate results in polydactyly.

Dysplasia and Deficiency

Necrosis of portions of the limb bud may be the result of local injury or ischemia. The resulting hand may have a corresponding area of dysplasia or deficiency. It has been suggested on the basis of experimental studies that disruption of the AER may lead to transverse defects, whereas loss of cells in the mesenchyme may result in longitudinal deficiency patterns. Poland's association, the occurrence of brachysyndactyly with absence of the sternal costal portion of the pectoralis major, may be related to unilaterally diminished vascular flow.

    Thalidomide provided a vivid demonstration of the potential effect of drug ingestion on limb morphogenesis. Thalidomide was marketed outside the United States in the late 1950s for the treatment of nausea associated with pregnancy. Administration of these drugs to pregnant rats has been demonstrated to result in fetal anomalies. The specific anomalies are related to the dose and timing of the drug administration.

Constriction Band Syndrome

Early amnion rupture sequence, also referred to as congenital constriction band syndrome, is usually the result of intrauterine injury to a normally developed hand. In response to the altered intrauterine environment, the fetus may be deformed, as fingers are forced together to create a secondary syndactyly. The mechanical constriction of amniotic tissue may disrupt or amputate fingers or toes.

IMPORTANT CLINICAL FACTS ABOUT COMMON ANOMALIES

The following discussion will describe the important clinical facts about some of the more common congenital anomalies based on the currently accepted classification system. Not all of the conditions listed in Box 2-1 will be presented.

FAILURE OF FORMATION OF PARTS

Failure of formation of parts may be transverse or longitudinal. Transverse failure is represented by congenital amputation that may occur from the shoulder region to the phalanx.

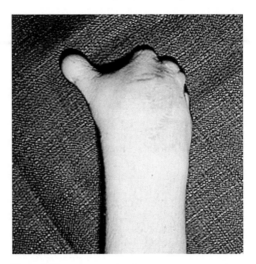

Figure 2-3   An example of transverse arrest at the metacarpal level.

Longitudinal failure of development is characterized by radial, central, ulnar or intersegmental deficiency. Examples of these deformities are complete or partial absence of the radius, cleft hand, complete or partial absence of the ulna, and phocomelia.

Transverse Arrest

The most common levels of amputation are proximal forearm and mid-carpal, followed by metacarpal and humerus. Figure 2-3 demonstrates the appearance of a transverse arrest at the level of the metacarpal region. The condition is believed to be associated with severe hemorrhage in the hand plate. These deficiencies differ from constriction ring amputations in that the proximal parts are hypoplastic and the amputation is usually at or near a joint.

Treatment

- Treatment of arm and forearm amputations involves prosthetic fitting of a dynamic or static device depending on the age of the patient and level of the amputation.
- Transcarpal deficiency and foreshortened fingers (nubbins) are often present.
- A palmar splint may provide rudimentary prehension.
- Digital lengthening of one or more digits may be considered.
- Separation of the radius and ulnar to form prehensile appendages may be considered in bilateral transverse arrest, especially if it is associated with visual impairment.

Longitudinal Arrest

Radial Ray Deficiency

This condition involves absence or hypoplasia of the thumb, radial carpal hypoplasia or absence and absence or

TABLE 2-3 RADIAL DEFICIENCY CLASSIFICATION

Type	X-ray Findings	Clinical Features
I. Short radius	Distal radial epiphysis delayed in appearance	Minor radial deviation of the hand
	Normal proximal radial epiphysis	Thumb hypoplasia is the prominent clinical feature
	Mild shortening of radius without bowing	requiring treatment
II. Hypoplastic	Distal and proximal epiphysis present	Miniature radius
	Abnormal growth in both epiphyses	Moderate radial deviation of the hand
	Ulna thickened, shortened, and bowed	
III. Partial absence	Partial absence (distal, middle, proximal) of radius	Severe radial deviation of the hand
	Distal one third to two thirds absence most common	Most common type
	Ulna thickened, shortened, and bowed	
IV. Total absence	No radius present	
	Ulna thickened, shortened, and bowed	Severe radial deviation of the hand

Taken from Kozin, S. Congenital anomalies. In: Trumble T, ed. Hand surgery update 3, hand, elbow and shoulder. Rosemont, IL: American Society for Surgery of the Hand, 2003:609.

hypoplasia of the radius. Four types have been classified and are described in Table 2-3. A more recent and global classification of radial longitudinal deficiency that includes carpal and thumb anomalies is presented in Table 2-4. The x-ray appearance of the four types listed in Table 2-3 is depicted in Figure 2-4. Ossification of the radius is delayed in radial deficiency and the differentiation between types III and IV may not be established until 3 years of age. The clinical appearance of a type III patient is seen in Figure 2-5. Syndromes associated with radial deficiency are presented in Table 2-5.

Treatment

- Treatment is aimed at improvement of appearance by correcting the radial deviation of the wrist, balancing the hand and wrist on the forearm, maintaining and improving wrist and finger motion, promoting growth of the forearm, and improving overall function of the upper extremity.

- This can be achieved by stabilizing the carpus on the end of the ulna by centralization or ulnocarpal fusion. This can be achieved with or without ulnar osteotomy and/or tendon transfers.
- These procedures work best in children, because functional patterns developed over many years in adults are best left unaltered.
- The radial deviation deformity allows the hand to reach the mouth. Bilateral conditions associated with noncorrectable stiff elbows should have only one side corrected.
- Surgery is most often needed in types II to IV.

Ulnar Ray Deficiency

This condition has four types; see Table 2-6 and Figure 2-6. The classification system in Table 2-6 is based on the status of the ulna and the humeral articulation. A more recent classification system based on the characteristics of

TABLE 2-4 GLOBAL CLASSIFICATION OF RADIAL LONGITUDINAL DEFICIENCY

Type	Thumb Anomaly	Carpal Anomaly	Distal Radius	Proximal Radius
N	Absent or hypoplasia	Normal	Normal	Normal
O	Absent or hypoplasia	Absent, hypoplasia or coalition	Normal	Normal, radioulnar or radial head dislocation synostosis
1	Absent or hypoplasia	Absent, hypoplasia or coalition	>2mm shorter than ulna	Normal, radioulnar synostosis, or radial head dislocation
2	Absent or hypoplasia	Absent, hypoplasia or coalition	Hypoplasia	Hypoplasia
3	Absent or hypoplasia	Absent, hypoplasia or coalition	Physis absent	Variable hypoplasia
4	Absent or hypoplasia	Absent, hypoplasia or coalition	Absent	Absent

Taken from Kozin, S. Congenital anomalies. In: Trumble T, ed. Hand surgery update 3, hand, elbow and shoulder. Rosemont, IL: American Society for Surgery of the Hand, 2003:610.

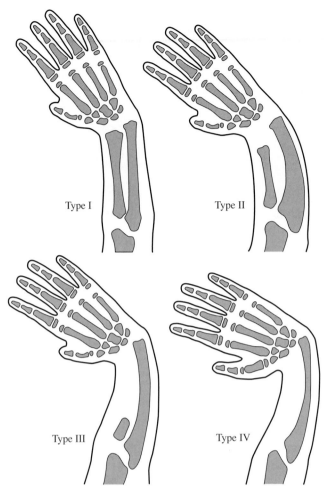

Figure 2-4 The osseous appearance of the four types of radial deficiency: type I, type II, type III, and type IV. See Tables 2-2 and 2-3 for details.

Type I

Type II

Type III

Type IV

the thumb and first web has been advocated due to the fact that most surgeries for this condition involved the thumb and first web (Table 2-7).

Treatment
- Principles of treatment include splinting to correct any significant ulnar deviation of the wrist and early excision of the fibrous anlage of the ulna if it is not possible to correct the ulnar deformity of the wrist.
- The radial head may be excised in those patients with minimal forearm rotation and elbow movement.
- Creation of a one-bone forearm using the proximal ulna and the distal radius may be indicated.
- Hand function may be significantly improved by corrective surgery to the thumb and first web when there is web deficiency, absence of the thumb or thumb hypoplasia, malposition, and loss of opposition.

Central Ray Deficiency

This includes typical cleft hand, which must be distinguished from atypical cleft hand, also known as brachysyndactyly. Figure 2-7 represents a typical cleft hand, and

Figure 2-8 an atypical cleft hand or, more accurately, brachysyndactyly. Table 2-8 compares the clinical features of these two conditions.

Clinical Features
- Typical cleft hand represents dysplasia of the central portion of the hand, and is not seen in conjunction with forearm or elbow anomalies.
- The deformity is characterized by a V-shaped cleft in the central aspect of the hand that may be associated with absence of one or more digits.
- Syndactyly may occur in the adjacent digits. The first web space may be compromised.
- Transverse bones may be noted on an x-ray, and there may be an absence of multiple digits with only one digit present (usually the little finger).
- Some cleft hands may be caused by the split hand/split foot gene localized on chromosome 7q21; see Table 2-1.

Treatment
- Treatment of cleft hands should improve any compromise of the first web space, close the cleft, and correct the syndactyly if present.
- Cleft closure may be achieved by transposition or translocation of the appropriate ray.
- In cases without a thumb, rotation of a radial ray, if present, should be considered.

Intersegmental Deficiency

This deficiency, also known as phocomelia because of its likeness to a seal limb, is distinguished from transverse deficiencies because of the presence of digital structures. Three types have been identified based on the presence or absence of an intermediate segment between the shoulder and hand. In type A, the hand is attached to the trunk, and there are no limb bones; type B is characterized by the absence or significant hypoplasia of the humerus so that the hand is attached to the trunk by the forearm; type C is characterized by absence of the forearm, with the hand attached to the humerus. Prosthetic or orthotic devices may be useful.

FAILURE OF DIFFERENTIATION OF PARTS

Soft Tissue Involvement

Disseminated

Arthrogryposis
The etiology of this condition is unknown. Although there are multiple forms of this disorder, the one most likely to be encountered on an orthopaedic service is known as amyoplasia congenita, or arthrogryposis.

Clinical Features
- The classic patient with arthrogryposis demonstrates adduction and internal rotation of the shoulders, extended elbows, and pronated forearms.

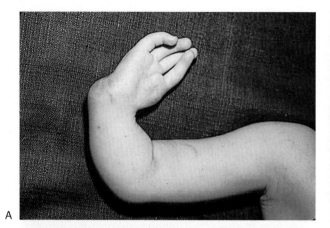

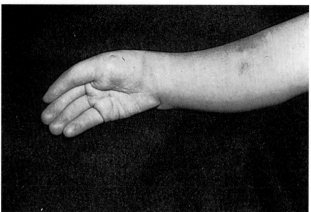

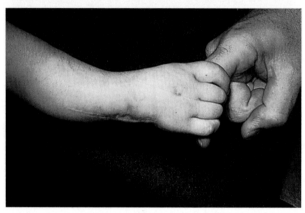

Figure 2-5   Type III radial deficiency. (**A**) Preoperative appearance. (**B**) Postoperative appearance following transposition of the ulna. (**C**) Improved appearance and function.

TABLE 2-5 SYNDROMES ASSOCIATED WITH RADIAL DEFICIENCY

Syndrome	Characteristics
Holt-Oram	Heart defects, most commonly cardiac septal defects
TAR	**T**hrombocytopenia **A**bsent **R**adius syndrome. Thrombocytopenia present at birth, but improves over time.
VACTERL	**V**ertebral abnormalities, **A**nal atresia, **C**ardiac abnormalities, **T**racheoesophageal fistula, **E**sophageal atresia, **R**enal defects, **R**adial dysplasia, **L**ower limb abnormalities
Fanconi's anemia	Aplastic anemia not present at birth, develops at about 6 years of age. Fatal without bone marrow transplant. Chromosomal challenge test now available for early diagnosis.

Taken from Kozin, S. Congenital anomalies. In: Trumble T, ed. Hand surgery update 3, hand, elbow and shoulder. Rosemont, IL: American Society for Surgery of the Hand, 2003:610.

TABLE 2-6 CLASSIFICATION OF ULNAR DEFICIENCIES

Type	Grade	Characteristics
I	Hypoplasia	Hypoplasia of the ulna with presence of distal and proximal ulnar epiphysis, minimal shortening
II	Partial aplasia	Partial aplasia with absence of the distal or middle one-third of the ulna
III	Complete aplasia	Total agenesis of the ulna
IV	Synostosis	Fusion of the radius to the humerus

Taken from Kozin, S. Congenital anomalies. In: Trumble T, ed. Hand surgery update 3, hand, elbow and shoulder. Rosemont, IL: American Society for Surgery of the Hand, 2003:608.

■ The wrists are palmar flexed and the hands ulnar deviated. The fingers are flexed and stiff. The thumb is flexed into the palm.
■ This classic posture is demonstrated in Figure 2-9.

Treatment
■ As with all congenital anomalies, treatment is directed toward the individual needs of each patient.

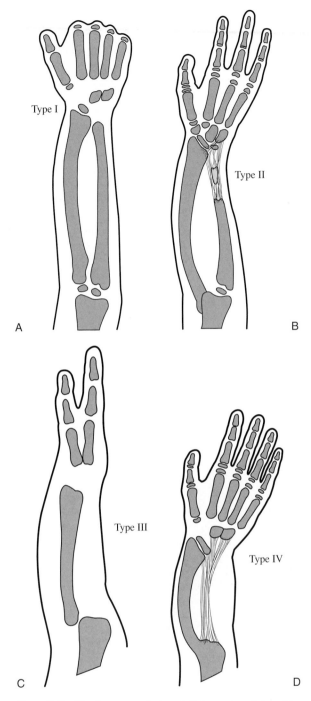

A

B

C

D

Figure 2-6   The four types of ulnar deficiency: type I, type II, type III, and type IV. See Table 2-6 for details.

Type I

Type II

Type III

Type IV

TABLE 2-7 CLASSIFICATION OF ULNAR DEFICIENCY ACCORDING TO FIRST-WEB SPACE ABNORMALITY

Type	Grade	Characteristics
A	Normal	Normal first web space and normal thumb
B	Mild	Mild first web deficiency and mild thumb hypoplasia, with intact opposition and extrinsic tendon function.
C	Moderate to severe	Moderate-to-severe first web deficiency and similar thumb hypoplasia with malrotation into the plane of the digits, loss of opposition, and dysfunction of the extrinsic tendons
D	Absent	Absence of the thumb

Taken from Kozin, S. Congenital anomalies. In: Trumble T, ed. Hand surgery update 3, hand, elbow and shoulder. Rosemont, IL: American Society for Surgery of the Hand, 2003:608.

■ Many of these children develop "trick motions" to meet their functional needs, and surgical intervention must be calculated to improve and not diminish function.

■ Tendon transfers such as triceps to biceps, and pectoralis major or latissimus dorsi to the front of the elbow, can restore active elbow flexion if a suitable muscle is available for transfer.

■ A recent study of various transfers to achieve elbow flexion revealed the following:

■ Exercises to obtain and maintain passive elbow flexion are initiated at birth.

■ If at least 90 degrees of flexion has not been achieved by 18 to 24 months of age after at least 6 months of supervised therapy, an elbow capsulotomy with triceps lengthening is recommended.

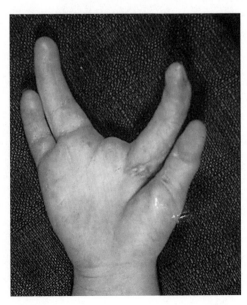

Figure 2-7   Clinical appearance of a true cleft hand deformity.

■ The classic treatment goals include independent toilet (perineal care) and self-feeding. In general, toilet care requires an extended elbow; self-feeding requires some degree of elbow flexion.

■ Early treatment is directed at passive movement and static progressive splinting of joints to promote what function may be present and as a useful precursor to surgical intervention in the form of joint releases and tendon transfers.

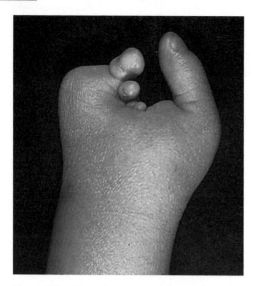

Figure 2-8   Clinical appearance of an atypical cleft hand or brachysyndactyly.

TABLE 2-8 CLINICAL FEATURES OF TYPICAL CLEFT HAND AND ATYPICAL CLEFT HAND

Typical Cleft Hand	Atypical Cleft Hand (Brachysyndactyly)
Familial, Autosomal dominant	Sporadic, spontaneous
1–4 limbs involved	1 limb involved (no feet)
V-shaped cleft	U-shaped cleft
No finger "nubbins"	Finger "nubbins" may occur
Syndactyly (especially first web)	Unusual
Bilateral	Unilateral

- After the age of 4 years, tendon transfers for elbow flexion on the dominant arm are recommended with triceps to biceps transfer giving the most predictable results.
- The muscle to be transferred should have muscle strength of at least grade 4.
- A persistent wrist flexion deformity may require surgical intervention. A proximal row carpectomy may be beneficial in mild to moderate deformities, but more severe flexion deformities may require a dorsal wedge mid-carpal osteotomy, along with a central transfer of the extensor carpi ulnaris (ECU) to help the wrist extend.
- The palm-clutched thumb may be repositioned, and the fingers realigned, by osteotomy.

Wrist and Hand

Cutaneous Syndactyly
The webbing of the fingers may be spontaneous, inheritable, or associated with a syndrome. The conditions currently known to be associated with syndactyly are given in Box 2-2. Inheritable syndactyly is associated with genetic defects on certain regions of the second chromosome

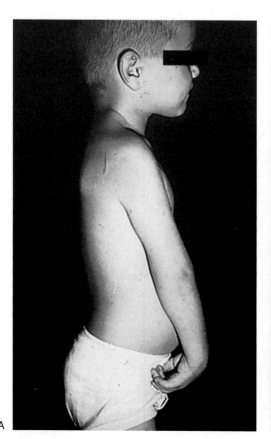
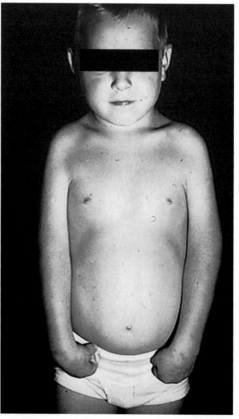

A   B

Figure 2-9   Clinical appearance of arthrogryposis in the upper extremities.

BOX 2-2 CONDITIONS ASSOCIATED WITH SYNDACTYLY

Chromosomal
 Trisomy 13
 Trisomy 14
 Trisomy 21
 Partial trisomy 10q
 Triploidy syndrome
Craniofacial Syndromes
 Aglossia adactylia syndrome
 Apert syndrome
 Carpenter syndrome
 Pfeiffer syndrome
 Cohen syndrome
 Cryptophthalmos syndrome
 Ellis-van Creveld syndrome
 Familial static Ophthalmoplegia syndrome
 Glossopalatine ankylosis syndrome
 Greig cephalopolysyndactyly syndrome
 Hanhart syndrome
 Hypertelorism and syndactyly syndrome
 Möbius syndrome
 Noack syndrome
 Oculodentodigital
 Oculomandibulofacial syndrome
 Oral-facial-digital
 Oto-palato-digital
 Pierre-Robin
 Saethre-Chotzen
Other Syndromes
 Acropectoral-vertebral dysplasia-F-form
  (F syndrome)
 Aarskog
 Bloom syndrome
 Brachydactyly A-2

Brachydactyly B
Chondrodysplasia punctata (Conradi) syndrome
Cornelia de Lange syndrome
EEC syndrome
Escobar syndrome
Fraser syndrome
Goltz focal dermal hypoplasia syndrome
Holt-Oram syndrome
Incontinentia pigmenti syndrome
Jarcho-Levin syndrome
Lawrence-Moon-Biedl syndrome
Lacrimoauriculodentodigital syndrome
Lenz-Majewski hyperostosis syndrome
Lenz microphthalmia syndrome
McKusick-Kaufman syndrome
Meckel syndrome
Miller syndrome
Neu-Laxova syndrome
Pallister-Hall syndrome
Pancytopenia dysmelia syndrome
Poland's anomaly
Popliteal pterygium syndrome
Prader-Willi syndrome
Roberts-SC phocomelia syndrome
Rothmund-Thomson syndrome
Sclerostenosis syndrome
Scott craniodigital mental retardation syndrome
Short rib-polydactyly (Saldino-Noonan) syndrome
Smith-Lemli-Opitz syndrome
Spondylothoracic dysplasia syndrome
Summit syndrome
Thrombocytopenia-absent radius syndrome
Wardenberg syndrome

Taken from Ezaki MB. Syndactyly. In: Green DP, Hotckiss RN, Pederson WC, eds. Green's operative hand surgery. 4th Ed. New York: Churchill Livingstone, 1999:414–428.

(2q34–q36). The mode of inheritable transmission is said to be autosomal dominant, with variable expressivity and incomplete penetrance.

Like most all congenital conditions, classification systems have evolved for syndactyly and the most simple system is *incomplete* versus *complete* and *simple* versus *complex*. In incomplete syndactyly, the interdigital web is extended, but soft tissue union does not extend as far as the distal aspect of the digits. Simple syndactyly involves only the skin and underlying soft tissues, whereas complex syndactyly also manifests some form of union of the underlying osseous terminal phalanx. Another classification system has been developed to guide the timing and extent of separation (Table 2-9). This system indicates the value of early (the first few months of life) separation of border digits (thumb-index and ring-little finger web space) or digits with marked differences in length. Separation prevents tethering of the longer digit and may prevent flexion contracture or rotational deformity. Surgery after 18 months of age has a lower incidence of complications such as web advancement. Figure 2-10 shows a case of complete, simple syndactyly, and Figure 2-11 is an example of complex syndactyly as seen in Apert's syndrome.

Clinical Features

- The most common site of webbing is between the middle and ring finger.
- Differential motion between the fingertips in complete syndactyly indicates absence of bony involvement.
- Confluence of the nails (synechia) or the absence of differential motion is most often associated with bony involvement as seen in complex syndactyly.
- Radiographs are an important part of the evaluation of syndactyly. They assist in differentiating between complex and simple syndactyly and in noting the presence or absence of a hidden polydactyly.
- The interdigital web has unique anatomy:
  - It is a three-dimensional space that allows normal finger movement in more than four planes.
  - It slopes from proximal to distal as viewed from the dorsal aspect of the hand. This slope is most noticeable when the digits are extended and abducted.
  - The web closes when the digits are flexed.
  - The web begins near the head of the metacarpal and ends near the mid-portion of the proximal phalanx.

TABLE 2-9 SYNDACTYLY CLASSIFICATION

Type	Description
Simple syndactyly (SS)	
Standard (SSs)	Straightforward, simple syndactyly of non-border digit. Surgery can be delayed until 18 months of age.
Complicated (SSc)	Simple syndactyly associated with additional soft tissue interconnections, syndromes (such as Poland's syndrome or central deficiency), or abnormal bony elements (such as hypoplasia). Treatment must be individualized. Beware of neurovascular anomalies.
Urgent (SSu)	Soft tissue syndactyly of borders digits or digits of unequal length, girth, or joint level. Requires early separation to prevent angular and rotational deformity of tethered digit.
Complex syndactyly (CS)	
Standard (CSs)	Complex syndactyly of adjacent phalanges without additional bony anomalies (such as delta phalanx or symphalangism).
Complicated (CSc)	Complex syndactyly associated with additional bony interconnections, (such as transverse phalanges, symphalangism, or polysyndactyly), or syndromes (such as constriction band syndrome). Treatment must be individualized, and digits may function better as a unit.
Unachievable (CSu)	Complex syndactyly with severe anomalies of the underlying bony structures, which often prohibits formation of a five-digit hand without extensive surgical intervention.

Taken from Kozin, S. Congenital anomalies. In: Trumble T, ed. Hand surgery update 3, hand, elbow and shoulder. Rosemont, IL: American Society for Surgery of the Hand, 2003:616.

■ Transversely oriented natatory fibers of the palmar fascia span the mid and distal aspects of the web, and are important support structures for the overlying skin and subcutaneous tissues.

Treatment
■ The goals of treatment are to improve the overall appearance of the hand and to improve function.
■ Contraindications include any condition that would preclude general anesthesia (in children), the lack of adequate vascular supply, soft tissue insufficiency, or lack of a potentially stable skeleton for each digit.
■ Early separation at 4 to 6 months of age is advised for complex syndactyly involving the border digits where continued growth may be expected to cause tethering or progressive deformity with growth.
■ Surgery is technically easier, and anesthesia is safer, after 1 year of age.

Surgical Techniques
■ Surgery is designed to try to reproduce this three-dimensional space. Many methods have been designed to achieve this, but the basic principles to achieve this goal are based on the formation of a dorsally based flap that is advanced to the palmar surface of the hand. The advancement will form a new web in association with zigzag incisions that run distally from the web area to the fingertips.
■ The zigzag incisions are used to prevent a linear scar and its resultant contracture.
■ The triangular flaps thus formed are applied to the opposing surfaces of the separated digits; the gaps that

inevitably result are covered with full thickness skin grafts from a suitable donor site such as the hairless aspect of the groin.
■ Figure 2-10 demonstrates the surgical technique used to separate a case of simple, complete syndactyly.
■ A four-tailed Z-plasty may also be used to deepen the first web, and is demonstrated in Figure 2-12.

Camptodactyly
Camptodactyly, meaning bent finger, is a congenital flexion deformity of the proximal interphalangeal (PIP) joint of the little finger. The term may be used less accurately to describe any congenital flexion deformity of a digit. This deformity has been noted in 70 or more syndromes.

Clinical Features
■ The finger assumes variable degrees of flexion contracture at the PIP joint. The neck and head of the proximal phalanx at the PIP joint may be deformed.
■ The clinical and x-ray appearance of the condition is presented in Figure 2-13.

Etiology
■ The etiology is unknown, although various anatomic abnormalities have been implicated, such as skin deficiency, intrinsic and extrinsic tendon contracture, and abnormal insertions, infection, and circulatory problems.
■ Abnormalities of insertion and contracture are most commonly found in the superficialis and or the lumbrical.

Treatment
■ Dynamic and static splinting may be useful if continued through adolescence.

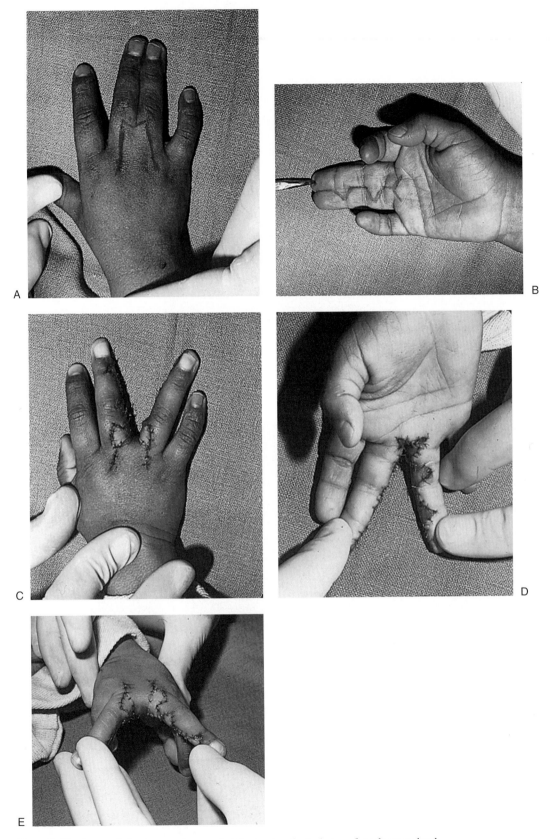

Figure 2-10   A case of simple, complete syndactyly showing the technique for release and web formation using a dorsal pantaloon flap developed by L.D. Howard.

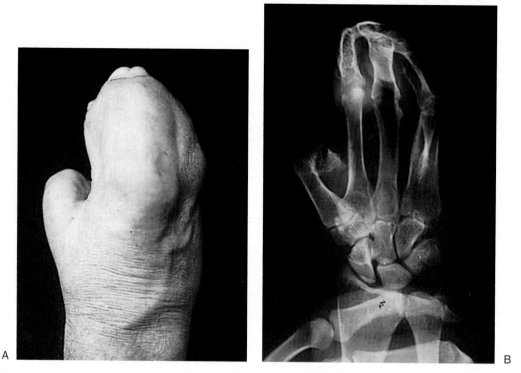

Figure 2-11 An example of complex syndactyly as seen in Apert's syndrome.

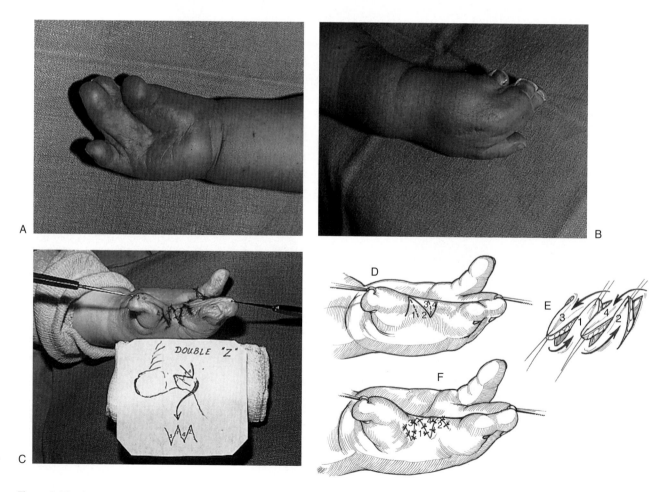

Figure 2-12 (**A–C**) Clinical appearance of a child with Apert's syndrome in which a 4-tailed Z-plasty was used to deepen the first web. (**D–F**) Details of surgical technique.

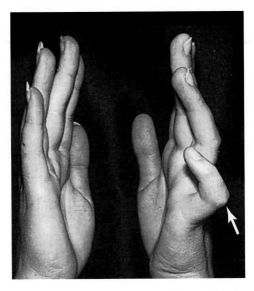

Figure 2-13 Clinical appearance of camptodactyly.

Elbow Synostosis

Humeral radial synostosis has been identified or found in three entities: as part of a systemic disorder manifested by multiple synostosis; dysgenesis of the ulna; and as a part of ulnar malformation and oligodactyly.

■ The position of the elbow may vary from full extension to 90 degrees of flexion, and there may be associated rotational deformities.

■ Treatment for this rare condition is directed at improving the placement of the hand, which is sometimes directed posteriorly.

■ A derotational osteotomy may be useful.

■ The exact procedure to be utilized will vary from patient to patient, depending on whether or not the condition is bilateral or unilateral.

■ The elbow is positioned to maximize hand function.

Forearm Synostosis

Forearm synostosis is often bilateral, and the forearm is fixed in pronation. Figure 2-14 demonstrates the clinical and x-ray appearance of a unilateral forearm synostosis in the left upper extremity, which is fixed in neutral rotation.

■ A proximal rotational osteotomy may be performed based on the functional needs of the patient (Figure 2-15). In this patient, no treatment was required because the synostosis on the left was in neutral, and the opposite extremity had full pronation and supination.

Carpal Synostosis

This condition is more common in black populations. Luno-triquetral coalitions are the most common. Figure 2-16 demonstrates the x-ray appearance of this condition. No particular treatment is indicated.

Metacarpal Synostosis

This condition occurs most commonly between the ring and little fingers, but may also present between the ring and middle finger metacarpals. The most common form is represented by fusion of the ring and little finger metacarpals, with abduction and hypoplasia of the little finger.

■ Splinting is usually continued only at night once correction has been obtained.

■ Surgical intervention is not always required. It is indicated for contractures of 30 degrees or more, or those digits that have failed to improve with splinting.

■ Corrective procedures for this condition are quite variable, but the basic principles relate to the release of the intrinsic or extrinsic contractures in and about the PIP joint. The principles also relate to the rebalancing of any deforming forces.

■ A full-thickness skin graft or local flap is usually required to treat the associated skin contracture.

Skeletal Involvement

Failure of differentiation as it relates to the skeleton is represented by synostosis. This condition may occur in the elbow, forearm, wrist, and hand.

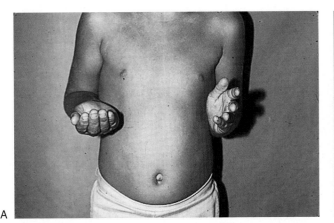
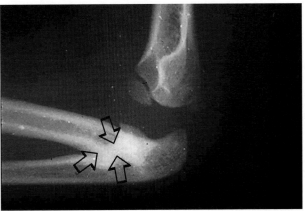

A   B

Figure 2-14 (A) Clinical appearance of left sided forearm synostosis in a young child with the forearm fixed in neutral. (B) X-ray showing coalition of the proximal radius and ulna (*arrows*).

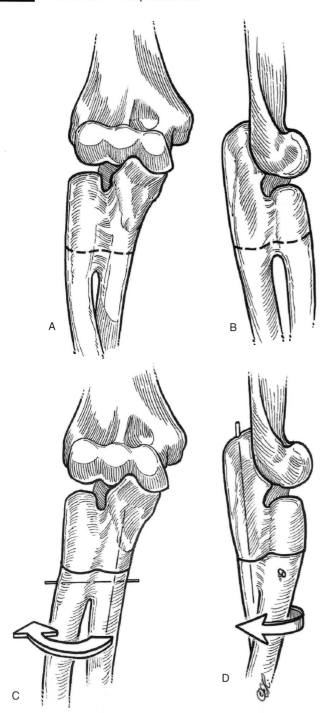

Figure 2-15 Surgical technique for proximal osteotomy in forearm synostosis after Green and Mital, showing a proximal osteotomy and reposition that is held in place by a longitudinal and a transverse K-wire through the synostosis mass.

■ Indications for surgery include the need to improve the appearance of the hand, but if severe little finger abduction is present this may interfere with function as the little finger may "catch" on things when the hand is used.
■ Osteotomy and realignment are designed to improve both function and appearance.

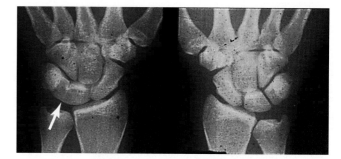

Figure 2-16 X-ray appearance of a luno-triquetral coalition in the wrist.

DUPLICATION

Digit

Polydactyly
Polydactyly may be divided into radial (preaxial), central, and ulnar (postaxial).

Radial Polydactyly
Two classification systems have been used to categorize thumb polydactyly. The first was by Wassel and the second was by Buck-Gramko and Behrens. Both systems classify the condition by the extent of bifurcation of the thumb. A comparison of these two systems is given in Figure 2-17. Wassel type IV thumbs are the most common. The preoperative and postoperative appearances of a type IV thumb polydactyly are shown in Figure 2-18.

Central Polydactyly
Polydactyly of the central rays is often associated with syndactyly. Ring ray involvement is the most common form.

■ Central polydactyly may be present in one hand, while cleft hand is noted in the opposite extremity.
■ A radiograph is needed to adequately diagnose the condition because the polydactylous digit may be concealed within a syndactyly.
■ Treatment varies with the form of polydactyly encountered, but the goal is improved function and appearance.
■ In some instances, separation or excision may result in lessened function and appearance.
■ The vascularity in synpolydacylous digits may be abnormal, and digital separation may be associated with digital ischemia.

Ulnar Polydactyly
Little finger polydactyly is common in black populations, and may represent one of the most common hand malformations.

■ Small digits with a narrow stalk may be ligated when seen in the newborn nursery. These digits will then necrose and fall off.
■ Small nubbins may be ignored or surgically removed.
■ More substantial and formed digits may require a more comprehensive approach to achieve better function and appearance.

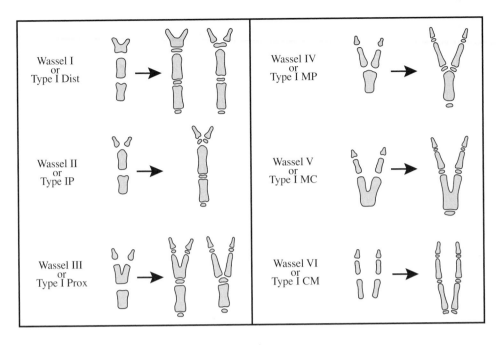

Figure 2-17 The classification systems for thumb polydactyly demonstrating the systems of Wassel and Buck-Gramcko and Behrens. The first column depicts immature thumbs, while the second shows maturing thumbs. The metacarpal or phalanges may partially or completely separate at the epiphysis, metaphysis, or diaphysis. (Taken from Light TR. Congenital anomalies: syndactyly, polydactyly and cleft hand. In: Peimer CA, ed. Surgery of the hand and upper extremity. New York: McGraw-Hill, 1996:2211–2144.)

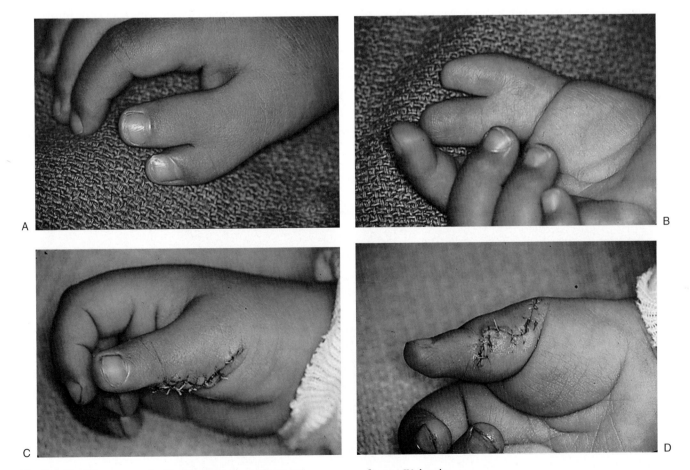

Figure 2-18 The preoperative (**A, B**) and postoperative (**C, D**) appearance of a type IV thumb polydactyly treated by removal of the less dominant appendage.

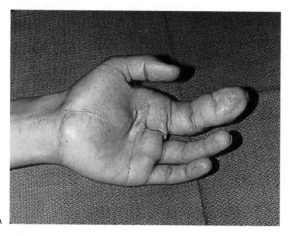
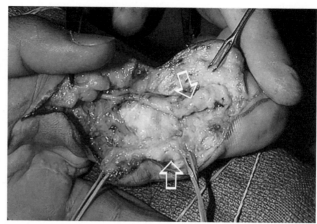

Figure 2-19   (**A**) Preoperative appearance of macrodactyly of the index finger (the middle finger was amputated previously; note scar). (**B**) Enlarged digital nerves (*arrows*) and generalized fibrofatty infiltration of the digit as seen at operation.

OVERGROWTH

Macrodactyly

The condition of enlarged fingers (macrodactyly) presents in two forms: static, with a single enlarged digit that is present at birth and that grows proportionately to the other digits; and progressive, with a digit that may not be enlarged at birth but begins to enlarge in early childhood. Growth in digits with this progressive type is much faster than the normal digits, and may demonstrate angular deviation. The progressive type is more common.

Clinical Features

- The index finger is most commonly involved, and multiple digits are frequently involved.

- Motion in the affected digits becomes diminished with age.
- Phalangeal enlargement occurs in transverse and longitudinal axes.
- The digital nerves are thickened by fibrofatty tissue, which renders identifying the conducting or functional portions of the nerve difficult.
- Both the median and ulnar nerve may enlarge proximal to the digital nerve involvement.

Treatment

- Treatment has included a variety of debulking, shortening procedures, including epiphyseal plate excision and osteotomies, to correct angular and rotational deformities.
- Debulking operations must be done in stages, and carry

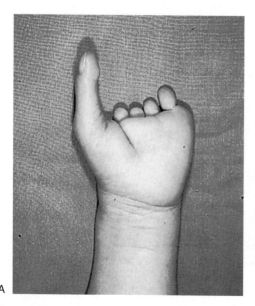
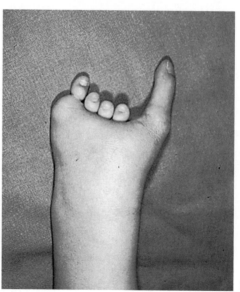

Figure 2-20   The clinical appearance of brachydactyly. Note the comparatively normal thumb, but the digits are represented as "nubbins."

the risk of vascular compromise if overly vigorous. Growth of these digits is relentless.
- Another form of treatment is amputation, usually in the form of a ray amputation.
- Amputation is often the last operation for a stiff, unsightly, and anesthetic digit.
- Figure 2-19 shows a classic index finger macrodactyly.

UNDERGROWTH

Undergrowth may involve the whole limb, whole hand, metacarpal, or digits. Brachysyndactyly and brachydactyly (short fingers with and without webbing, respectively) will be discussed. As previously noted, these two conditions should not be confused with true cleft hand. Table 2-8 lists the features that differentiate atypical and typical cleft hand.

Clinical Features

- The affected hand is smaller in patients with brachydactyly, which is a unilateral condition.
  - The thumb and little finger are often present and the central digits are represented by "nubbins" of tissue rather than fingers. Figure 2-20 depicts the clinical appearance of brachydactyly in a child.
- Brachysyndactyly is similar to brachydactyly in that the condition is unilateral and the affected hand smaller.
  - The fingers are shorter than normal, and the webbing of the digits may be simple and incomplete, or complex.
  - Figure 2-21 is an example of brachysyndactyly as seen in Poland's syndrome.
  - Figure 2-22 represents a more complex form of brachysyndactyly.

Treatment

- In brachydactyly, treatment is directed at obtaining an adequate first web and thumb reconstruction, if needed. The thumb may be reconstructed by a toe transplant or by lengthening, and the digits may be lengthened by free toe phalangeal transfers into the small nubbins or skin pockets.
- In brachysyndactyly, if a thumb and adequate web are present, treatment is focused on the release of the webbed fingers.

CONSTRICTION BAND SYNDROME

Etiology

- This condition is said to be a defect in the amnion (the innermost layer of the placenta).
- Strands or threads of this membrane detach and wrap around digits or limbs.

Clinical Features

- The end result of these constricting bands is intrauterine amputation, constriction rings, and syndactyly.

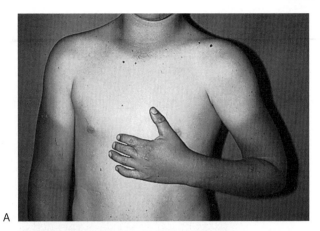

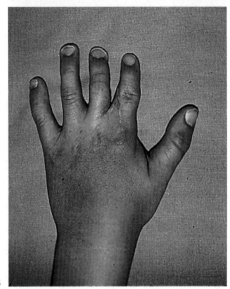

Figure 2-21   Brachysyndactyly as seen in Poland's syndrome. (**A**) The pectoralis muscle is absent on the left side. (**B**) The index and middle fingers are foreshortened, and the second and third web spaces have partial (incomplete) webbing.

- Secondary syndactyly results from abnormal tissue between the digits, which does allow separation.
- If the ring does not result in amputation, the clinical findings are present in the soft tissues.
- Some rings are comparatively superficial, but some extend to the underlying osseous structures.
- In the digits, the ring is deepest on the dorsal aspect.

Treatment

- The surgeon must distinguish between shallow and deep rings, because deep rings may have little or no venous or lymphatic drainage. In these cases, the only venous drainage is the vena comitantes of the digital arteries.
- Minimal rings of little or no cosmetic consequence require no particular treatment, but deep rings are treated with excision of the ring and closure by a series of continuous or interconnected Z-plasties.

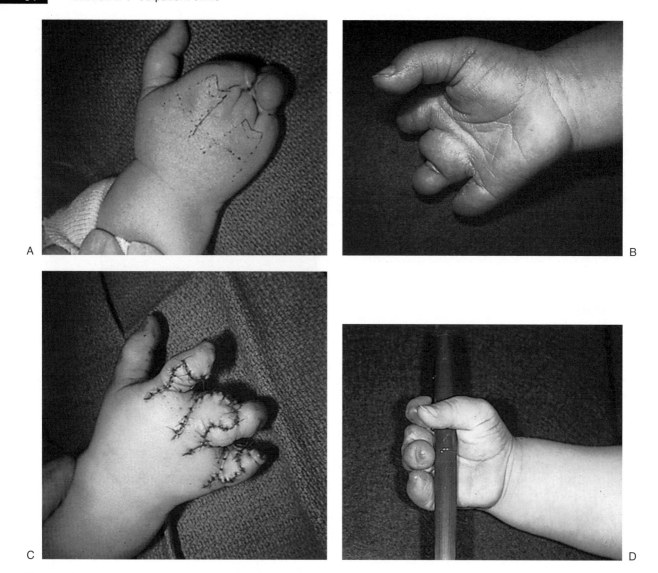

Figure 2-22   (**A–B**) A more complex form of brachysyndactyly. (**C**) Initial treatment by release of the border fingers by dorsal flaps and skin grafts. (**D**) The early result.

■ Although some surgeons have corrected the deformity in a one-stage procedure, it is customary to excise and correct no more than half the ring at the first procedure.

■ The technique involves excision of the ring, followed by mobilization of the skin and soft tissues as one composite layer. This extends down to the level between the fat and underlying fascia or vital structures.

■ A series of Z-plasties at angles of 60 degrees are then laid out.

■ The length of each limb of the Z-plasty should be equal to one-third to one-half the diameter of the digit or limb being treated.

■ The flaps should be contoured and/or thinned to produce a smooth nonbulging contour. Skin closure is with 5-0 or 6-0 chromic catgut (Fig. 2-23).

GENERALIZED SKELETAL ABNORMALITIES

Madelung's Deformity

Etiology

■ Most cases of Madelung's deformity are caused by hereditary dyschondrosteosis in the form of a lesion in the volar-ulnar zone of the distal radial physis. This retards growth asymmetrically, especially in late childhood.

Clinical Features

■ The condition is seen most often in females.

■ The distal ulna is very prominent.

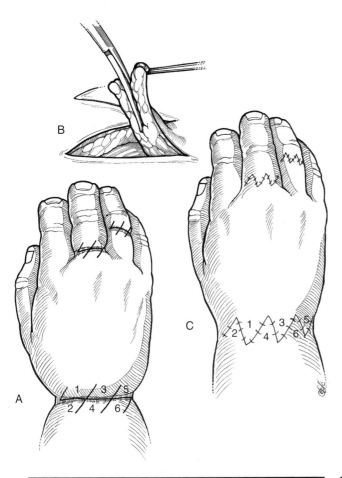
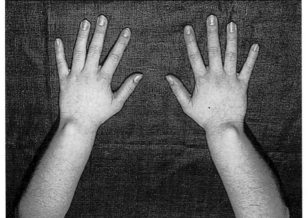
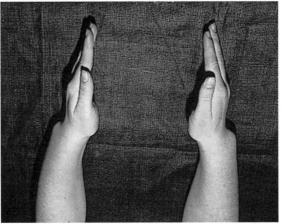

Figure 2-23 Z-plasty technique for constriction ring syndrome. (**A**) The constriction ring is excised down to the interval between the fat and underlying vital structures or fascia. Redundant fat is excised from the deep side of the flaps to achieve the appropriate contour. (**B**) Sixty-degree interconnected Z-plasties are laid out and the major arteries, veins, and nerves identified and preserved. (**C**) The flaps are rotated and sutured in place with 5-0 or 6-0 chromic catgut. (Taken from Doyle JR. Constriction ring reconstruction. In: Blair WF, Steyers CM, eds. Techniques in hand surgery. Baltimore: Williams and Wilkins, 1996.)

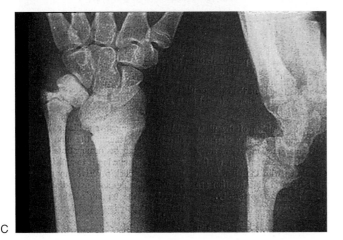

Figure 2-24 Clinical and x-ray appearance of Madelung's deformity.

- The hand is displaced palmarward along with the carpus, and is pronated in reference to the long axis of the forearm.
- The clinical and x-ray appearance is seen in Figure 2-24.

Treatment

- Surgical treatment is indicated in those patients with a significant and symptomatic deformity who are unresponsive to conservative management.
- In the adolescent, performing a physiolysis procedure in the ulnar aspect of the distal radius and then filling the defect created with fat may be considered as a possible prophylactic procedure.
- In the adult, surgical treatment is in the form of corrective osteotomy of the distal radius, with shortening or resection and stabilization of the distal ulna as needed.

SUGGESTED READING

Bayne LG, Klug MS. Long-term review of the surgical treatment of radial deficiencies. J Hand Surg 1987;12A:169–179.

Beatty E. Upper limb tissue differentiation in the human embryo. Hand Clin 1985;1:391–404.

Cole RJ, Manske PR. Classification of ulnar deficiency according to the thumb and first web. J Hand Surg 1997;22A:479–488.

Ezaki M. Treatment of the upper limb in the child with arthrogryposis. Hand Clin 2000;16:703–711.

Harley BJ, Carter PR, Ezaki M. Volar surgical correction of Madelung's deformity. Techniques in Hand and Upper Extremity Surg 2002;6:30–35.

James MA, McCarroll HR Jr, Manske PR. The spectrum of radial longitudinal deficiency: a modified classification. J Hand Surg 1999;24A:1145–1155.

Jones KL. Smith's recognizable patterns of human malformation. 5th Ed. Philadelphia: WE Saunders, 1997.

Kozin S. Congenital anomalies. In: Trumble T, ed. Hand surgery update 3, hand, elbow and shoulder. Rosemont, IL: American Society for Surgery of the Hand, 2003:599–624.

Light TR. Congenital anomalies: syndactyly, polydactyly and cleft hand. In: Surgery of the hand and upper extremity. New York: McGraw-Hill, 1996:2211–2144.

Light TR. Development of the hand. In: Green DP, Hotckiss RN, Pederson WC, eds. Green's operative hand surgery. 4th Ed. New York: Churchill Livingstone, 1999:333–338.

McCarroll HR Jr. Congenital anomalies: a 25 year review. J Hand Surg 2000;25A:1007–1037.

Moore KL. The developing human: clinically oriented embryology. Philadelphia: WB Saunders, 1988.

Ogino T. Teratogenic relationship between polydactyly, syndactyly and cleft hand. J Hand Surg 1990;15B:201–209.

Taussig HB. A study of the German outbreak of phocomelia: the thalidomide syndrome. JAMA 1962;180:1106–1114.

Van Heest A, Waters PM, Simmons BP. Surgical treatment of arthrogryposis of the elbow. J Hand Surg 1998;23A:1063–1070.

Vickers D, Nielsen G. Madelung deformity: surgical prophylaxis (physiolysis) during the late growth period by resection of the dyschondrosteosis lesion. J Hand Surg 1992;17B:401–407.

Zaleske DJ. Development of the upper limb. Hand Clin 1985;1:383–390.

TUMORS

In this chapter, the word *tumor* is used to describe any abnormal mass, or neoplastic growth or erosion, involving soft tissue or bone that may be present in the hand or wrist. Thus, benign soft tissue growths such as ganglion cysts, giant cell tumors of the tendon sheath, pyogenic granulomas, gouty deposits, and aneurysms will be discussed, along with malignant lesions of soft tissue such as melanoma, squamous cell carcinoma, and sarcomas of soft tissue and bone.

All of these conditions are considered tumors under the broad definition that a tumor is any swelling, tumefaction, or erosive lesion of skin, soft tissue, or bone. The tumors that will be discussed are representative of many of the lesions that may be commonly encountered. But this does not represent a comprehensive compilation.

Tumors of the hand and wrist are more often than not benign, but the wise practitioner will always be aware of the need to consider all possibilities. This chapter will be divided into benign and malignant categories, including lesions of the skin, soft tissue, and bone, as well as tumor-like conditions.

The most important feature of this chapter is the section on the basic principles of diagnosis, including imaging techniques, tumor classification, biopsy, and staging of soft tissue sarcomas.

PRINCIPLES OF DIAGNOSIS

- Tumors that present with a history of rapid enlargement, aching discomfort, or exceed 3 to 4 cm in size, warrant a careful evaluation of the mass and overlying skin, and require palpation for enlarged lymph nodes in the epitrochlear and axillary regions.
- A plain radiograph is an appropriate initial study to obtain. For suspicious soft tissue tumors, magnetic resonance imaging (MRI) is advised with T1, T2, and short tau inversion recovery (STIR).
  - T1 images are useful for anatomic detail.
  - T2 images show fluid collections, such as purulent material and hematomas.
  - Gadolinium contrast may enhance the appearance of soft tissue tumors.

- If a malignancy is diagnosed, the workup should include a chest radiograph and total-body scintigraphy (radioisotope scans) to rule in or out metastatic spread.
- Computed axial tomography (CT) of the chest, abdomen, and pelvis is also utilized, along with routine hematology, chemistry panel, and coagulation studies.
- A medical oncologist and radiation therapist may be used as indicated.

TUMOR CLASSIFICATION

The classification system developed by Enneking and adopted by the Musculoskeletal Tumor Society is based on the location (site) and extent of the lesion, and the histologic grade. The site of the lesion can be either intracompartmental (T1) or extracompartmental (T2). The extent of the tumor refers to the presence or absence of metastatic lesions. The histologic grade may be benign (G0), low grade (G1), or high grade (G2).

The Enneking system for staging of soft tissue and bone sarcomas is given in Table 3-1.

BIOPSY

It has been recommended that the biopsy be performed at the institution where subsequent treatment will be given, as studies have suggested that this increases the ultimate survival. Four dissection methods have been employed for biopsy and are given in Table 3-2. All biopsies should be carefully planned, and open biopsies are preferred over needle biopsies.

- The biopsy is performed under tourniquet control, and the limb is elevated *but not exsanguinated with an Esmarch bandage* prior to inflation of the tourniquet.
- The resultant biopsy tract becomes a contaminated tract of tumor cells, and will require removal en bloc if the lesion is malignant.
- Thus, the biopsy incision should be placed in such a way that it facilitates future surgery. In general, longitudinal incisions are preferred over transverse incisions.

TABLE 3-1 ENNEKING SYSTEM FOR STAGING OF SOFT TISSUE SARCOMA AND SARCOMA OF THE BONE

Stage	Grade	Site	Metastases
IA	G1	T1	M0
IB	G1	T2	M0
IIA	G2	T1	M0
IIB	G2	T2	M0
IIIA	G1–G2	T1–T2	M1
IIIB	G1–G2	T1–T2	M1

Characteristics

Grade (G)	
G1	Low
G2	High
Site (T)	
T1	Intracompartmental
T2	Extracompartmental
Metastases (M)	
M0	No regional or distant metastases
M1	Regional or distant metastases present

Taken from Enneking WF, Spanier SS, Goodman MA. A system for the surgical staging of musculoskeletal sarcoma. Clin Orthop Rel Res 1980;153:106–120.

■ Frozen sections may be used to determine that adequate tissue has been removed for study, or for determining margins. However, permanent sections are required for definitive treatment.

CAVEATS ABOUT TUMOR TREATMENT

The brief discussion under each tumor presented is meant to introduce the reader to some current concepts regarding treatment options.

The following comments may be applied to all tumors, but especially to malignant tumors and those tumors that are benign but behave aggressively, such as giant cell tumor of the bone.

■ The treatment options are not inclusive of all recommended treatments, and are intended as an introduction to the subject.

TABLE 3-2 MUSCULOSKELETAL TUMOR DISSECTION METHOD

Type	Description
Intralesional	Dissection plane is through tumor
Marginal	Dissection plane is through tumor "reactive zone"
Wide	Dissection plane well away from tumor in normal tissue but within the compartment
Radical	Dissection plane is extracompartmental

■ The treatment options may change as further experience and knowledge are applied to a given tumor.
■ A team approach is ideal, and may include surgical specialists, pathologists, diagnostic and therapeutic radiologists, and oncologists.
■ In suspicious lesions, referral of the patient to a team or center of experience for evaluation and treatment, even before a biopsy is performed, may be considered.

BENIGN SOFT TISSUE TUMORS

Ganglion Cyst

Incidence and Location

■ Ganglion cysts are probably the most commonly encountered benign soft tissue tumor in the wrist and hand.
■ They occur most commonly over the dorsal aspect of the wrist, the palmar and radial aspects of the wrist, the flexor tendon sheath in the region of the A-1 pulley, and over the distal interphalangeal (DIP) joint of the fingers and the interphalangeal (IP) joint of the thumb.
■ In the flexor tendon sheath, they are termed volar retinacular ganglia. Over the DIP joint of the digits and IP joint of the thumb, they are termed mucous cysts.
■ Less common sites are about the PIP joint, the carpal and ulnar canal, in the substance of extensor tendons, from the extensor retinaculum, and in carpal bones.

Diagnosis

Clinical Features

■ At the wrist, ganglion cysts may present as a firm, non-tender mass that can be up to several centimeters in diameter (Figure 3-1). These cysts may transilluminate when a bright light source, such as a penlight, is pressed against them.
■ The size of the cyst may vary from time to time, and may be related to physical activities.
■ The lesions are fixed to the underlying structures, and do not move with flexion or extension of the wrist or digits.
■ At the wrist, the diagnosis may be confirmed by aspiration that yields a thick, jelly-like material that has no color.
■ At the radial and palmar aspects of the wrist, the ganglion cyst may lie beneath the radial artery and push it up beneath the skin into a more prominent position. This displacement of the radial artery must be remembered if the ganglion cyst is treated by aspiration or excision (Figure 3-2).
■ In the flexor sheath, they present as firm masses in the palm at the level of the metacarpophalangeal joint, and become more prominent with hyperextension of the fingers (Figure 3-3).
■ In the digits, they may be seen as thin walled cysts that overlie the DIP and IP joints and may often be associated with osteoarthritis (Figure 3-4 and Figure 3-5).
■ Examples of a ganglion cyst in the carpal canal and in the substance of the extensor tendon, respectively, are seen in Figure 3-6 and Figure 3-7.

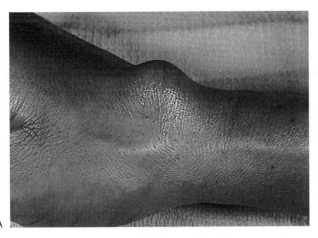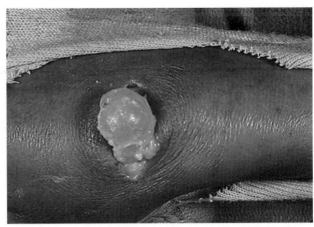

A B

Figure 3-1 (**A**) View of the dorsal aspect of the right wrist, showing a large cystic mass. (**B**) The mass had the characteristic appearance of a ganglion cyst and was removed, along with a suitable portion of the dorsal capsule.

Differential Diagnosis

- At the dorsal aspect of the wrist, the ganglion should not be confused with a carpal boss, rheumatoid synovitis, or an accessory muscle called the extensor digitorum brevis manus (EDBM).
- The correct diagnosis is aided by noting that a carpal boss occurs at the base of the middle finger metacarpal and the adjacent capitate, is hard like bone, and is more distal than the dorsal carpal ganglion that arises from the region of the scapholunate capsule (Figure 3-8). For a complete discussion of a carpal boss, see the section on benign bone tumors.
- Rheumatoid synovitis is usually softer to palpation than the ganglion, and moves distal and proximal as the fingers are flexed and extended. It flattens out when a complete fist is made and presents with a "tuck sign" when the fingers are extended (Figure 3-9).

- The EDBM is a fusiform-shaped mass that occurs over the metacarpals, does not transilluminate, and maintains its shape with finger flexion and extension (Figure 3-10).
- An intratendinous ganglion of an extensor tendon may occur over the wrist and hand, and is diagnosed by the fact that it moves with flexion and extension of the fingers and maintains its shape. Rheumatoid synovitis, however, does not (see Figure 3-7 and Figure 3-9).

Treatment

Treatment for these lesions may be in the form of observation, aspiration (with or without an injection of cortisone), multiple puncture technique, or surgical excision. While the specifics of treatment are beyond the scope of this text, note that for surgical intervention of the ganglion, current

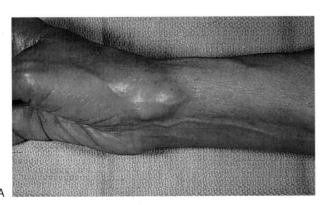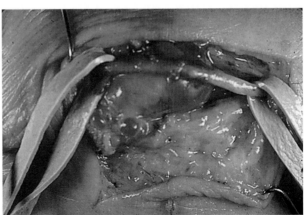

A B

Figure 3-2 (**A**) View of the radial and palmar aspect of the right wrist showing a prominent mass. (**B**) The mass arose beneath the radial artery; rubber bands have been placed about the artery proximal and distal, to retract the artery out of harms way so that the ganglion may be excised. Remember that the radial artery may be misidentified as a vein. It should be protected and preserved.

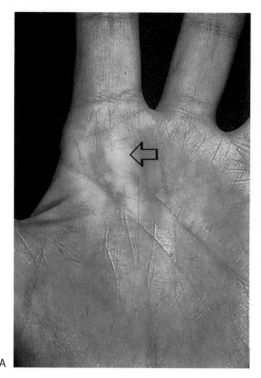 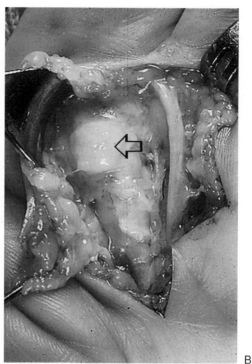

A   B

Figure 3-3   (**A**) Mass (*arrow*) at the base of the left index finger ray. (**B**) The volar retinacular ganglion cyst (*arrow*) is arising from the first annular pulley and will be excised along with a small portion of the pulley.

conventional wisdom recommends excision of a small portion of the wrist capsule along with the cyst.

- Excision of a recurrent or multilocular cyst may be aided by careful injection of a dilute solution of methylene blue into the cavity of the cyst using a 30-gauge needle.
  - The dye provides for excellent contrast of the cyst from the surrounding structures, and aids in its complete removal (Figure 3-11).
- The intratendinous ganglion can usually be removed from the substance of the extensor by longitudinally splitting its fibers and shelling out the cyst (see Figure 3-7).
- A word of caution is warranted when aspirating or removing a volar carpal ganglion:
  - The radial artery is in close proximity, and is often applied to the wall of the ganglion.
  - A preoperative assessment of the status of the radial and ulnar arteries with an Allen's test and/or Doppler device will allow you to make appropriate decisions should the radial artery be injured during the procedure.
- These lesions have no malignant potential, and may be observed. Cosmetic rather than functional factors, or concerns about cancer, may play a significant role in the patient's decision to remove a large cyst from the wrist.
- In contrast, the volar retinacular cyst may interfere with grip, and one or two punctures of the cyst often result in its disappearance.
- Patients may try to needle a mucous cyst at home, and should be cautioned against this. Because the lesion

connects to the joint, any resulting infection may be difficult to treat.

Pathology
- The diagnosis is seldom in doubt, based on the clinical appearance and microscopic demonstration of a fibrous capsule. That structure is often lined with a flattened layer of epithelial-like cells and contains a mucinous material that usually stains a pale blue on hematoxylin and eosin sections.

Giant Cell Tumor of the Tendon Sheath

Incidence and Location
- Aside from the ganglion cyst, this is probably the most common benign soft tissue tumor encountered in the upper extremity.
- Giant cell tumor may not be a suitable term for this lesion, because it does not always contain giant cells and is not always associated with the tendon sheath. This lesion has also been called a fibrous tissue xanthoma.
- It is the most common tumor in the palm and digits, and appears to have a propensity for the radial three digits and the DIP joint region.
- It is usually on the palmar surface of the hand and fingers, but may occur dorsally.

Clinical Features and Diagnosis
- These tumors are slow growing, firm, nodular, and nontender.

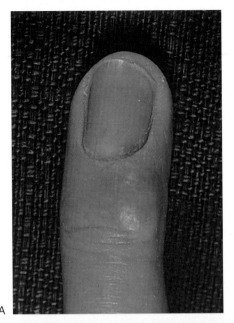

A

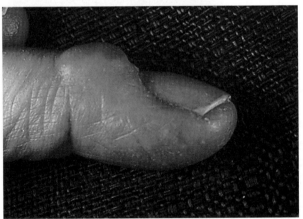

B

Figure 3-4 Characteristic appearance of the ganglion cyst (mucous cyst) at the distal interphalangeal joint.

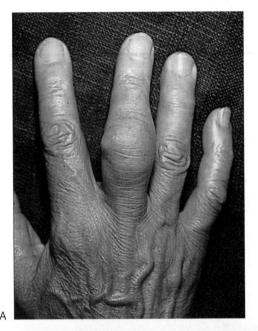

A

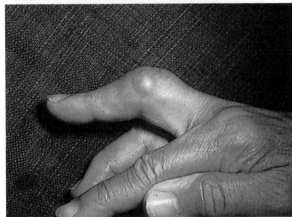

B

Figure 3-5 Ganglion cyst arising from the PIP joint. Radiographs (not shown) demonstrated significant degenerative arthritis in this joint.

■ They are brown-yellow. In some instances, portions of the lesion may lie just beneath the skin; a hint of this color may show through in a thin-skinned patient.
■ In contrast to the ganglion, they do not transilluminate.
■ They may occur as compound multinodular lesions.
■ Radiographs may demonstrate a soft tissue mass. In some instances there may be erosion of the adjacent osseous phalanx, or extension into the joint space.

Treatment
■ Treatment is surgical through an appropriate incision.
■ Because of their slow growth, these lesions may wrap around nerves and other vital structures, and care must be exercised in their removal. Figure 3-12 shows the preoperative, intraoperative, and microscopic appearance of such a lesion.
■ At surgery, the lesions are moderately easy to remove.

■ Failure to identify all satellite extensions or discover an extension into the joint space, however, may be associated with a higher than normal recurrence rate. The same comments would apply if the tumor has invaded the flexor tendon sheath.

Pathology
■ The microscopic appearance often, but not always, reveals collections of giant cells in a dense and cellular fibrous tissue matrix.
■ Hemosiderin collections are prominent, and may explain the coloration of these lesions (Figure 3-12D).

Epidermal Inclusion Cyst

Incidence and Location
■ These cysts are found most commonly in the distal phalanx, most often in males. They may be found following amputation or injury of the fingertip.

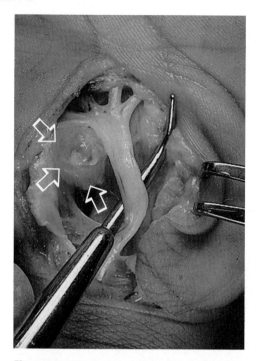

Figure 3-6 This large ganglion cyst arose from the volar aspect of the carpal canal, and caused median nerve complaints. The ganglion is to the left (*arrows*) and the probe is deflecting the median nerve.

■ They are most commonly found on the palmar surface of the digits, in contrast to sebaceous cysts (due to obstructed sebaceous glands) that occur on the dorsal aspect of the hand. Epidermal inclusion cysts are believed to result from the traumatic implantation of epithelial cells into the underlying soft tissue.

Clinical Features and Diagnosis
■ These slow-growing masses in the distal phalanx of the fingers or thumb are firm and slightly moveable.
■ They are thick-walled white lesions that contain a white, thick, "cheesy" material.
■ A history of trauma is not always present.
■ If the cyst has been present for a long time, it may produce a pressure defect on the adjacent osseous phalanx that is visible on radiograph.
■ The typical appearance is shown in Figure 3-13.

Treatment
■ Epidermal inclusion cysts are easily removed from the surrounding soft tissue.
■ They may often recur, and some surgeons have claimed a lower recurrence rate by excising an ellipse of skin over the cyst that may contain the site of the original traumatic implantation.

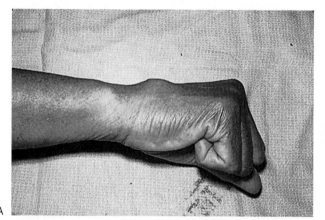

A

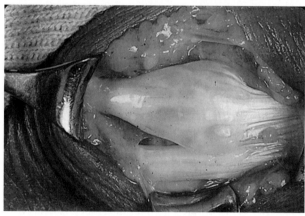

B

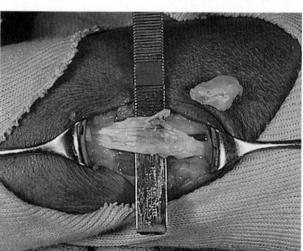

C

Figure 3-7 (**A**) Ganglions may arise in the substance of extensor tendons, and present as a mass that moves distally with flexion of the fingers. (**B**) The ganglion cyst is fusiform in shape. (**C**) It can be removed without loss of integrity of the extensor tendon.

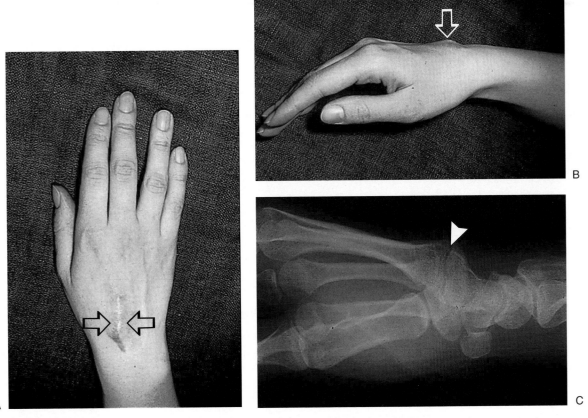

Figure 3-8   The carpal boss is often mistaken for a ganglion cyst. (**A–B**) Prominent mass and scar (*arrows*) following an attempted removal of a "ganglion." (**C**) A radiograph clearly demonstrates the true nature of this mass.

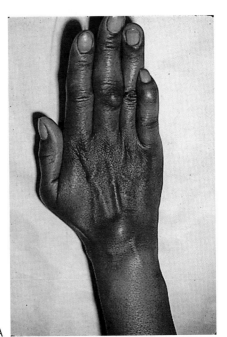

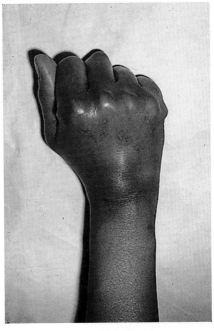

Figure 3-9   This patient with rheumatoid synovitis demonstrates the fact that synovial lesions "bunch-up" and become more prominent when the fingers are extended (**A**), and flatten out when a fist is made (**B**).

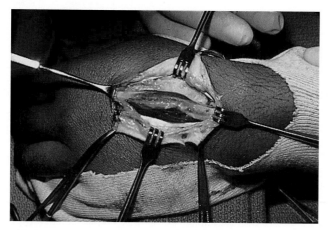

Figure 3-10 This anomalous muscle called the extensor digitorum brevis manus (EDBM) may also mimic the ganglion cyst; it is distal to the typical ganglion location, and is more fusiform in shape.

Pathology

- They have a wall of fibrous tissue on microscopic section, and the white, "cheesy" material is keratin.
- These lesions have no malignant potential.

Lipoma

Incidence and Location

- Although lipoma is the most common benign soft tissue tumor in the body, it is relatively uncommon in the wrist or hand.

- It may occur in any location in the hand and wrist, including Guyon's canal or the carpal tunnel—where it may produce nerve symptoms.

Clinical Features and Diagnosis

- The typical lipoma is represented by a soft to firm non-tender mass that does not transilluminate.
- It may be firm if it has been growing for a long time in a confined anatomic space.
- It may be diagnosed on radiograph by its comparatively diminished density (it appears darker) than the surrounding tissues.
  - This finding, called Bufalini's sign, demonstrates the comparative diminished radio-density of fatty tissue.
- Figure 3-14 demonstrates the preoperative, intraoperative, and x-ray appearance of a large lipoma in the hand.

Treatment and Pathology

- Lipomas are well demarcated and easily removed, and recurrence is unusual.
- Typical fat cells are seen on the histological sections, with minimal amounts of fibrous tissue.
- There is no malignant potential.

Neurilemmoma (Schwannoma)

Incidence and Location

- Neurilemmoma is the most common benign nerve tumor of the hand and wrist, and most often involves the median nerve at the wrist.
- It is most often seen in the 4th to 6th decades.

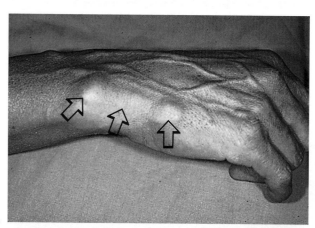

A

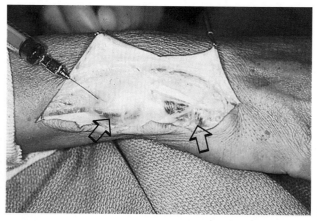

B

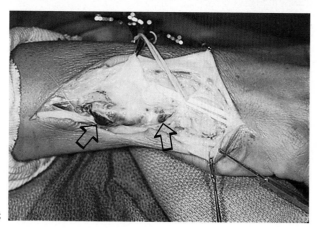

C

Figure 3-11 (**A**) This elongated compound ganglion cyst spanned a considerable distance across the wrist and hand (*arrows*). (**B**) An injection with a dilute solution of methylene blue demonstrated its true extent. (**C**) That made its complete removal easier.

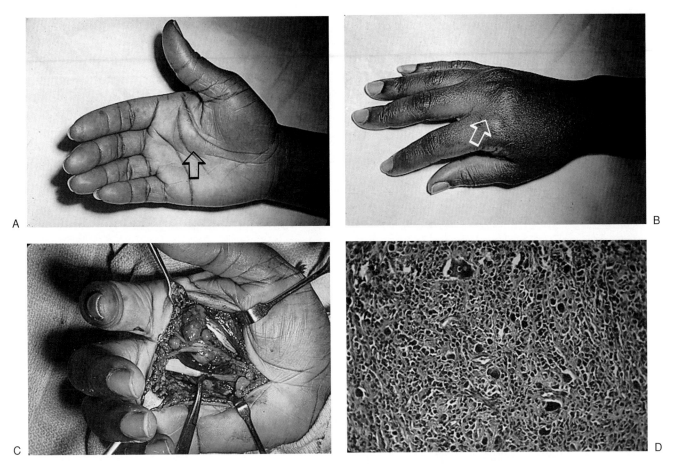

Figure 3-12 (**A**) This compound giant cell tumor of the tendon sheath presented as a palmar hand lesion (*arrow*). (**B**) It also presented as dorsally. (**C**) It was associated with several vital structures in the palm, and invaded the metacarpophalangeal joint of the middle finger. (**D**) The characteristic histologic features of giant cells in a cellular matrix with scattered hemosiderin deposits are noted. (Hematoxylin and eosin, original magnification ×160.)

Clinical Features and Diagnosis
- Most often, patients present with a pain free mass on the flexor side of the wrist.
- Percussion over the mass may produce some distal paresthesias.
- The mass is mobile side-to-side, but not longitudinally. It does not transilluminate.
- It is more medial in the wrist than the usual volar carpal ganglion.

Treatment and Pathology
- This lesion is easily differentiated from other nerve tumors by the fact that it may be removed from the nerve involved by shelling it out of the nerve.
- The nerve fibers are separated longitudinally, and the mass is removed (Figure 3-15A-D).
- It is surprising to note that little or no nerve deficit is present following its removal.
- The histological appearance in Figure 3-15E is characteristic, and recurrence is uncommon.

Neurofibroma

Incidence and Location
- Neurofibromas are benign nerve lesions that arise from nerve fasciculi.
- They may be single or multiple, and are most common in neurofibromatosis (von Recklinghausen's disease).
- They may present as subcutaneous masses about the hand and wrist.

Clinical Features and Diagnosis
- These lesions may be associated with café-au-lait spots seen in neurofibromatosis.
- The typical appearance of this lesion in a patient with neurofibromatosis is shown in Figure 3-16.

Treatment
- In contrast to the neurilemmoma, these lesions have a nerve that enters and exits the mass, and that cannot be freed from the mass.

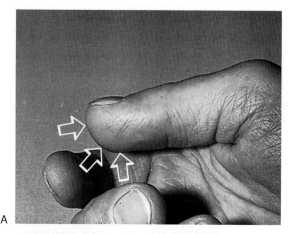

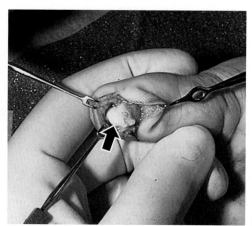

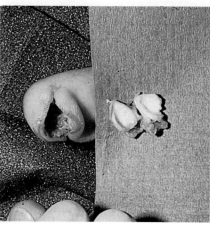

Figure 3-13 (**A**) The enlarged terminal phalanx (*arrows*) of this carpenters thumb revealed a thick-walled cyst. (**B**) It was filled with keratin material. (**C**) It was easily shelled out of the pulp of the terminal phalanx.

■ If a small sensory nerve is involved, it may be excised along with the lesion—and little or no residuals will be encountered. Note the afferent and efferent nerve fibers from the neurofibroma in Figure 3-16C.

■ Progressively enlarging lesions that are symptomatic may require removal.

Pathology

■ The characteristic histology is demonstrated in Figure 3-16D.

■ Malignant degeneration is possible in patients with neurofibromatosis.

Digital Fibroma of Infancy

Incidence and Location

■ This is a benign but very aggressive lesion that occurs almost exclusively in the fingers and toes of children before the age of one year.

■ In the hand, it is most often seen in the region of the IP joint.

Clinical Features and Diagnosis

■ These lesions present as small raised masses that are nontender.

■ With growth, joint contracture and deformity may be seen.

■ The lesions may grow at an alarming rate, and may mimic a malignancy (Figure 3-17).

Treatment

■ Treatment may include observation, limited and wide excision, and amputation.

■ Observation is indicated because spontaneous resolution may occur. Progressive deformity may require surgical intervention.

■ Wide excision and skin grafting may give the best local control but recurrence is high (Figure 3-18).

Pathology

■ Intracytoplasmic inclusion bodies are present in the histologic section, which suggests a viral or myofibroblast origin.

Juvenile Aponeurotic Fibroma

Incidence and Location

■ This childhood and adolescent condition is a benign but aggressive lesion seen most often in the palm.

Clinical Features and Diagnosis

■ The lesion presents as a small, pain free mass that may be closely applied to the underlying vital structures in the palm.

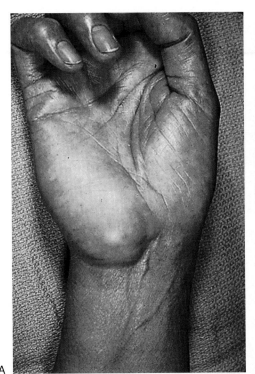
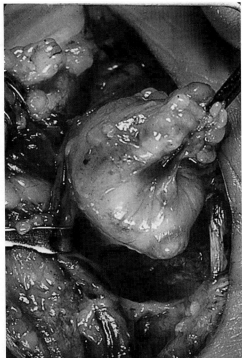

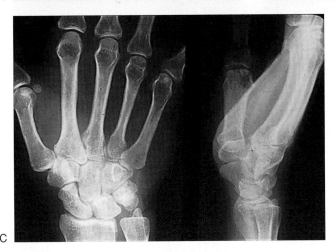

Figure 3-14   (A) This patient presented with a slow-growing, pain-free mass in the palm of her right hand. (B) It was a classic lipoma. (C) The diagnosis was made preoperatively, based on the radiolucent nature of the lesion on a radiograph (Bufalini's sign).

Treatment
- Wide excision with sparing of the associated vital structures is the treatment of choice. Use skin grafts or flap coverage as needed.

Pathology
- The histologic appearance resembles fibrosarcoma; the recurrence rate may be 50% or more.

Nodular Fasciitis

Incidence and Location
- This condition is also known as pseudosarcomatous fasciitis, subcutaneous pseudosarcomatous fibromatosis, and infiltrative fasciitis.

- The lesion begins as a small nodule in the forearm or hand.

Clinical Features and Diagnosis
- The lesion is characterized by a small but rapidly growing nodule that was only recently noted.
- Figure 3-19 shows the intraoperative and histologic appearance of this lesion.

Treatment
- The natural history of this lesion appears to be self-limited, and even partially excised lesions do not reoccur.
- The key to treatment of this lesion is to differentiate it from a soft tissue sarcoma, and to avoid inappropriate and aggressive treatment.

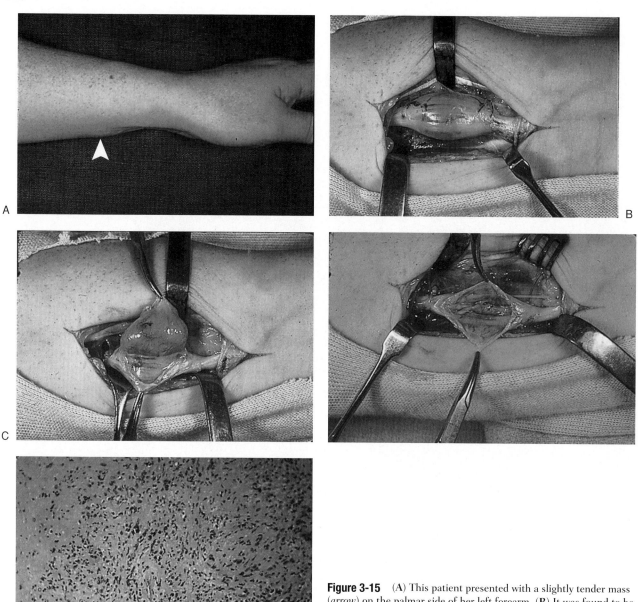

Figure 3-15　(**A**) This patient presented with a slightly tender mass (*arrow*) on the palmar side of her left forearm. (**B**) It was found to be a large tumor involving the substance of the median nerve. (**C**) The lesion was "shelled-out" under loupe magnification. (**D**) No residual nerve deficits were noted following excision of this schwannoma. (**E**) Microscopic view of the schwannoma. Note the dense and irregular cellular pattern. (Hematoxylin and eosin, original magnification ×160.)

Pathology
■ Its histologic appearance may resemble that of a fibrosarcoma and myxoid liposarcoma.

Pyogenic Granuloma

Incidence and Location
■ These lesions most often involve the contact surface of the digits.

Clinical Features and Diagnosis
■ These lesions present as dark red, raised, and small spherical masses that are often associated with a history of injury to the site of presentation.

■ They may appear to be sessile, but are usually pedunculated and bleed easily.
■ Figure 3-20 shows two examples of pyogenic granuloma.

Treatment
■ In most cases, the condition is cured by severing the stalk or pedicle flush with the skin, followed by applying silver nitrate to the base of the pedicle on the digit.
■ Some have suggested that a small ellipse of skin be excised with the lesion, but this may not be necessary.

Pathology
■ This condition represents "run-away" angiogenesis, and has no malignant potential. The histologic sections reveal a collection of blood vessels.

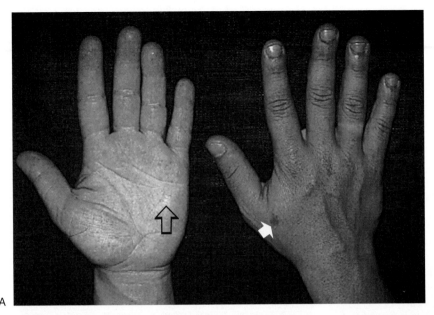
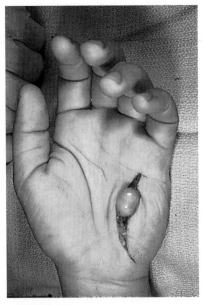
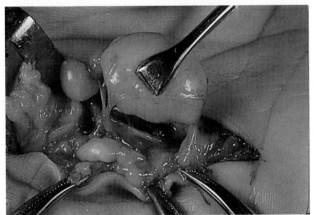
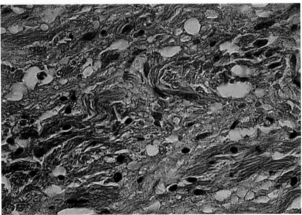

Figure 3-16   (A) This woman, age 24, presented with a small subcutaneous mass in the hypothenar eminence of the left hand (*arrow*), which was associated with a café-au-lait spot on the dorsum of the opposite hand (*arrow*). (B–C) The lesion was a neurofibroma that arose from a small sensory fiber, and complete removal was possible without significant deficit. (D) Histologic appearance of the neurofibroma, demonstrating a moderately cellular matrix. (Hematoxylin and eosin, original magnification ×400.)

Glomus Tumor

Incidence and Location
- This is a relatively uncommon lesion that occurs in the distal phalanx and often under the fingernail.
- It represents a neoplastic proliferation of the smooth muscle cells of the normally occurring glomus, which is a temperature regulating shunt.

Clinical Features and Diagnosis
- The patient with this tumor presents a classic history of pain that is often severe, cold sensitivity, and tenderness over the distal phalanx.
- Physical findings may include discoloration (reddish-blue) beneath the fingernail, if the lesion is subungual; ridging or deformity of the nail plate; and point tenderness.

- Radiographs may reveal a bony defect in the osseous phalanx because of pressure from the glomus tumor.
- Although often subungual, any painful and tender subcutaneous area in the digit with the above noted history should be considered to be a glomus tumor.
- Figure 3-21 demonstrates a patient with a longstanding glomus that was being treated as an infection (note the changes in the finger nail), and the intraoperative appearance of the lesion. Figure 3-21C shows the intraoperative appearance of another glomus tumor, which is smaller.

Treatment
- Excision of the lesion is the treatment of choice. It is performed through a window in the nail, or by elevating the nail proximally to expose the lesion.
- Many of the lesions are in the soft tissues proximal to the nail plate, and may be removed through an incision in

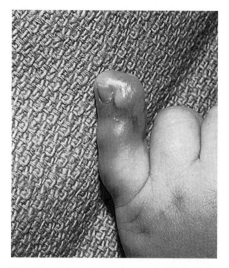

Figure 3-17   A clinical example of digital fibroma of infancy. This lesion enlarged rapidly in this infant of 1 year of age. Note the enlarged little finger and the alarming appearance of the lesion.

this region without disturbing the nail plate (see Figure 3-21C).

Pathology
■ Histologic findings include endothelial pericyte and non-myelinated nerve fibers.

Hemangioma

Incidence and Location
■ The majority of these tumors are seen within the first 4 weeks of life.
■ Females are affected three times as frequently as males.
■ Rapid growth may be noted in the first year of life, followed by slower growth thereafter.
■ The final stage is represented by involution; by age 7, 70% of the lesions have involuted.
■ Noninvoluting lesions are capillary or cavernous.

■ The *capillary* hemangiomas are represented by the port-wine stain.
■ The *cavernous* hemangiomas are represented by arteriovenous connections that may be either low or high flow in nature.

Clinical Features and Diagnosis
■ The capillary hemangioma is represented by a minimally raised port-wine stain lesion of variable size.
■ It presents as a bluish, raised subcutaneous mass that is nontender, soft, and often multiloculated.
■ An MRI offers the diagnostic advantage of being noninvasive, and may delineate the proximity of neural structures. It is especially useful in visualizing skeletal muscle hemangiomas.
■ Radiographs of cavernous hemangiomas may show phleboliths (calcific deposits in a vein wall or thrombus).
■ The preoperative and intraoperative appearance of a cavernous hemangioma is seen in Figure 3-22.

Treatment
■ Management of hemangiomas is usually conservative, since most will involute by 7 years of age.
■ Surgical management may be indicated in noninvoluting lesions if the diagnosis is in question, or if ulceration, bleeding, or recurrent infection is a problem.
■ Surgery involves ligation of feeder vessels and complete excision of the lesion.
■ Cryosurgery and YAG laser treatment has been used.

Keratoacanthoma

Incidence and Location
■ This is a fast-growing skin tumor that mimics the appearance of squamous cell carcinoma.
■ It most often occurs on the hair-bearing dorsal skin of the forearm, wrist, and hand.
■ In 1 to 2 months, it may grow from a small papule to a raised lesion that is 2 to 3 cm in diameter.

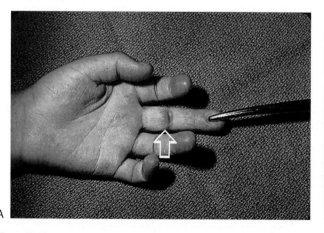

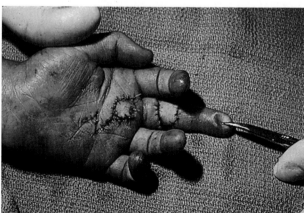

Figure 3-18   Another example of digital fibroma of infancy (proximal phalanx of the middle finger) in another slightly-older child (**A**) who was treated with an excision and skin graft (**B**).

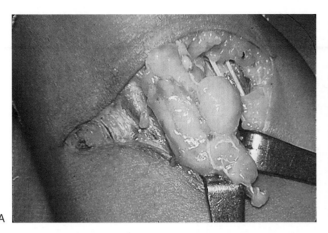

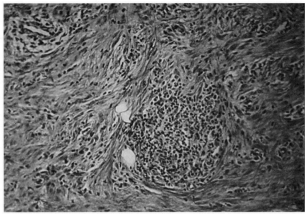

Figure 3-19 (**A**) Intraoperative appearance of this example of nodular fasciitis in the forearm. (**B**) Histologic appearance of this benign lesion. Note the cellular "nodule" in the lower right. (Hematoxylin and eosin, original magnification ×160.)

Clinical Features and Diagnosis

■ The history of rapid growth, and its size and alarming appearance, may make it difficult to distinguish it from squamous cell carcinoma.

■ However, the central keratin plug in this lesion is in contrast to the small area of central necrosis seen in squamous cell carcinoma.

■ Their rapid growth is in marked contrast to the slower growth of squamous cell carcinoma.

■ Figure 3-23A demonstrates the clinical appearance of the lesion.

Treatment

■ Although the natural history of this lesion is spontaneous regression after a latent phase of variable duration, the lesion should be excised for an accurate diagnosis.

■ The resultant defect may be closed by skin grafts as needed, and the resultant scar will, more often than not, be less noticeable than the original lesion.

■ Figure 3-23B demonstrates the postoperative appearance of this lesion following excision and split-thickness skin grafting.

Pathology

■ The entire tumor must be evaluated. A pathologist experienced in skin tumors is useful in distinguishing this lesion from squamous cell carcinoma.

■ Figure 3-23C shows the histologic appearance of the lesion at ×35 magnification.

SOFT TISSUE TUMOR-LIKE CONDITIONS

Aneurysms (True and False)

Incidence and Location

■ Although not a neoplasm, an aneurysm may be appropriately included in a discussion of tumors of the hand

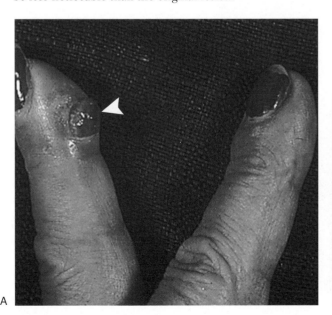

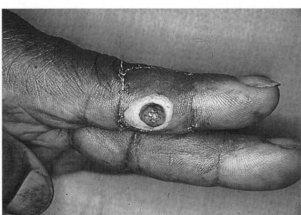

Figure 3-20 Two examples of pyogenic granuloma, both of which were excised without recurrence.

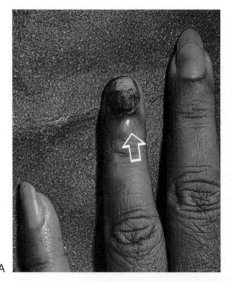

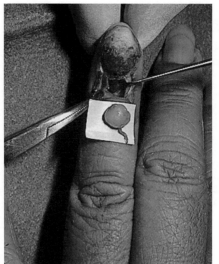

A

B

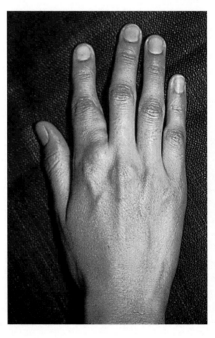

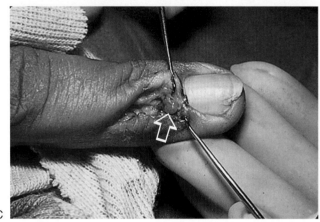

C

Figure 3-21   (**A**) A soft tissue mass (*arrow*) proximal to the fingernail, with deformity of the fingernail. (**B**) Surgery revealed a classic glomus tumor. (**C**) Another example (*arrow*) of a glomus tumor.

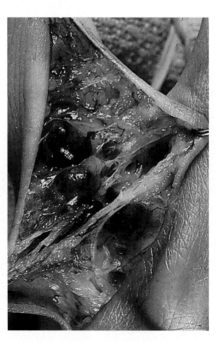

A

B

Figure 3-22   (**A**) This patient presented with a long-standing history of a soft and pain-free mass over the index finger. (**B**) At surgery, the grape-like clusters of a cavernous hemangioma were noted and excised.

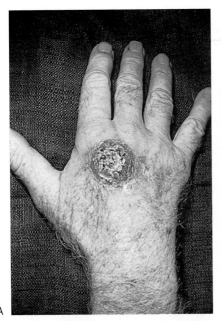
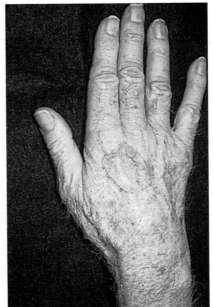

A

B

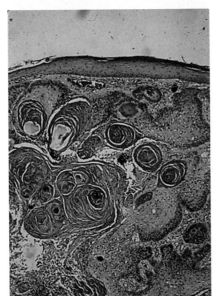

C

Figure 3-23 (A) This elderly man presented with this ominous-looking lesion that he said began as a small bump only 6 weeks before. (B) The rapid growth of this lesion indicated the probability that the lesion was a keratoacanthoma, and excision followed by skin graft was performed. (C) Note the histologic appearance of the keratoacanthoma. (Hematoxylin and eosin, original magnification ×35.)

and wrist since it must be differentiated from a true neoplasm.

- Aneurysms may be *false* or *true*.
  - *False* aneurysms result from a penetration of the blood vessel wall, with subsequent hemorrhage and hematoma formation that organizes to form a lumen in continuity with the injured vessel. This often global-shaped lesion does not have a true vascular endothelial lining.
  - A *true* aneurysm results from an injury to the vessel wall that permits gradual expansion or dilatation of the vessel wall, and has a true vascular epithelial lining.
- *True* aneurysms occur most frequently in areas subjected to repetitive trauma, such as the ulnar artery and the superficial arch in the palm. Mechanics, bakers, or others that use their hypothenar eminence as a tool for forceful pounding or pushing may experience such injuries.
- *False* aneurysms are most often seen after penetrating injuries, and are most common at the palmar side of the wrist. They may occur in the radial artery in the anatomical snuffbox, the palmar arch, and the digits. Aneurysms of the ulnar and digital vessels are evenly distributed between the *false* and *true* types.

Clinical Features and Diagnosis

- Large aneurysms may present as visible and palpable masses at the wrist, or in the palm of the hand.

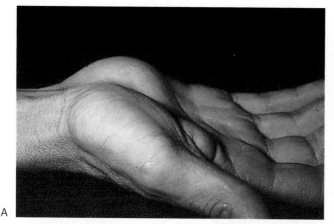

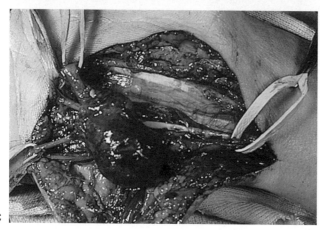

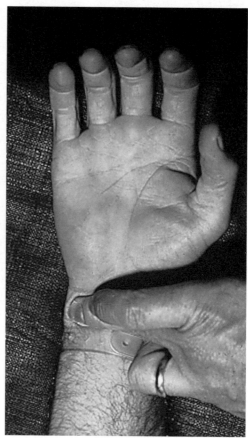

Figure 3-24 (**A**) This baker noted a slowly growing mass on the ulnar aspect of his right hand for several months. It was believed that repetitive impact over the hypothenar eminence may have been associated with the lesion. (**B**) Occlusion of the radial and ulnar arteries at the wrist diminished the size of the mass. (**C**) At surgery, an aneurysm of the ulnar artery was identified and excised, and the resultant arterial defect was bridged by a vein graft.

- *True* aneurysms are usually fusiform-shaped, whereas *false* aneurysms are global- or spherical-shaped.
- Neurologic deficits may occur due to pressure on adjacent nerves.
- Large aneurysms may have a bruit that is audible with a stethoscope.
- Doppler ultrasonography and arteriography are useful diagnostic aids.
- Arteriography aids in preoperative planning and defines the nature of collateral blood flow and thus may aid in the method of treatment.
- Figure 3-24 demonstrates a true aneurysm of the ulnar artery in a 34-year-old baker.

Gouty Tophus

Incidence and Location
- Gouty tophi, although not true neoplasms, may occur throughout the hand and wrist, and may be associated with joint and tendon dysfunction.

Clinical Features and Diagnosis
- Gouty deposits may be small or large, and may often erode through the skin over the extensor surfaces of the hand.

- They are chalky white collections of a toothpaste-like material that is unmistakable in appearance.
- Figure 3-25 shows the clinical, x-ray, and intraoperative appearance of gout in the left hand.

Treatment
- Treatment is directed at the medical control of the gout.
- Surgical intervention is directed at removal of large deposits that may compromise joint and/or tendon function.

MALIGNANT SOFT TISSUE TUMORS

Skin Tumors

Basal Cell Carcinoma

Incidence and Location
- These lesions are located on the dorsum of the hand and wrist in the areas of sun exposure.
- They ultimately present as raised erosions, with an occasional "pearly" border.

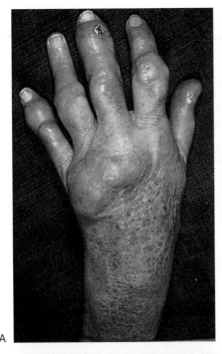

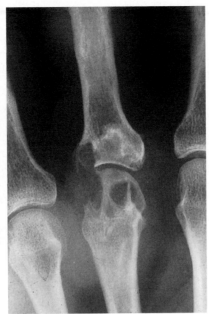

A

B

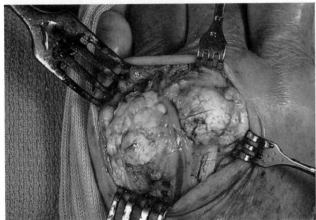

C

Figure 3-25 (**A**) This patient with a longstanding history of gout presented with gouty tophi and skin erosion over the middle finger distal interphalangeal joint. (**B**) Radiographs revealed bone erosions at the metacarpophalangeal joint. (**C**) Clinical appearance of the tophi at the time of excision.

■ They are slow growing but may invade deeper tissues over time.

Clinical Features and Diagnosis
■ There are many variations in the appearance of this tumor, and they may present as areas of skin atrophy, pink discoloration, or telangiectatic changes. They also may have a scar-like quality to their advancing edges.

Treatment
■ Surgery is by excision of the lesion with a sufficient margin, followed by immediate histologic confirmation of the adequacy of excision.
■ Closure may be by direct means in small lesions, or by skin grafts or flaps in larger cases.

Squamous Cell Carcinoma

Incidence and Location
■ These lesions are the most common malignant tumor in the hand.
■ They have the capacity to expand locally and to metastasize via the lymphatic or blood vessels.

Clinical Features and Diagnosis
■ They may vary from wart-like, slow-growing lesions under or near the fingernail, to large, ulcerated, or exophytic growths most commonly over the dorsum of the finger and hand.
■ They may also present as a red, scaly, and sometimes ulcerated area. Figure 3-26 demonstrates the clinical and

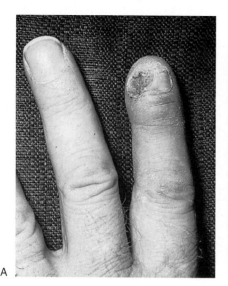
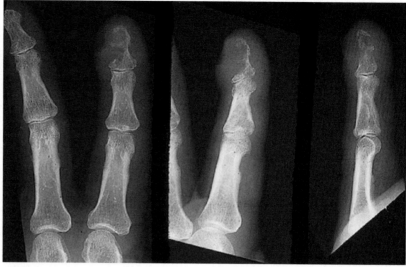

Figure 3-26 (A) This patient was being treated for a chronic infection about his left index finger. (B) X-rays demonstrated an erosion of the osseous phalanx, and surgery confirmed the presence of squamous cell carcinoma of the nail bed.

x-ray appearance of this lesion that was treated initially as an infection.

Treatment
- Treatment will vary depending on the location, size, and extent of the lesion, and presence or absence of metastatic lesions.
- In those lesions confined to the terminal phalanx, amputation at, or proximal to, the DIP joint may be an effective treatment.

Malignant Melanoma

Incidence and Location
- The incidence of these dangerous and insidious tumors continues to increase, and a significant percentage of these lesions involve the upper extremity.
- They represent 5% of skin cancers, but are responsible for 75% of deaths from skin cancer.
- Sun exposure is considered to be the major cause for this increase.
- Four major types have been described.

Clinical Features and Diagnosis
- Melanomas are cancers of the melanocytes.
- Half arise from atypical moles; the other half arise de novo.

Classification

Superficial Spreading Melanoma
- This is the most common type in Caucasians, and represents 70% of all melanomas.
- It is most likely to arise from, or adjacent to, a pre-existing nevus.

- It begins as a pigmented plaque, and has a radial growth phase of months to years before vertical growth begins.
- Metastatic spread is associated with the vertical growth phase.

Nodular Melanoma
- This type represents 15% of all melanomas, and has little or no radial growth phase. It may metastasize early.
- It grows rapidly, and usually arises de novo.
- It is usually dark blue-black in color, but may be gray or pink. If it is, it is called an amelanotic melanoma.

Acral Lentiginous Melanoma
- This type represents 2% to 8% of all melanomas, and is found on palmar surfaces and the fingernail.
- It does not appear to be associated with sun exposure, and is seen in all ethnic groups.
- In those groups where melanoma is uncommon (African American and Hispanics), it is the most common variant found.
- A slow-growing radial growth phase occurs before vertical growth. Because of its location, it is an area not routinely examined—so the diagnosis may be delayed.
- The subungual melanoma is in this category, and usually affects the matrix of the thumbnail or great toenail.
- Acral lentiginous melanomas must be differentiated from subungual hematomas. A subungual hematoma is usually associated with a history of injury, and may progress distally as nail growth occurs.

Lentigo Maligna Melanoma
- This type represents 4% to 10% of all melanomas, and is a type of de novo growth that is associated with long-term sun exposure.
- It is sometimes associated with actinic keratoses, and is most common on the dorsal surface of the forearm.

TABLE 3-3 BRESLOW SYSTEM FOR STAGING MALIGNANT MELANOMA

Depth of Lesion (mm)	5-Year Survival Rate (%)
<0.76	89
0.76–1.49	75
1.5–2.49	58
2.5–3.99	46
>3.99	25

■ It begins as a tan, flat lesion that may have a radial growth phase of 1 to 2 decades.

Surgical Staging

The Breslow system (Table 3-3) is based on the depth of the lesion in millimeters, and 5-year survival rates are based on this system.

Treatment

■ The depth of invasion of the malignant melanoma determines the recommended treatment.

■ Melanoma *in situ* that has not gone beyond the basement membrane is excised with a 0.5 to 1.0 cm margin.

■ Tumors less than 1.0 mm deep should be excised with a 1 cm margin. In the subungual location, this means amputation at, or just proximal to, the DIP joint.

■ Melanomas 1 to 4 mm in depth should be excised with a 2 cm margin, and the proximal lymph nodes should be evaluated with scintigraphy and biopsy as indicated. If a lymph node is positive, consideration may be given to a chemotherapy protocol. That is beyond the scope of this chapter.

■ Melanomas greater than 4 mm in depth have a very high incidence of lymph node involvement.

   ■ Excision with a 3 cm margin is advised, and clinically involved nodes should be resected.

   ■ Chemotherapy may be considered based upon the patient's general medical condition.

Soft Tissue Sarcomas

Incidence and Location

■ Soft tissue sarcomas are relatively uncommon in the hand.

Clinical Features

■ Most soft tissue sarcomas present as a painless mass that has been present for a long time but has recently grown.

■ An epithelioid sarcoma is a notable exception, and may present as an ulcerated nodule that has been treated as an infection.

Diagnosis

■ In general, soft tissue sarcomas may be misdiagnosed as infection, ganglion, or lipoma.

■ In addition to assessment of size, location, depth, and mobility, the lymph nodes should be evaluated.

■ Plain radiographs may demonstrate regional calcification and bone involvement.

■ An MRI is useful for determining abnormal anatomy and the extent of disease. It also may lead to a suitable pre-operative diagnosis and aid in pre-operative planning.

■ Although very small lesions may be excised with a surrounding cuff of tissue, larger lesions may be evaluated with an incisional biopsy.

■ The biopsy incision must be planned to meet the needs of more extensive treatment later on, and transverse, oblique, or similar incisions should be avoided.

■ It should be considered that biopsies will contaminate all adjacent tissue planes.

Staging

■ After the diagnosis of a sarcoma has been established, systemic staging should be performed with CT of the chest and axilla, as upper extremity sarcomas commonly spear to the lungs and regional lymph nodes.

■ Staging is based on grade, size, and the presence or absence of metastatic lesions, as well as the histologic grade.

■ A useful guide is the system developed by Enneking and adopted by the Musculoskeletal Tumor Society (see Table 3-1).

Treatment

The management of soft tissue sarcomas is under constant study, and changes to current recommendations and new modalities may emerge as new or modified treatment protocols are developed and evaluated. Surgery is the primary form of local treatment for soft tissue sarcoma. It is planned as two distinct parts, and consists of resection and reconstruction.

■ Excision is the initial form of treatment. Primary consideration is for an appropriate resection, while secondary consideration is for reconstruction.

■ The goal of surgery is to achieve complete resection of the tumor, with a surrounding cuff (2 to 3 cm) of normal tissue.

■ If these margins cannot be achieved, then amputation should be considered.

■ Following wide excision of a large, high-grade lesion, external radiation or radiation implants (brachytherapy) therapy may be performed.

■ The role of chemotherapy in the preoperative or postoperative period is still under investigation.

■ Patients with metastases may be treated by chemotherapy and/or resection of lung lesions.

Epithelioid Sarcoma

Incidence and Location

■ This tumor is said to be the most common soft tissue sarcoma of the hand.

Clinical Features and Diagnosis

■ This tumor presents as a slow-growing, benign-looking, firm nodule that may occur in the digits, palm, or volar forearm in a young adult.

- The nodule may ulcerate. It tends to spread proximally along the course of tendons, lymphatics, and fascial planes, and does not respect fascial boundaries.
- It is often misdiagnosed, and has a propensity for recurrence and regional lymph node involvement.

Treatment

- This lesion must be treated aggressively, with a wide excision, radical resection, or amputation.
- Lymph node biopsy is indicated even without clinical evidence of involvement.
- Marginal excision is not advised.
- Radiation may be considered after wide excision of large lesions; chemotherapy may be considered in those patients with lymph node involvement, recurrence, or metastatic lesions.

Pathology

- Histologic features include formation of discrete nodules of epithelial cells with areas of central necrosis.

Synovial Sarcoma

Incidence and Location

- Synovial cell sarcoma is one of the more common sarcomas in the hand and wrist.
- They typically occur over the wrist, are seldom seen in the finger, and occur in the 15 to 40 age group.
- They typically arise around joints, tendons, and bursae.

Clinical Features and Diagnosis

- These tumors often present as slow growing, painless, and firm masses that may have been present for several years.
- Soft tissue calcification may be seen on plain radiographs.

Treatment

- Surgery is the initial form of treatment. Primary consideration is for an appropriate resection. Reconstruction is a secondary consideration.
- The goal of surgery is to achieve complete resection of the tumor, with a surrounding cuff (2 to 3 cm) of normal tissue.
- If these margins cannot be achieved, amputation should be considered.

Pathology

- Small size may not be associated with a more favorable prognosis.
- Histologic sections reveal two cell types: epithelial cells and spindle cells.

BENIGN BONE TUMORS

Enchondroma

Incidence and Location

- These bone lesions are the most common primary bone tumors of the hand, and 35% of all enchondromas arise in the hand.

- The proximal phalanx is the most common site of occurrence, followed by the metacarpal and middle phalanx.
- Most lesions occur in patients 10 to 40 years of age.

Clinical Features and Diagnosis

- The usual presentation is with a painless swelling over a phalanx or metacarpal.
- Pain and deformity may be the presenting complaint due to a pathologic fracture through the enchondroma.
- Pathological fractures in the hand are most often associated with enchondroma.
- X-rays reveal a well-defined lytic lesion, with calcification of the matrix in some cases.
- The vast majority of cases may be diagnosed without CTs or MRIs.
- X-ray appearance, intraoperative findings, and histologic appearance are depicted in Figure 3-27.

Treatment

- Small lesions that are incidental findings on a radiograph may be treated by observation.
- Larger lesions, or those associated with fractures, may be treated by curettage and bone grafting.
- In patients with a pathologic fracture, it is best to reduce the fracture as needed and allow the fracture to heal before curettage and bone grafting.
- The osseous phalanx is often thin at the site of the lesion, and attempts at open reduction, fixation, and bone grafting may be difficult because of the lack of sufficient bone for anatomic reduction and fixation.
- Shortening or deformity may be the end result.
- After healing of the fracture, however, good bone stock is present, and definitive curettage and bone grafting may be achieved.

Pathology

- Histologic sections reveal a characteristic cartilage matrix with scattered lacunae that contain cartilage cells.

Multiple Enchondromatosis (Ollier's Disease) and Maffucci's Syndrome

- Multiple enchondromatosis is an uncommon and nonhereditary disorder manifested by multiple enchondromas in the metaphysis and diaphysis of the long bones and of the short, tubular bones of the hands and feet.
  - These benign lesions may become malignant chondrosarcoma or osteosarcoma in 30% of the patients, so careful monitoring is indicated.
- Maffucci's syndrome is a rare condition, and its x-ray findings are similar to Ollier's disease. However, patients may also have multiple hemangiomas.
  - These patients may also develop sarcomas of the bone and of the soft tissue.

Aneurysmal Bone Cyst

Incidence and Location

- This lesion accounts for about 5% of all benign bone tumors, but only 3% to 5% of these lesions occur in the hand.

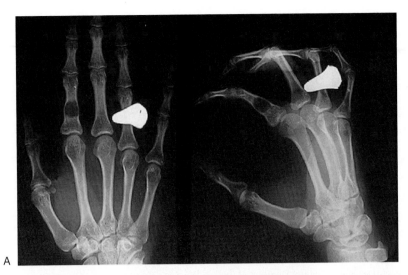
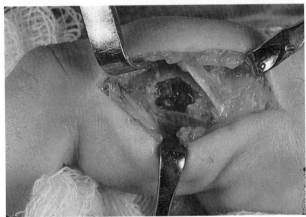
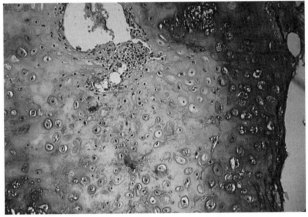

Figure 3-27   (**A**) This patient's hand radiograph revealed an incidental finding of a lytic lesion of the proximal phalanx of the index finger. (**B**) Biopsy, followed by curettage, revealed an enchondroma. (**C**) The histologic appearance of an enchondroma. (Cartilage stain, original magnification ×160.)

■ Hand lesions are most common in the second decade, and metacarpal involvement is more common than involvement of the phalanx.

Clinical Features and Diagnosis
■ These lesions often present as a rapidly enlarging, alarming-appearing mass.
■ Radiographs demonstrate an expanding lesion on the bone metaphysis/diaphysis, with thinning of the cortex.
■ An MRI may suggest a fluid-filled lesion.
■ Soft tissue extension is uncommon, and metastasis has not been reported.
■ This lesion is demonstrated in Figure 3-28.
■ A biopsy and limited curettage was performed shortly after this depiction, and the lesion gradually diminished in size over the next several months.

Treatment
■ An incisional biopsy is performed followed by curettage, cryosurgery, and bone grafting, if sufficient bone stock is available.

■ If bone stock is not available, wide excision and reconstruction may be indicated. Cryosurgery may be associated with damage to the physis and subsequent growth arrest.

Giant Cell Tumor of Bone

Incidence and Location
■ This lesion accounts for about 5% of all benign bone tumors, but only 2% of these lesions occur in the hand.
■ This tumor occurs most commonly in the 4th decade and may involve the distal radius, the metacarpals and phalanges, and, rarely, the carpal bones.

Clinical Features and Diagnosis
■ The usual clinical presentation is with pain and swelling in the affected region.
■ Radiographs demonstrate a lytic lesion with no matrix and indistinct borders.
■ Cortical expansion, destruction, and soft tissue extension are common.

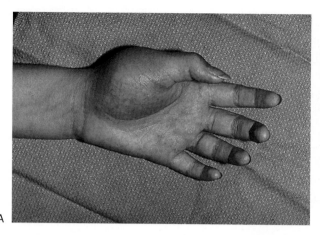
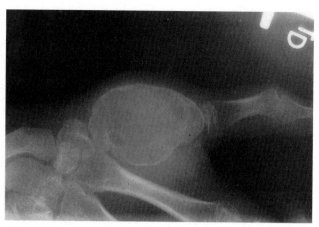

A   B

Figure 3-28   (A) This otherwise healthy teenager presented with a rapidly enlarging mass in her left thumb. (B) X-ray examination revealed an expanding osteolytic lesion of the thumb metacarpal. Biopsy revealed an aneurysmal bone cyst, and curettage resulted in involution of the lesion.

Treatment

- Giant cell tumors of bone, although considered to be benign bone lesions based on their histology, behave aggressively, may metastasize, and may ultimately result in death.
- Lesions in the hand have a higher risk of local recurrence. These lesions should be approached as malignant lesions, and should be staged following an incisional biopsy with chest radiographs and a bone scan.

- Lesions in the metacarpals or phalanges that have penetrated the cortex may be treated with wide excision and reconstruction, or amputation.
- Distal radius lesions confined within the cortex may be treated with curettage, burring, cryosurgery, and cementation if sufficient bone stock is available.
- Those lesions that have pathologic fracture or cortical perforation are treated by wide excision of the distal radius, and reconstruction. Figure 3-29 depicts such a lesion that was treated by wide soft-tissue and bone

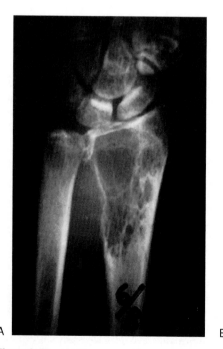
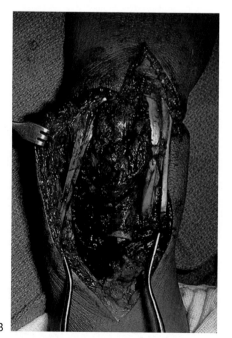
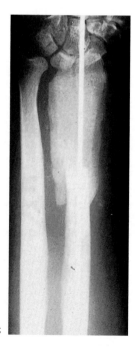

A   B   C

Figure 3-29   (A) This giant cell tumor of bone had been initially treated by curettage, followed by recurrence as noted here. (B) Wide excision of soft tissue and bone was performed. (C) The resultant defect was treated with a large iliac crest bone graft and wrist fusion.

resection, followed by an immediate bone graft from the iliac crest, and wrist fusion.

Osteoid Osteoma

Incidence and Location
- About 5% to 15% of these benign bone lesions appear in the hand and wrist.
- This lesion is most often seen in the carpal bones or proximal phalanx. It mostly presents in the 2nd or 3rd decade.

Clinical Features and Diagnosis
- Patients with this lesion often present with a history of a dull ache in the affected region, which is often relieved by nonsteroidal anti-inflammatory medication.
- Swelling and tenderness is usually present. Radiographs may demonstrate reactive and sclerotic bone, with or without a small nidus surrounded by a radiolucent area.
- A CT scan may further delineate the lesion.
- Lesions in the distal phalanx may result in swelling in the pulp and nail deformity.
- The clinical and preoperative x-ray appearance, as well as the intraoperative radiograph, are depicted in Figure 3-30A-C.

Treatment
- Surgery in the form of excision of the nidus often results in a cure.
- Some have argued that treatment may be nonsurgical, since nonsteroidal anti-inflammatory medication may relieve the pain. Also, the natural history of this reactive and benign bone lesion is one of gradual involution over a several-year period.

Pathology
- The histologic appearance of the dense bone is illustrated in Figure 3-30D.

Carpal Boss

Incidence and Location
- Although not a true neoplasm, this bony prominence is often misdiagnosed as a ganglion cyst or other tumor over the dorsal aspect of the wrist.
- It is an osteophytic lesion that develops at the base of the index and middle finger metacarpals and the adjacent carpal capitate.
- Carpal boss is most common in women, and usually presents in the 3rd and 4th decades.

Clinical Features and Diagnosis
- The lesion is bony, hard, nonmobile, and sometimes-tender mass that is most noticeable when the wrist is flexed.
- Radiographs profiling the mass (30 to 40 degrees of supination and 20 to 30 degrees of ulnar deviation) reveal a prominent, raised triangular bony mass that arises from the opposing dorsal aspect of the metacarpal and capitate.
- An irregular and narrow pseudo-articulation is noted between the two opposing halves of the mass. The abutment

of the two opposing surfaces may be likened to an osteoarthritic joint, and may explain some of the symptoms of tenderness and discomfort.
- A small, thin-walled, bursa-like sac may develop over the boss, and may be confused with a ganglion cyst.
- This lesion is depicted in Figure 3-8.

Treatment
- In patients with significant symptoms, the two sides of the boss are removed down to normal articular cartilage.
- Care is taken to avoid detachment of the extensor carpi radialis brevis (ECRB) tendon insertion on the base of the middle finger metacarpal.

MALIGNANT BONE TUMORS

Osteogenic Sarcoma

Incidence and Location
- This is the most common malignant bone tumor in children and adolescents, but is rarely seen in the hand.
- When it does appear in the hand, it is usually in patients in the 4th to 6th decades.
- It is most often found in the proximal phalanges and metacarpals, and rarely in the carpus.

Clinical Features and Diagnosis
- The usual presentation is that of a rapidly enlarging mass that is firm and painful.
- Radiographs may reveal an expanding sclerotic tumor with new bone formation or a lytic lesion and an associated soft tissue mass.

Treatment
- Incisional biopsy should be performed with the anticipated need for limb salvage and amputation.
- In the finger, wide excision or ray amputation may be entertained along with neoadjuvant chemotherapy.

Chondrosarcoma

Incidence and Location
- This lesion is the most common primary malignant bone tumor that occurs in the hand.
- The lesion occurs mainly in the proximal phalanges and metacarpals in patients over the age of 60 years.

Clinical Features and Diagnosis
- The lesion often presents as a firm, slow-growing, and sometimes painful mass.
- Radiographs show a lesion with poorly defined borders and with areas of lysis and stippled calcification.
- Cortical breakthrough and extension into the soft tissues helps to distinguish it from enchondroma.
- Chondrosarcomas are slow growing.
- Metastasis of about 10% may be seen after local recurrence following intralesional treatment.

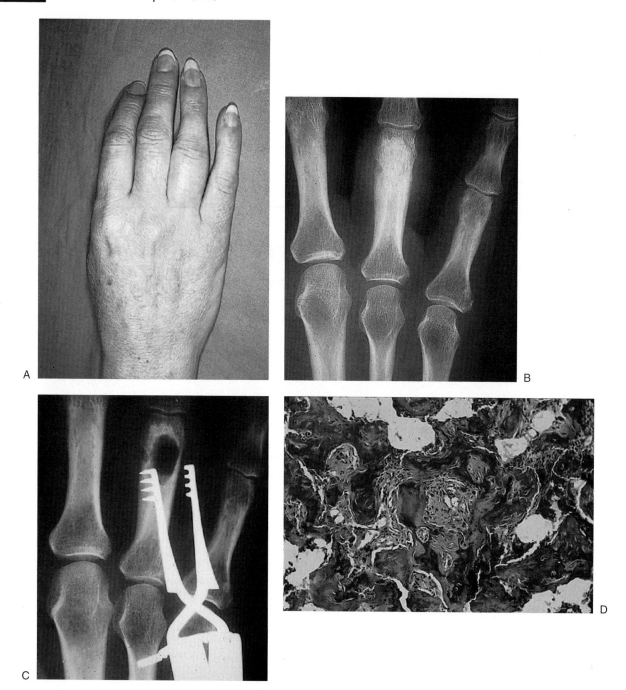

Figure 3-30 (**A**) This patient noted pain and progressive swelling in the proximal phalanx of the right ring finger, which was relieved by aspirin. (**B**) X-rays revealed an osteoblastic lesion that appeared to have a segment (nidus) that was denser in its distal aspect. (**C**) This dense area was removed using a high-speed burr, and the symptoms resolved. (**D**) Review of the specimen by the pathologist confirmed the preoperative diagnosis of osteoid osteoma. (Hematoxylin and eosin, original magnification ×160.)

Treatment

- Incisional biopsy is performed and reviewed by a pathologist very familiar with cartilage lesions.
- Preoperative treatment includes a chest CT, because these lesions most often metastasize to the lungs.
- Treatment is by wide excision, including digit or ray amputation.

Metastatic Tumors

Incidence and Location

- Metastatic lesions in the hand (acrometastases) are uncommon and the incidence is less than 0.3%.
- When it does occur, the phalanges and metacarpals are equally involved, and involvement of the carpal bones is said to be rare.

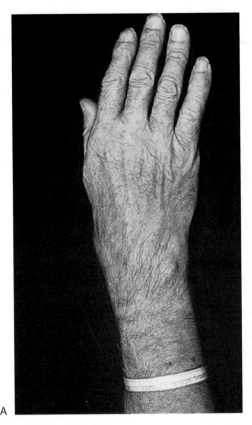

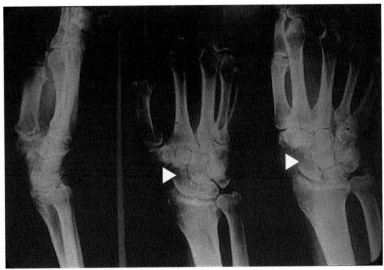

A   B

Figure 3-31   Metastatic carcinoma of the wrist. (A) This man, age 62, with bronchogenic carcinoma of the lung complained of pain and swelling in the right wrist. (B) Radiographs demonstrated an osteolytic metastatic lesion (*arrows*) in the radial aspect of the wrist.

- Bronchogenic carcinoma of the lung is said to be the primary malignancy in about 50% of the cases.
- Other primary sources are renal, esophageal, breast, colon, prostate, thyroid gland, and bone cancer.

Clinical Features and Diagnosis

- Clinical findings sometimes mimic an infection with pain, swelling, and erythema being present.
- Radiographs usually reveal a lytic lesion, although metastatic prostate cancer can appear as a sclerotic lesion.
- If the metastatic lesion appears without a history of prior tumor, then a suitable workup is performed to identify the primary site.
- Biopsy and cultures of the lesion will usually confirm the diagnosis.
- Figure 3-31 shows clinical and x-ray views of a 62-year-old man with bronchogenic carcinoma of the lung that has metastasized to the wrist.

Treatment

- Treatment is usually palliative and is based on the needs of the patient.

SUGGESTED READING

Aletikiar K, Leung D, Zelefsky M, et al. Adjuvant brachytherapy for primary high-grade soft-tissue sarcoma of the upper extremity. Ann Surg Oncol 2002;9:41–56.

Al-Qattan MM. Giant cell tumors of tendon sheath: classification and recurrence rate. J Hand Surg 2001; 26B:72–75.

Athanasian, E. Tumors. In: Trumble, TE, ed. Hand surgery update 3, hand, elbow, shoulder. Rosemont, IL: American Society for Surgery of the Hand, 2003:555–588.

Carroll RE, Bowers WH. Keratoacanthoma: an unusual hand tumor. Clin Orthop 176;118:173–179.

Cheng CY HN, Su KY, Hsu RWW. Treatment of giant cell tumor of the distal radius. Clin Orthop 2001;383:221–228.

Enneking WF, Spanier SS, Goodman MA. A system for the surgical staging of musculoskeletal sarcoma. Clin Orthop 1980;153:106–120.

Gustafson P, Arner M. Soft-tissue sarcoma of the upper extremity: descriptive data and outcome in a population-based series of 108 adult patients. J Hand Surg 1999;24A:668–674.

Kang HJ, Shin SJ, Kang ES. Schwannomas of the upper extremity. J Hand Surg 2000;25B:604–607.

Marcuzzi A, Acciaro A, Landi A. Osteoid osteoma of the hand and wrist. J Hand Surg 2002;27B:440.

Stephen AB, Lyons AR, Davis TR. A prospective study of two conservative treatments for ganglia of the wrist. J Hand Surg 1999;24B:104–105.

Warso M, Gray T, et al. Melanoma of the hand. J Hand Surg 1997;24A:354–360.

DUPUYTREN'S DISEASE

Dupuytren's disease (DD) is a well-known but poorly understood clinical entity involving the palmar and digital fascia of the hand. From the patient's perspective, this disease begins as small nodules or lumps in the palm or fingers, which may eventually develop into longitudinally oriented cords or bands that contract. When this happens, a condition known as *Dupuytren's contracture* results (Figure 4-1).

HISTORICAL FEATURES

Henry Cline in 1777 was the first to recognize that the disease involved the palmar fascia. He recommended fasciotomy—as did his student, Astley Cooper of London. However, it was in 1831, at the Hotel Dieu in Paris, that Dupuytren presented a lecture, later transcribed by one of his students, that described the disease within the palmar fascia. Dupuytren recommended open fasciotomy through a transverse incision, and also recommended it be left open to heal.

EPIDEMIOLOGY AND ETIOLOGY

The condition is most often seen in patients with Northern European and Scandinavian ancestry, and is more common in males than females. It has a genetic etiology and has been associated with seizure disorders, alcohol and tobacco use, and HIV. Hormones such as peptides (cytokines) may play a role in the development of DD and may promote transformation of fibroblasts into myofibroblasts.

PATHOPHYSIOLOGY

DD begins in the perivascular fibroblasts within the fibrous bundles of the fascia. During the active stage of the disease when progressive joint contracture occurs, myofibroblasts are the predominant cells. These cells demonstrate cell-to-cell and cell-to-stroma attachments. The myofibroblasts contain contractile elements called alpha smooth muscle actin. Figure 4-2 depicts the cellular model of contracture in DD.

Histologically, DD resembles scar tissue, and the collagen found in DD is type III. That's the same type of collagen identified in scar tissue. Normal palmar fascia is mainly type I collagen with only small amounts of type III collagen. Type IV and VI collagen with fibronectin are seen in early stages of DD, when myofibroblasts proliferate.

NORMAL ANATOMY

Palmar Aponeurosis (PA)

The PA is the specialized structure in the central portion of the palm with longitudinal, transverse, and vertical fibers. It is distinguished from the covering of the thenar and hypothenar eminences by its triangular shape and greater thickness. The longitudinal fibers of the palmar fascia represent the distal continuation of the palmaris longus (when present). These fibers, which begin as a conjoined apex at the base of the palm, form bundles in the middle and distal palm that run to the corresponding four fingers and, in some instances, to the thumb. The longitudinal fibers are essentially parallel to the deeper flexor tendons; because of this arrangement, they are sometimes called *pretendinous* bands. The four bundles of longitudinally oriented fibers overlay *transverse fibers* in the palm, which are located at the junction of the middle and distal thirds of the palm and over the metacarpophalangeal (MCP) joints. The transverse fibers of the PA course beneath the longitudinal cords, from the ulnar side of the small finger to the radial side of the index finger. In the thumb-index finger web space, the *proximal commissural ligament* (PCL) is the radial continuation of these transverse fibers. The more distal counterpart of the PCL is the *distal commissural ligament* (DCL), which is more longitudinally oriented and which spans the space between the MCP joint of the thumb and index finger. Both the PCL and DCL course toward the thumb's MCP joint, where they send attachments to the undersurface of the skin. The deep portion of the DCL sends fibers to attach on both sides of the flexor pollicis longus (FPL) sheath. The more longitudinal orientation of the DCL may be a factor in its more likely involvement in DD, although both the DCL and PCL may be involved in Dupuytren's contracture. The PCL and DCL

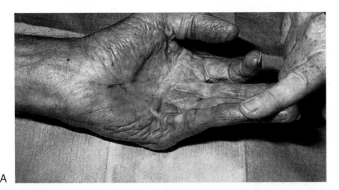

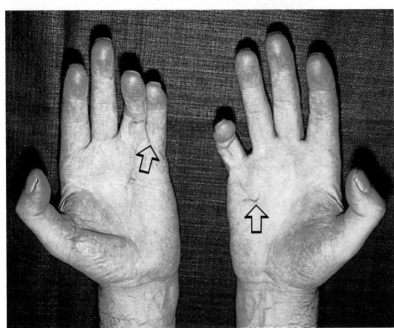

Figure 4-1 Clinical appearance of Dupuytren's disease. (**A**) An elderly male with a several year history of progressive "drawing down" of his left little finger. Note the prominent cord that begins in the palm and extends into the finger and that limits passive and active extension of the finger. (**B**) Another patient with recurrent Dupuytren's disease showing contracture of the web space between the left ring and little finger (*arrow*), and "dimpling" of the skin (*arrow*) in the palm on the right hand.

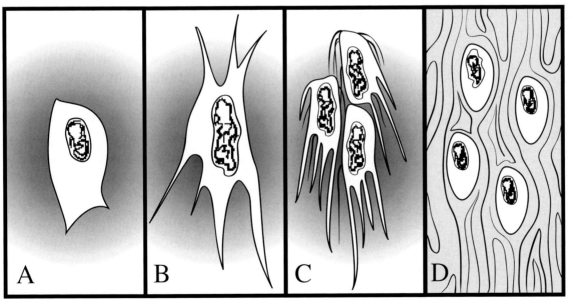

Figure 4-2 Diagrammatic depiction of the pathogenesis of Dupuytren's disease. (**A**) The perivascular fibroblast in an early nodule, surrounded by fibrillary material penetrating into the palmar fascia. (**B**) The myofibroblast that appears when clinical contracture is apparent. (**C**) The myofibroblasts have cell-to-cell and cell-to-stroma connections. (**D**) The mature cord consists of longitudinally oriented type III collagen, with a few residual cells of fibroblasts and myofibroblasts. (Redrawn after Chiu HF, McFarlane RM. Pathogenesis of Dupuytren's contracture: a correlative clinical-pathological study. J Hand Surg 1978;3A:1–10.)

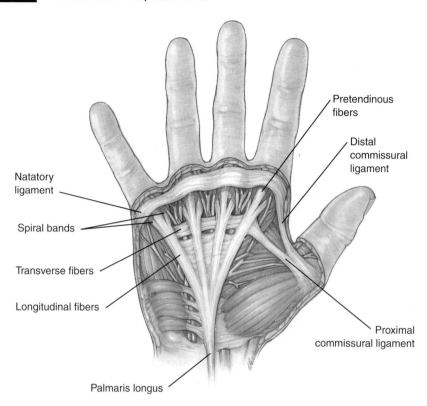

Natatory ligament

Spiral bands

Transverse fibers

Longitudinal fibers

Pretendinous fibers

Distal commissural ligament

Proximal commissural ligament

Palmaris longus

Figure 4-3 The palmar fascia and its associated ligaments. See the text for details.

are usually thinner and less noticeable than the transverse fibers between the fingers. Both the longitudinal and transverse fibers course through the vertical septa to reach the transverse metacarpal ligament. The third component of the palmar fascia consists of the nine vertical (sagittal) septa, called the fibers of Legueu and Juvara, which are located deep to the transverse fibers. They form the sides of eight canals, four of which contain the underlying finger flexor tendons, and four adjacent ones that contain the lumbrical muscles and neurovascular bundles. These paratendinous septa, along with the transverse palmar aponeurosis, form a fibrous tunnel system that has been described as the palmar aponeurosis pulley. These nine vertical septa are anchored to the transverse metacarpal ligament, palmar interosseous, and adductor fascia, and they divide the distal portion of the central palmar space into eight canals. The normal anatomy of the palmar fascia is depicted in Figure 4-3.

Function

Compression Loading/Shock Absorbing. Any discussion of the role of the palmar retinacular structures must note that these structures are only a part of a complex tissue consortium designed to meet a variety of functional demands. This complex three-dimensional network may be considered a fibrous skeleton or framework designed to assist in the hand's mechanical functions. Compression loading is a common force applied to the hand, and requires a system of shock absorption. In the hand, one method of shock absorption is to contain somewhat compliant tissues, such as fat or muscle, in compartments that can change shape but not volume. This is amply demonstrated in the palm, with its various layers of multidirectional fascia that contain and compartmentalize fat and muscle while

conforming to the shape or contour of the object being grasped or manipulated.

Skin Anchorage. Skin is retained by fascial elements that allow the hand to flex while maintaining the skin in position. The skin folds at prominent creases that are minimally anchored; this contrasts to the skin on the adjacent sides of the crease, which possess multiple strong anchor points. This allows the relatively unanchored skin to fold, while the anchored skin is held in place. These fascial anchors may be vertical, horizontal, or oblique, depending on the specific need of the skin envelope. A good example is the horizontal attachments of the superficial fibers of the pretendinous bands, which attach to the dermis of the distal palm. This arrangement resists horizontal shearing forces in gripping actions, such as holding a hammer or a golf club. The PA, which includes the nine vertical septa anchored to the deep transverse metacarpal ligament, is tensed with power grip and thus anchors the skin to the skeleton of the hand.

Skeletal Stability. Although not a part of the palmar fascia, the previously mentioned transverse metacarpal ligament that attaches to the palmar plates of the MCP joints plays a role in maintaining the transverse metacarpal arch, as do the transverse fibers of the palmar fascia and the natatory ligaments.

Joint Stability. The fascial ligaments in the web space of the finger and thumb may play a role in limiting abduction, and thus may indirectly limit the impact of potentially destabilizing forces that might be applied to the digits.

Pulley Function. The transverse fibers of the palmar fascia, supported by the vertical septa, form what is called the palmar aponeurosis pulley.

Vascular Protection and Pumping Action, and Nerve Protection. Vascular structures in the palm are protected by surrounding substantial fibrous tissue and fat pads. When the hand is compressed, as in making a fist, the incompressible fascia may act as a venous pumping mechanism. This is in contrast to the large dorsal veins on the dorsum of the hand, which are surrounded by loose areolar tissue. The nerves in the palm are protected by fascial structures; those near the base of the fingers are protected by fat pads.

Distal Palmar and Digital Fascia

The longitudinal fibers of the PA divide into *three layers* in the distal palm. *Layer one*, the most superficial, inserts into the skin of the distal palm and onto the proximal aspect of the flexor sheath. *Layer two* splits and passes on each side of the flexor sheath, where it continues distally as the *spiral band* beneath the neurovascular bundle and natatory ligaments. It then inserts on the *lateral digital sheet*. *Layer three* passes on each side of the flexor sheath to the region of the MCP joint. The natatory ligaments have transverse as well as curved fibers that follow for the contour of the webs. The curved or distal continuations of these fibers join the lateral digital sheet. The lateral digital sheet is a condensation of the superficial digital fascia on each side of the finger; it receives fibers from the natatory ligament, the spiral band, and *Grayson's ligament*. The retaining skin ligaments of Grayson and *Cleland* stabilize the skin during flexion and extension of the finger. Grayson's ligaments are palmar to the neurovascular bundles, and pass from the skin to the flexor tendon sheath. These ligaments form a tube from the proximal aspect of the finger to the distal interphalangeal joint, where the digital nerves and vessels always can be found during surgical dissection. The distal palmar and digital fascia is depicted in Figure 4-4.

PATHOLOGIC ANATOMY

In this discussion the word *band* is used to describe a normal palmar or digital fascial structure and the word *cord* to describe its pathological counterpart. Thus, a diseased band is a cord.

- DD begins in the palm as a *nodule* that represents the early manifestation of the disease in the longitudinal fibers of the PA.
- Histologically, nodules are a collection of fibroblasts and myoblasts in a fibrous tissue matrix.
- These nodules may coalesce to form cords that contract and produce the characteristic contracture deformity.
- This may appear clinically as a nontender nodule in the palm, or a skin dimple of retracted skin.
- The nodules form in and along the longitudinal axis of the rays. The ring and little finger are most commonly involved.

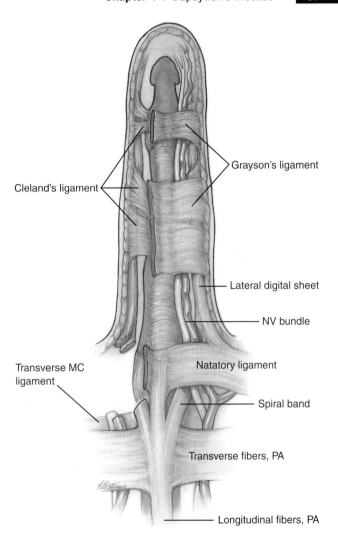

Figure 4-4 Distal palmar and digital fascia. See the text for details.

Labels: Cleland's ligament; Grayson's ligament; Lateral digital sheet; NV bundle; Transverse MC ligament; Natatory ligament; Spiral band; Transverse fibers, PA; Longitudinal fibers, PA

- As the disease progresses, it spreads to the fingers and produces the typical contracture of the MCP and often the proximal interphalangeal (PIP) joints.
- Recognition of the distinct anatomic separation of the longitudinal (involved) and transverse (noninvolved) fibers of the PA, and the distal separation of the longitudinal fibers into three layers, allows the surgeon to selectively excise the diseased tissue instead of all fascial tissue.

Pretendinous Bands

- The *pretendinous bands* of the PA are the most common places for Dupuytren's contracture to occur.
- A palpable nodule may progress to a prominent *pretendinous cord*, which may produce a flexion contracture of the MCP joint.
- Although the pretendinous cord is the primary cause of flexion contracture of the MCP joint, it may join the *central cord* of the finger that extends well beyond the PIP joint.

- The central cord originates from the superficial fibrofatty digital fascia on the flexor side of the finger.
- The central cord always is in continuity with the pretendinous cord.

Transverse Fibers

- Only the longitudinal fibers (*pretendinous bands*) of the PA are involved; the transverse fibers are ideally left behind during excision of the diseased palmar fascia.
- The transverse fibers to the thumb web, the PCL, and the DCL, which are more obliquely oriented and subject to tension, may contract. The loss of abduction and extension of the thumb can result.

Natatory Ligament

- The natatory ligaments frequently are diseased. Because they not only span the finger web space but also send fibers distally into the fingers, they may be responsible for web space contracture as well as PIP joint contracture.

Finger Fascia

The fibers in the finger that may become diseased are the fibrofatty fascia on the flexor aspect of the fingers; the distal continuation of the pretendinous fibers, called the *spiral band*; the distal (longitudinal) extension of the natatory ligaments; Grayson's ligament (as terminal attachment for the spiral bands); and the lateral digital sheet.

Fibrofatty Fascia

- This tissue forms the central cord in the finger, joining the pretendinous cord of the palm to form a continuous cord from the palm to the middle phalanx.
- It often divides into two tails that attach to the flexor sheath and osseous middle phalanx.

Spiral Band

- The fibers (layer two) are the deep and distal continuation of the pretendinous band on each side of the flexor sheath.
- They pass deep to the neurovascular bundle as they proceed to the lateral side of the finger, and then migrate superficial to the neurovascular bundle to attach to the middle phalanx by means of Grayson's ligament.
- This configuration progressively displaces the neurovascular bundle with increasing PIP joint contracture, first toward the midline, then proximally, and then superficially. This places the neurovascular bundle at considerable risk during surgery because the neurovascular bundle spirals around this fascial structure, called the spiral cord.
- The spiral cord is either a continuation of the spiral band or arises from the musculotendinous junction of an intrinsic muscle; it attaches distally to the flexor sheath and bone in the middle phalanx.

Natatory Ligament

- Disease and contracture of the transverse elements of the natatory ligaments form the natatory cords that produce contracture of the finger web spaces, with loss of abduction of the fingers.
- The distal digital extension of the natatory ligament joins the spiral band, and these two bands subsequently join the lateral digital sheet to form the lateral cord.

Grayson's Ligaments

- Grayson's ligaments, located in the middle and proximal phalanges, pass from the digital flexor sheath, palmar to the neurovascular bundle, to the lateral digital sheet. They are in the same fascial plane as the natatory ligaments.
- They provide attachment for the spiral cords to the middle phalanx.

Lateral Digital Sheet

- The lateral digital sheet is a condensation of the superficial fascia on either side of the finger.
- It receives fibers from the natatory and spiral ligaments, as well as from Grayson's and Cleland's ligaments.
- When diseased, it is known as the *lateral cord*.

Lateral Cord

- The lateral cord runs from the natatory ligament to the lateral digital sheet.
- It usually does not cause PIP joint contracture, except on the ulnar side of the small finger. There it attaches to an abductor cord overlying the ADM and can cause PIP joint contracture.

Retrovascular Cord

- This cord lies deep to the neurovascular bundle. It arises from the periosteum of the lateral base of the proximal phalanx, passes close to the PIP joint, and ends at the lateral aspect of the distal phalanx.
- It is the usual cause of DIP joint contracture, and an occasional cause of PIP joint contracture.

Isolated Digital Cord

- Isolated cords may arise in the fingers as single or double cords without any attachments in the palm.
- These cords arise from the periosteum at the base of the proximal phalanx in conjunction with adjacent ligaments.
- They pass distally to displace and then cross the neurovascular bundle, inserting on the tendon sheath or bone of the middle phalanx.
- These cords may result in a significant loss of extension of the PIP joint, and cause isolated contractures.
- Figure 4-5 demonstrates the pathologic tissues in the distal palm and finger in DD.

First Web Space

- Although only the longitudinal fibers (pretendinous bands) of the palmar fascia are involved in the hand, the transverse fibers to the thumb web, PCL, and DCL are more obliquely oriented and are subject to tension.
- If diseased, they may contract and be responsible for loss of abduction and extension of the thumb (Figure 4-6).

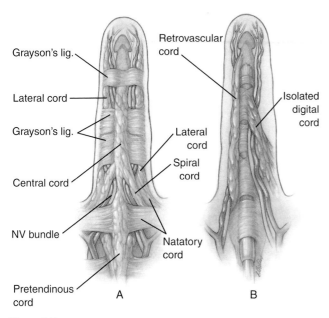

Grayson's lig.

Lateral cord

Grayson's lig.

Central cord

NV bundle

Pretendinous cord

Retrovascular cord

Isolated digital cord

Lateral cord

Spiral cord

Natatory cord

A   B

Figure 4-5   Pathological anatomy of the distal palmar and digital anatomy. (**A**) The more superficial diseased elements. (**B**) The deeper diseased elements.

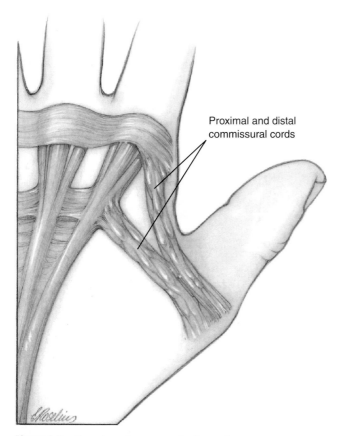

Proximal and distal commissural cords

Figure 4-6   Fascial involvement in the first web.

Table 4-1 summarizes the relationship between fascial bands/ligaments, cords, and the clinical result of cord formation. The convention adopted here is that fascial bands or ligaments are normal structures and that cords are their pathological counterparts.

TREATMENT

DD cannot be cured by surgery or any other means currently available. Recurrence is likely, and surgery may be associated with complications such as vascular compromise to a digit, skin necrosis, hematoma, infection, nerve injury, failure to completely relieve the contracture, and irreversible stiffness with or without reflex sympathetic dystrophy. DD that presents at an early age carries a greater potential for recurrence. Contractures in younger patients are often more severe, and repeated surgery is often required. The long-term prognosis for a suitable result is diminished when the disease begins at an early age.

Operative indications must be clearly understood by both the surgeon and the patient, and are based on the progression of the disease and the loss of function. Manifestations of functional loss may include difficulty or embarrassment while shaking hands, placing the hand in tight places, such as the pocket, or a variety of functional activities related to everyday use. Some surgeons use a certain or set degree of contracture to propose surgery. This may be useful in some circumstances, but must be tailored to the individual needs of the patient.

In terms of prognosis, contracture of the PIP joint is the most difficult to treat and obtain a satisfactory release. However, the MCP joint seldom manifests a permanent contracture after release. An experienced DD surgeon has noted that when the PIP joint contracture was less than 30 degrees, *the patient was more often made worse with surgery than made better.*

The current and accepted treatment for DD is a surgical approach employing *fasciotomy* or *partial fasciectomy.* The effect of *clostridial collagenase injection* into the cords that are causing contracture is currently under study. The technique involves injection of the material into the substance of the cord, followed by passive extension of the affected joint to stretch or rupture the cord.

It may be argued that *fasciotomy* is not a definitive procedure. It may, however, serve the needs of some selected patients. It can serve as a preliminary procedure to release a finger from the palm for hygiene purposes prior to a more comprehensive *fasciectomy.* Fasciotomy may also be used as a definitive procedure in those patients who have associated medical problems that would dictate a less comprehensive approach. A fasciotomy may be performed under local anesthesia and the wound left open followed by early motion. This approach may serve the needs of some patients better than a more comprehensive procedure. Although closed or blind fasciotomy was used in the past, open fasciotomy is more commonly used today.

Total fasciectomy has been abandoned in favor of limited or *partial fasciectomy.* Prophylactic removal of normal or nondiseased fascia is not indicated, and may increase the probability of postoperative complications.

TABLE 4-1 DUPUYTREN'S DISEASE: FASCIAL BANDS THAT MAY FORM CONTRACTURE CORDS

Fascial Bands/Ligaments	Cords	Result
Palm		
Pretendinous bands of palmar fascia	Pretendinous cord	MCP joint contracture
Commissure		
Natatory ligaments	Natatory cords	Digital web contracture
Proximal commissure ligament	First commissure cords	Thumb web contracture
Distal commissure ligament	First commissure cords	Thumb web contracture
Finger		
Spiral band	Spiral cord	Displaces neurovascular bundle, PIP contracture
Fibrofatty fascia	Central cord	PIP joint contracture
Natatory ligament and lateral digital sheet	Lateral cord	PIP joint contracture
Periosteum of proximal phalanx	Retrovascular cord	DIP contracture
Periosteum of proximal phalanx	Isolated digital cord	PIP contracture

PIP, proximal interphalangeal; MCP, metacarpophalangeal; DIP, distal interphalangeal.

The surgeon must have a comprehensive plan for dealing with DD in each patient. Such plans must include management of the skin, of the diseased fascia, and of joint contracture. Various techniques will be used based on the surgeon's experience and the needs of the patient. Open techniques, skin grafts, Z-plasties, and PIP joint release may be required.

Surgical Technique

Fasciotomy

■ The diseased fascia is *incised* rather than *excised,* and the wounds are left open to heal by secondary intention.
■ Sterile dressings protect the incisions and healing usually occurs within 3 weeks.
■ Immediate closure of the incisions would result in a recurrence of the flexion posture, especially at the MCP joints.

■ Exercises are initiated immediately after surgery.
■ An open fasciotomy is illustrated in Figure 4-7.

Open (McCash) Technique

■ This technique was first published in 1964, and has proved to be a useful method for dealing with apparent skin loss following palmar, or even digital, fasciotomy or fasciectomy.
■ Closure of these incisions often results in a flexed posture at the MCP and/or the PIP joints because of skin contracture.
■ Leaving the incisions open avoids this problem of, or the necessity for, a skin graft.
■ The method is used based on the experience of the surgeon and the needs of the patient.
■ Figure 4-8 depicts the preoperative and postoperative healing sequence using this method.

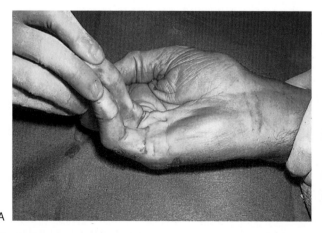 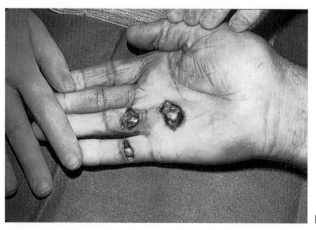

A   B

Figure 4-7   Open fasciotomy. (**A**) Preoperative appearance showing significant contractures at the MCP and PIP joints of the ring and little fingers. (**B**) Release of the contractures. The incisions were *left open,* and kept covered with nonadherent sterile dressings until healed at 3 weeks. This technique is useful for patients that may not tolerate a more comprehensive procedure.

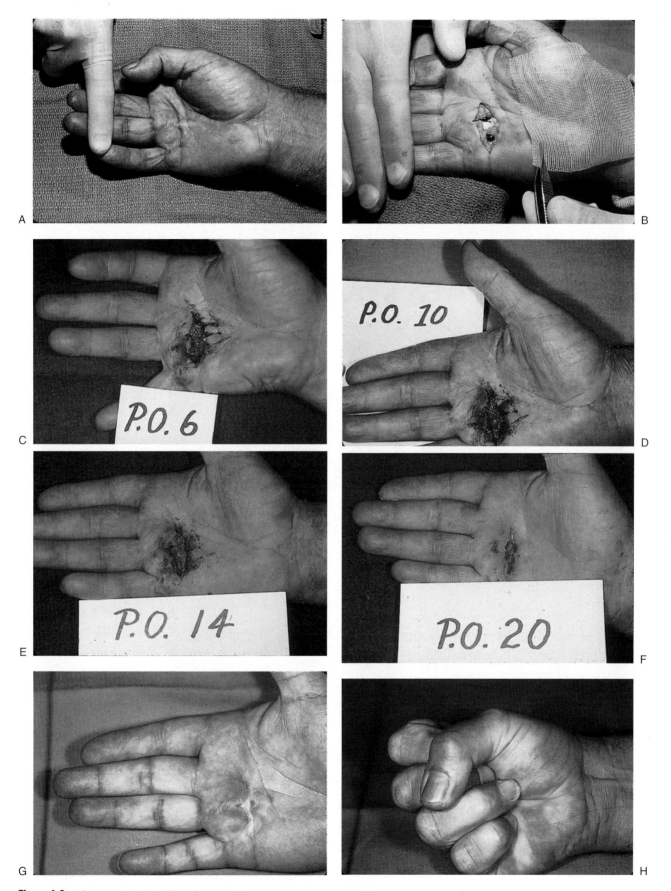

Figure 4-8 The open (or McCash) technique. (**A**) Preoperative appearance. (**B**) Appearance immediately after fasciectomy and just before application of the non-adherent sterile dressing. (**C**) Appearance at postoperative day 6, (**D**) day 10, (**E**) day 14, and (**F**) day 20. (**G–H**) Postoperative appearance at 2 months showing good extension and flexion.

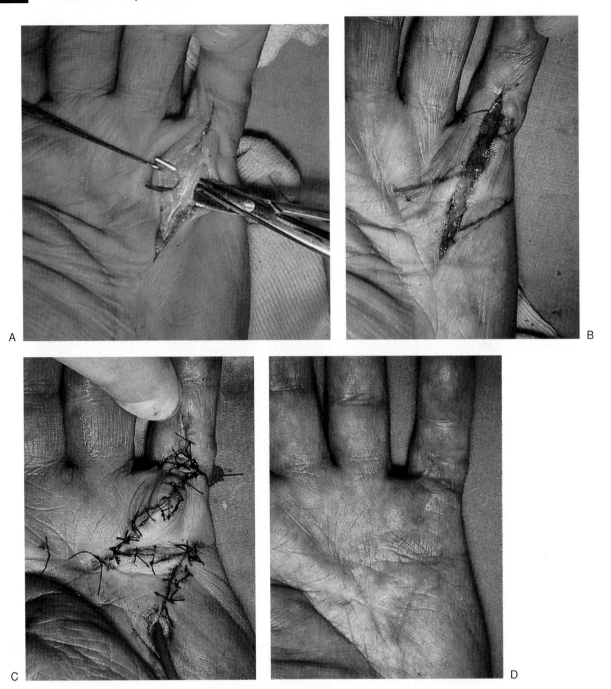

Figure 4-9 The longitudinal skin incision with Z-plasty closure. (**A**) Note the isolated diseased cord of palmar fascia elevated by the scissors. (**B**) A double-running Z-plasty has been laid out in proximity to the distal palmar crease and the MCP flexion crease of the little finger. (**C**) The flaps are rotated and sutured in place. (**D**) The result 2 months postoperatively.

Longitudinal Incision with Z-Plasty Closure

- In addition to the transverse incisions previously noted in Figures 4-7 and 4-8, longitudinal incisions with Z-plasty closures may be used to excise the diseased fascia in the palm and digit.
- Such incisions are ideally suited for *single ray involvement* (Figure 4-9).
- The longitudinal incision with a Z-plasty closure may also be used for more than one ray involvement of disease confined to the palm.

- Figure 4-10 illustrates the use of a longitudinal incision in the palm, with Z-plasty closure for involvement of two rays.
- The Z-plasty should be laid out with reference to the palmar and digital flexion creases.
- Surgeons should handle the flaps carefully, keeping them as thick as possible to preserve their blood supply.
- *These longitudinal incisions that cross the flexion creases should never be used without Z-plasty closure, because a pronounced scar that is associated with significant contracture will result.*

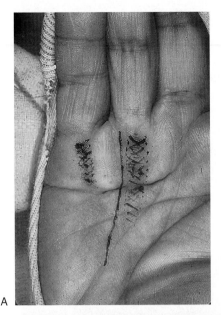
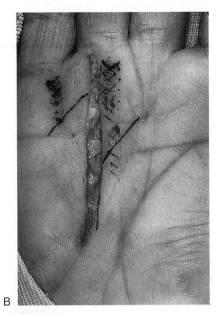
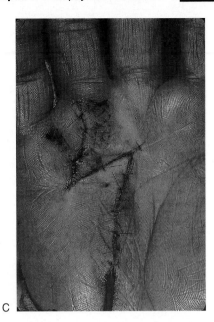

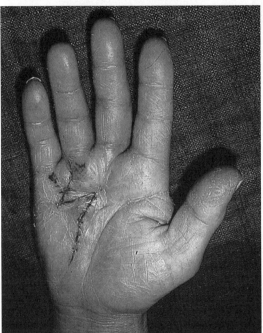

Figure 4-10 The longitudinal incision and Z-plasty closure for disease encompassing two rays in the palm. (**A**) The longitudinal incision is laid out between the ring and little finger rays. The cross-hatched marks denote the underlying fascial cords. (**B**) The cords have been removed and the Z-plasty is laid out centered about the distal palmar crease. Note that the oblique limbs of the Z are carried to the distal palmar crease, and that the incision axis and two oblique limbs are equidistant. (**C**) The flaps are rotated and the distal palmar crease is restored. (**D**) The result at 8 days postoperative, showing that the flaps are viable and healing satisfactorily.

Zigzag Incision

- This incision is widely used to expose palmar and digital diseased cords.
- Although it resembles a longitudinal incision, its multidirectional configuration avoids longitudinal tension lines and is well tolerated by the palmar and digital tissues. Figure 4-11 shows the zigzag incision and the postoperative result.

Skin Grafts

- Skin grafts may be used to replace badly diseased skin or to fill a skin defect following fasciectomy.
- Full-thickness skin grafts are used most often because they are less likely to contract.

- Figure 4-12 shows a patient with severe contracture in whom skin closure was facilitated by full thickness skin grafts.

The Skoog Principle

In 1967, Skoog published his findings and recommendations regarding the noninvolved nature of the transverse elements of the palmar fascia in patients with DD. This concept focused the attention of surgeons on the need to remove only those tissues that are diseased. In many instances, this results in less trauma to the hand, and preserves the parts of the palmar fascia that could continue to play an important role in the hand. Figure 4-13

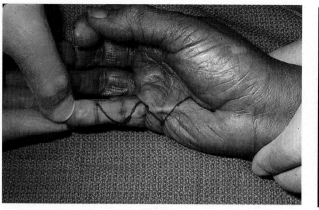
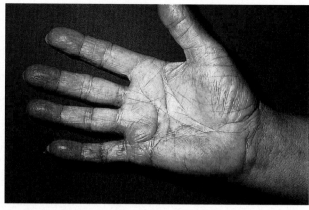

Figure 4-11 The zigzag incision for Dupuytren's disease. (**A**) Comprehensive incision from the proximal palm to the DIP joint for removal of the single-ray palmar and digital cords in Dupuytren's disease. (**B**) The end result at 3 months with nearly full extension and good skin healing in the palm and finger.

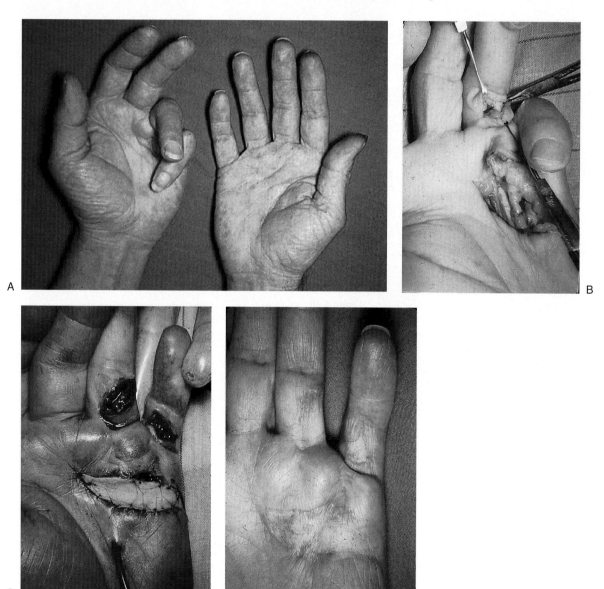

Figure 4-12 Full-thickness skin graft to facilitate closure in Dupuytren's disease. (**A**) The preoperative appearance of severe Dupuytren's disease, with contracture in the left hand. (**B**) Intraoperative appearance as the procedure progresses. (**C**) A palmar skin graft has been applied in the palm, while a second graft (not shown) will be applied to the defect in the proximal phalanx of the little finger. The ring finger was left open. (**D**) The end result at 3 months.

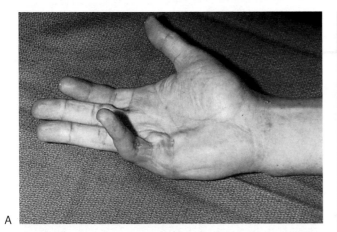

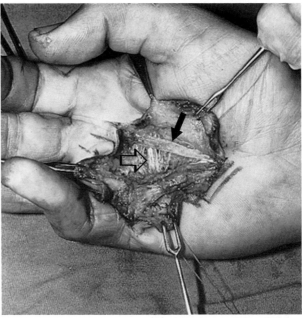

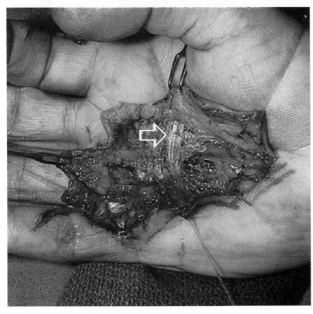

Figure 4-13   The Skoog principle of preservation of the transverse fibers of the palmar fascia in fasciectomy. (**A**) Clinical appearance of Dupuytren's disease in the right little finger ray. (**B**) The transverse fibers (*open arrow*) can be seen between and *beneath* the longitudinal cords (*solid arrow*) of the palmar fascia. (**C**) The end result after removal of the longitudinal cords. Note the preserved transverse fibers (*arrow*) and the underlying nerves and vessels.

demonstrates the relationship of the diseased longitudinal cords to the underlying transverse fibers of the palmar fascia.

Structures at Risk During Surgery

One of the principles in DD surgery is to begin the dissection in relatively normal tissue and progress to the site of maximum disease involvement. Thus, dissection often begins in the proximal palm, where the cords are more easily identified and their relationship to associated structures is more evident. Wise and experienced surgeons look for vital structures such as the common and proper digital vessels and nerves in the palm. Surgeons focus on this as the dissection enters the region of the distal palm and fingers, in order to avoid injury to these structures.

A review of the normally occurring bands in the distal palm and finger is appropriate here. The pretendinous band splits into two spiral bands just proximal to the first annular pulley. These bands then continue distally as the spiral band, where they join the lateral digital sheet. That sheet in turn may join the fibers of Grayson's ligament (Figure 4-14).

With contracture the spiral band, lateral sheet and Grayson's fibers join to form the *spiral cord*. It is this composite structure that "spirals" around the digital nerve and vessel and, with increasing contracture, progressively draws the neurovascular bundle toward the midline, proximally and superficially (Figure 4-15). It is here, in the region of the proximal phalanx and PIP joint, that the neurovascular bundle is at risk. The digital nerve and cord are not easily distinguished because they are similar in color. The nerve is soft compared to the firmer nature of the cord, and the color of the blood vessel (even under tourniquet control) may provide some distinguishing features. A useful technique is to identify the nerve and vessel in the distal palm, and then trace them distally.

Other cords adjacent to the neurovascular bundles in the finger are the *lateral* and *central cord*, which may also produce PIP joint contracture, along with the *spiral cord*.

Figure 4-16 shows the clinical appearance of the neurovascular bundle and adjacent cords in the fingers of two patients.

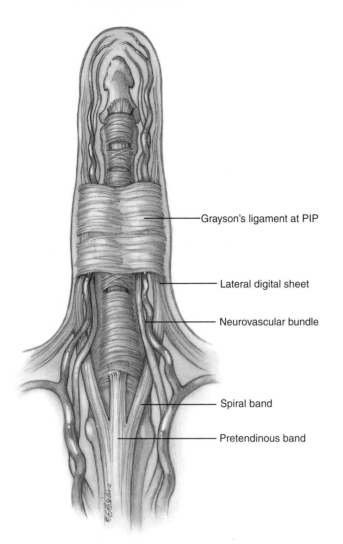

Grayson's ligament at PIP

Lateral digital sheet

Neurovascular bundle

Spiral band

Pretendinous band

Figure 4-14 The anatomy of the normal tissues that may form the spiral cord: Pretendinous band; spiral band; lateral digital sheet; and Grayson's ligament.

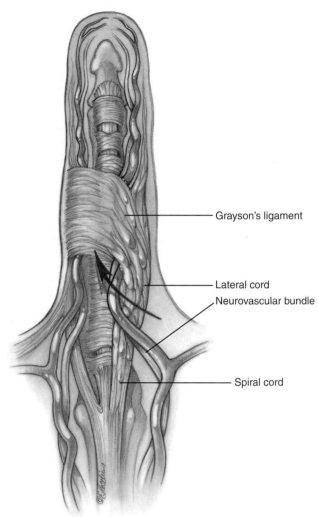

Grayson's ligament

Lateral cord

Neurovascular bundle

Spiral cord

Figure 4-15 The spiral cord and its relationship to the neurovascular bundle.

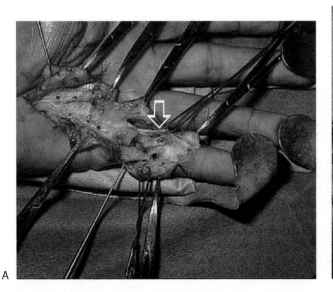

A

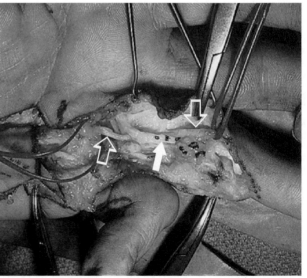

B

Figure 4-16 Clinical examples of cords and their relationship to the neurovascular bundles in the finger. (**A**) Note the proximity of the digital nerves (retraction loops) to the cords (*arrow*) in this little finger. (**B**) Note the proximity of the digital nerves and vessels (*open arrows*) to the digital cord (*closed arrow*) in this ring finger.

SUGGESTED READING

Baldalamente MA, Hurst LC. Enzyme injection as nonsurgical treatment in Dupuytren's disease. J Hand Surg 2000;25A:629–636.

Chiu HF, McFarlane RM. Pathogenesis of Dupuytren's contracture: a correlative clinical-pathological study. J Hand Surg 1978;3A:1–10.

Doyle JR. Palmar Hand. In: Doyle JR, Botte MJ, eds. Surgical anatomy of the hand and upper extremity. Philadelphia: Lippincott Williams & Wilkins, 2002:532–641.

McCash CR. The open palm technique in Dupuytren's contracture. Br. J Plastic Surg 1964;17:271–280.

McFarlane RM. On the origin and spread of Dupuytren's disease. J Hand Surg 2002;27A:385–390.

McGrouther DA. The microanatomy of Dupuytren's contracture. Hand 1982;14:215–236.

McGrouther DA. Dupuytren's contracture. In: Green DP, Hotchkiss RN, Pederson WC, eds. Green's operative hand surgery. 4th Ed. New York: Churchill Livingstone, 1999:563–591.

Skoog T. The transverse elements of the palmar aponeurosis in Dupuytren's contracture. Their pathological and surgical significance. Scand J Plast Reconstr Surg 1967;1:51–63.

Tomasek J, Rayan GM. Correlation of alpha-smooth muscle actin expression and contracture in Dupuytren's disease fibroblasts. J Hand Surg 1995;20A:450–455.

Lubahn, JD. Dupuytren's disease. In: Trumble, TE, ed. Hand surgery update 3, hand, elbow, shoulder. Rosemont, IL: American Society for Surgery of the Hand, 2003:393–401.

Zachariae L. Dupuytren's contracture. The aetiological role of trauma. Scand J Plast Reconstr Surg 1971;5:116–119.

INFECTIONS

This chapter will present the basic principles involved in the diagnosis and treatment of common infections in the hand. Discussion will begin with the more common bacterial infections involving soft tissue and bone that may be seen in an acute situation.

Prior to the antibiotic era, infections in the hand and their sequelae could be disabling, and in some cases fatal. Antibiotics have changed that, but early diagnosis and treatment is a necessary part of the management equation in order to minimize the potential disability that result from infections that are diagnosed late or treated inappropriately. The specifics of the pertinent anatomy as it relates to each infection will be addressed under each type of infection.

The effect of antibiotics is most pronounced in the early phases of an infection. Antibiotics may in some instances cure certain types of infections if they are administered early and are organism specific. Many infections, however, do not present in a timely fashion. Some infections may begin as cellulitis; at this stage a more serious or deep infection may be averted by prompt treatment including antibiotics, and elevation and rest of the affected part.

The patient's history of injury or onset is often critical to making the correct diagnosis. Not all patients will be forthcoming with the true details of the circumstances surrounding the infection. Human bite wounds are a prime example: most patients will not admit that the problem occurred from a fistfight, but rather say it resulted from a fall.

A basic principle of the treatment of deep or closed-space infections is to provide open drainage in a suitable and timely fashion. Drainage of an infection is accompanied by a culture of the material obtained, and includes routine bacterial and fungal cultures. A smear and gram stain of the drained material may allow a presumptive or tentative identification of the organism involved. Antibiotics are started based on the most likely organism involved. Table 5-1 includes examples of selected antibiotic agents, and their class, spectrum, use, and cost.

Immobilizing the affected part and allowing it to rest are also important aspects of treatment. Elevation means that the affected part is at least 30 cm above the level of the heart, a posture that is most easily obtained by recumbency. *Sitting in a chair with the hand at or below the level of the heart is not elevation.* Immobilization by use of a splint or cast

provides rest to the part and will also prevent inappropriate inspection or manipulation of the lesion by the patient.

Remember that infections in diabetic, debilitated, malnourished, or immunocompromised patients will be more difficult to treat, and will sometimes present as chronic, rather than acute, infections. Infections in these patients sometimes require amputation of digits.

The following discussion will include some of the more common infections that may be encountered in the outpatient clinic or the emergency department.

Felon

The felon is a subcutaneous infection that occurs in the distal pulp of the fingers or thumb.

Pertinent Anatomy

The distal pulp of digits is covered by thick skin that is tethered to the osseous phalanx by multiple fibrous tissue septae. This three-dimensional space is filled with fat, and contains numerous vessels and nerves and their specialized end organs. These septae stabilize the pulp for pinching and grasping, and form compartments that may prevent adequate drainage unless incised (Figure 5-1).

Clinical Appearance and Diagnosis

- The felon presents as a swollen, red, painful, and tender terminal phalanx that may or may not have a history of a penetrating injury (Figure 5-2).
- Spontaneous drainage or pointing of the abscess may occur (Figure 5-3). This indicates a late and neglected infection, and diagnosis and treatment should have been started in a more timely fashion.
- The felon may also migrate to the distal interphalangeal (DIP) joint and to the adjacent flexor sheath in untreated cases.

Treatment

- Treatment is aimed at decompression of the abscess, which is often under tension.
- Surgical drainage is indicated if there is evidence of a purulent collection under pressure. This may occur within 2 to 3 days of the onset of the condition.

TABLE 5-1 CLASS, SPECTRUM, USE, AND COST OF SELECTED ANTIBIOTIC AGENTS

Class		Spectrum	Notes	Cost[a]
Penicillins				
Natural penicillins	Penicillin G, penicillin V	Most *streptococci*, gram(+) anaerobes, some *Staphylococci*; poor gram(−)	Effective for *S. viridans, Pasteurella* in bite infections	$–$$
Penicillinase-resistant	Nafcillin, methicillin, dicloxacillin	Similar to natural penicillins, but better *Staphylococcus* coverage	Nafcillin effective for septic arthritis, osteomyelitis	$$$
Extended spectrum	Ampicillin, amoxicillin	Similar to natural penicillins, but better gram(−) coverage		$
With β-lactamase inhibitors	Amoxicillin/clavulanate (Augmentin), ampicillin/ sulbactam (Unasyn)	Similar to extended-spectrum penicillins, but better coverage of β-lactamase-producing *Staphylococci*, gram(−)	Good first line coverage for diabetic hand infections	$$$
Cephalosporins				
First generation	Cephalexin (Keflex), cefazolin (Ancef, Kefzol)	Similar to penicillinase-resistant penicillins against gram(+); some gram(−)	Recommended prophylaxis against wound infections	$–$$
Second generation	Cefuroxime, cefotetan	Similar to penicillinase-resistant penicillins against gram(+); more gram(−)		
Third generation	Ceftriaxone, ceftazidime	Similar to second generation but including *Pseudomonas*	Ceftriaxone effective against gonococcus	$$$
Fourth generation	Cefepime	Similar to third generation cephalosporins		
Other β-lactams				
Carbapenems	Imipenem, meropenem	Broad-spectrum against most gram(+) and gram(−) bacteria, some *Pseudomonas*	Reserved for severe, polymicrobial infections	$$$$$
Monobactam	Aztreonam	Some gram(−), no anaerobes or gram(+) cocci		$$$$$
Glycopeptides	Vancomycin	Gram(+), including MRSA; no gram(−) coverage	IV only, can cause red-man syndrome if infused quickly	$$$
Polypeptides	Bacitracin, polymyxin	Bacitracin covers only gram(+), polymyxin only covers gram(−)	Topical use only	$
Aminoglycosides	Gentamicin, tobramycin, amikacin	Gram(−), including *Pseudomonas*	Monitor levels, screen for nephrotoxicity, ototoxicity	$$$
Tetracyclines	Tetracycline, doxycycline	Most gram(+), some gram(−)	Do not use in children (stains teeth, bones)	$
Macrolides	Erythromycin, clarithromycin	Most gram(+), some gram(−), clarithromycin active against mycobacteria	GI side effects common	$–$$
Oxazolidinones	Linezolid (Zyvox)	All *Staphylococci* (incl MRSA, all *Streptococci,* all enterococci (incl. VRE)	Good PO bioavailability, bone/joint penetration	$$$$
Lincosamides	Clindamycin	*Staphylococci*, some gram(−) anaerobes	High incidence of GI side-effects	$$
Streptogramins	Quinupristin-dalfopristin (Synercid)	*Staphylococci, Streptococci,* enterococci (including VRE)	IV only, good bone/joint penetration	$$$$$
Fluoroquinolones Broad-spectrum	Ciprofloxacin (Cipro), levofloxacin (Levaquin)	Broad gram(+) and gram(−) coverage	Good PO bioavailability for bone and joint infections	$$–$$$$
Expanded-spectrum	Gatifloxacin (Tequin), moxifloxacin (Avelox)	Similar to broad-spectrum fluoroquinolones, but better gram(+) coverage	Good PO bioavailability, limited FDA approval	$$$$$

(continued)

TABLE 5-1 Continued

Class		Spectrum	Notes	Cost[a]
Other β-lactams				
Metronidazole	Metronidazole (Flagyl)	Parasites, anaerobes, including *C. difficile*	Drug of choice for *C. difficile*	$
Sulfonamides	Trimethoprim-sulfamethoxazole (TMP-SMX, Bactrim)	Broad range of gram(+) and gram(−)	Commonly used for urinary tract infections	$
Antimycobacterials	Isoniazid (INH), ethambutol, cycloserine, rifampin, pyrazinamide (PZA)	Mycobacteria; rifampin also effective against gram(+) cocci	Usually used in combinations; consult infectious disease specialist	$–$$$$

[a] Costs for recommended courses of treatment: $, $1–10; $$, $10–50; $$$, $50–200; $$$$, $200–1000; $$$$$, $1000–20,000; FDA, US Food and Drug Administration; GI, gastrointestinal; gram(−), gram negative; gram(+), gram positive; IV, intravenous; MRSA, methicillin-resistant *Staphylococcus aureus*; PO, by mouth; VRE, vancomycin-resistant *Enterococcus*. (From Cornwall R, Bednar MS. Infections. In: Trumble, TE, ed. Hand surgery update-3, hand, shoulder & elbow. Rosemont, IL: American Society for Surgery of the Hand, 2003:433–457.)

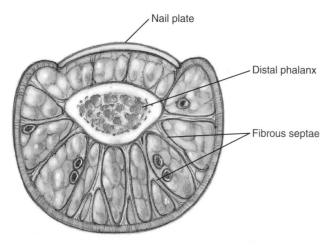

Nail plate
Distal phalanx
Fibrous septae

Figure 5-1 The anatomy of the terminal phalanx.

- The aim of surgery is to produce immediate and continuous drainage of the abscess.
- The usual organism is *Staphylococcus aureus*, although opportunistic gram-negative and mixed organisms may be encountered in the immuno-compromised patient.
- This requires an appropriate incision and division of the fibrous septae to promote drainage.
- Appropriate and inappropriate incisions for drainage of the felon are depicted in Figure 5-4.
- Incisions that extend on both sides of the pulp (fish-mouth incisions) are to be avoided. They result in unsuitable scars, may result in vascular or neurological compromise of the resultant flap, and in general alter the shape and function of the pulp.
- The preferred surgical incision is a lateral midaxial incision that begins distal to the DIP joint flexion crease and continues distally at a level adjacent to the free edge of the nail plate.

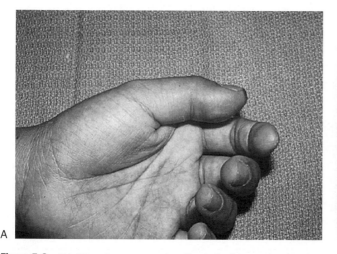
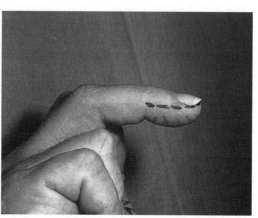

A
B

Figure 5-2 (**A**) Clinical appearance (swelling) of a felon in the thumb. The pulp was firm and tender to palpation. (**B**) Felon of the left middle finger. Note the swelling in the pulp and the proposed midlateral incision of the noncontact side of the digit.

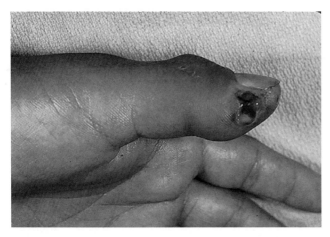

Figure 5-3 A felon that was neglected and drained spontaneously (or *pointed*).

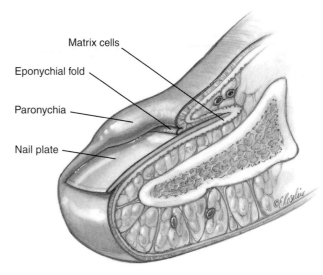

Figure 5-5 The anatomy of the distal phalanx showing the finger nail components, nail plate, matrix, and eponychium, with an artist's depiction of a lateral fold infection called a *paronychia*.

- This incision maintains the architectural integrity of the pulp, while at the same time providing adequate exposure and drainage.
- Oblique or longitudinal volar incisions may be used if the abscess is pointing in that direction (volar), but should be relatively short and should avoid injuring the underlying digital nerves.
  - This volar incision may be most suitable when the abscess has spontaneously drained in that direction.
  - These incisions should not cross the flexion crease.
- The incisions are placed on the *non-contact* side of the digit.
  - In the index, middle, and ring fingers, the incisions are on the ulnar side and in the thumb and little finger they are on the radial side.

Drains, Antibiotic Therapy and Splints

- A small drain is inserted into the wound to keep it open and promote drainage.

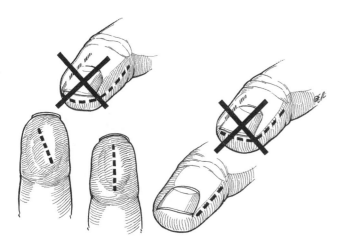

Figure 5-4 Inappropriate (marked with an X) and appropriate incisions for drainage of the felon.

- An alternative to this drain is to place a small catheter in the wound for irrigation and drainage.
- Antibiotic therapy, along with rest (a plaster splint is effective) and elevation of the extremity, is instituted.
- Prompt drainage, suitable incisions, and antibiotic therapy usually result in a satisfactory outcome that will preserve the function of the pulp and avoid a disabling scar. These actions also tend to prevent the spread of the infection to bone or to the flexor tendon sheath.

Acute Paronychia

Pertinent Anatomy
A paronychia is an infection of the lateral soft tissue fold surrounding the nail plate. The interface between the nail plate and the overlying skin is a unique anatomic arrangement that allows for growth of the nail plate from matrix cells (Figure 5-5). This interface or seal however may be penetrated by foreign bodies that introduce bacteria into an otherwise sterile interface. Over-vigorous manicures and nail biting may be associated with these infections.

Clinical Appearance and Diagnosis
- The initial infection usually involves half or less of the eponychia fold, and in such instances is called an *eponychia*.
- A neglected infection may involve the entire fold, and is called a *run-around infection* (Figure 5-6A).
- These neglected lesions may spread to the insertion of the adjacent extensor tendon. This can result in a mallet finger deformity and can deform the fingernail secondary to injury to the germinal nail matrix (Figure 5-6B).
- *Staphylococcus aureus* is the usual organism involved, but *Streptococcus* and oral anaerobes may be seen in infections caused by nail biting.

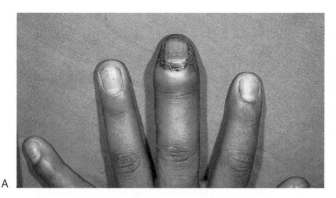

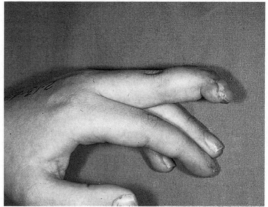

A

B

Figure 5-6   (A) The "run-around" form of paronychia. (B) The end result of delayed treatment of a severe paronychium with chronic mallet finger and nail deformity.

Treatment

- Early cases (before fluctuance and an abscess have developed) may be treated by warm water soaks, splinting, and cephalosporins.
- If an abscess is identified, it must be drained by one of several methods, including elevation of the eponychial fold to drain the purulent material, followed by insertion of a small drain; or an oblique incision in the eponychial fold centered over the site of maximum involvement. In more chronic cases, a margin of the nail plate is removed, followed by a drain insertion.

Chronic Paronychia

Clinical Appearance and Diagnosis

- The term *chronic paronychia* is used to describe nonbacterial infection of the eponychial fold caused, most commonly, by a *Candida albicans* infection. Other organisms such as tuberculosis, syphilis, atypical mycobacteria, gram-negative rods, and cocci have also been identified, however.
- It is most often associated with chronic maceration, and occurs in patients such as dishwashers, homemakers, bartenders, and others that have their hands in water that contain irritants.
- Some have concluded that this condition is a type of hand dermatitis and not onychomycosis.

Treatment

- Treatment is difficult and not always successful.
- *Nonsurgical treatment* includes topical corticosteroids and systemic antifungal agents.
- Treatment that removes the patient from constant exposure to water may be as important as medications.
- In patients who do not respond to conservative treatment, *surgical marsupialization* with or without plate removal may be effective.
- A crescent of skin that is 3 to 4 mm wide is excised proximal and parallel to the eponychium, which includes skin, fat, and nail plate—but not the nail matrix (Figure 5-7).

Herpes Simplex (Herpetic Whitlow)

Clinical Appearance and Diagnosis

- This condition represents an important differential diagnosis of both *pyogenic* paronychia and felon.
- It is an infection caused by the herpes simplex virus (types 1 or 2) and is usually seen in medical and dental personnel.
- The affected digit is swollen, painful, and red.
- The infection may involve more than one digit and is often less tender than a bacterial lesion.
- Figure 5-8 shows the typical appearance of the herpes simplex lesion in the digit.
- Small vesicles may appear early on, and the fluid in them is clear and not purulent.
  - These lesions then involute and desquamate, and the cycle resolves in 3 to 4 weeks.
  - The diagnosis is usually made by taking a history and performing an examination.

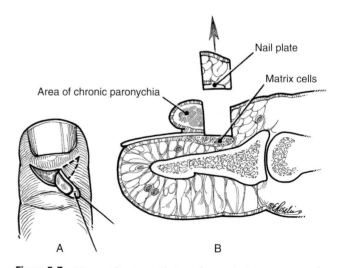

Nail plate

Matrix cells

Area of chronic paronychia

A

B

Figure 5-7   Marsupialization technique for surgical management of chronic paronychia.

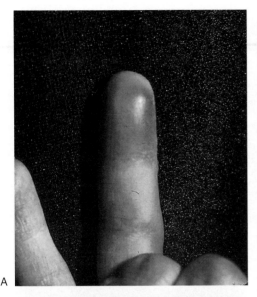

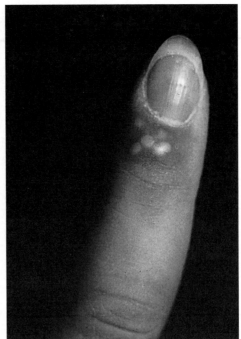

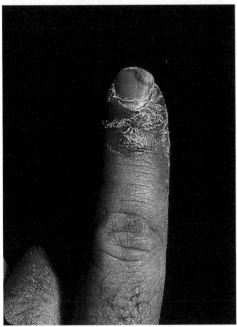

Figure 5-8   The clinical appearance of a herpes simplex infection in the digit. (**A**) The erythematous phase. (**B**) The pustular phase. (**C**) The desquamation phase. (Courtesy of Dean S. Louis, University of Michigan.)

Treatment

■ Surgery is not necessary and is *contraindicated* since bacterial infections may contaminate the incision site. Systemic dissemination with a secondary viral encephalitis can also occur.

Pyogenic Flexor Tenosynovitis

Pertinent Anatomy

The flexor tendons are enclosed in a double-walled synovial sheath that extends from the region of the DIP joint to the midpalm in the index, middle, and ring fingers; from the DIP joint to the wrist in the little finger; and from the interphalangeal (IP) joint to the wrist in the thumb. The most common arrangement of the synovial sheath of the digits

is shown in Figure 5-9. This sheath represents a closed space that, if infected, can produce severe disability in the digit. Such infections require early diagnosis and appropriate treatment. The relationship of the pulley system that must be preserved during surgical drainage is depicted in Figure 5-10.

Clinical Appearance and Diagnosis

■ Kanavel described four characteristic findings in pyogenic flexor tenosynovitis:

■ Flexed posture of the finger.

■ Swelling of the finger (Figure 5-11).

■ Tenderness along the course of the sheath.

■ Significant pain with passive extension of the flexed finger.

■ The most common organism is *Staphylococcus aureus*.

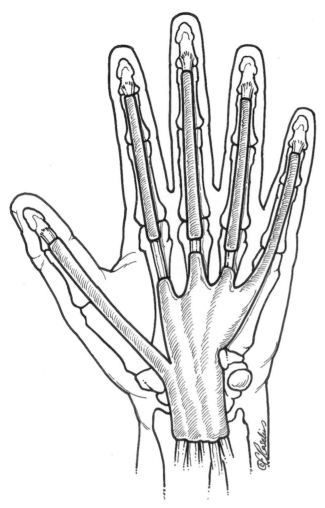

Figure 5-9 The most common arrangement of the synovial sheaths in the hand. This configuration gives anatomic support to the concept of the "horseshoe abscess," which is a flexor sheath synovial infection that may communicate from thumb to little finger and vice versa through Parona's space. See Figure 5-12 for depiction of Parona's space.

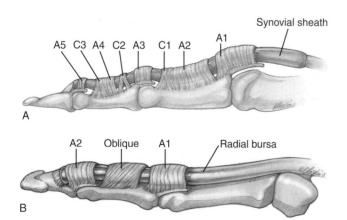

Figure 5-10 The digital pulley system. (**A**) The finger pulleys. (**B**) The thumb pulleys.

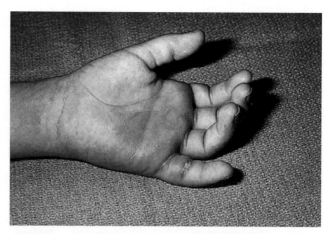

Figure 5-11 The clinical appearance of pyogenic flexor tenosynovitis in the little finger following an untreated laceration at the PIP flexion crease. Note the swelling and erythema in the finger and palm.

Treatment

- If seen early (within 24 to 48 hours), it may be feasible to treat to the condition by hospitalization with intravenous antibiotics, bed rest and elevation of the hand, and immobilization with a splint—with the hand and wrist in the position of function (wrist in moderate extension and the fingers slightly flexed).
  - The patient should be evaluated twice daily; if the condition is not resolved within 24 to 48 hours, surgical drainage should be performed.
- Most cases will be in the late category. Surgical drainage is performed along with the modalities listed for early conservative treatment.
- Open drainage through midaxial and palmar incisions has been employed in the past for these infections, but when compared to closed catheter irrigation, the former technique may be associated with a higher incidence of complication and reoperation.
- The current trend for recommended treatment is for closed catheter irrigation.
- Closed catheter irrigation consists of insertion of a 16-gauge polyethylene catheter into the sheath just proximal to the first annular pulley through a transverse, oblique, or zigzag incision.
- The catheter is passed under the A1 pulley distally for about 2 cm (see Figure 5-10).
- The catheter is sutured to the skin, and the wound is closed.
- A second incision is made distally, either on the noncontact side of the digit in the midaxial plane or volarly distal to the A4 pulley.
- The sheath distal to the A4 pulley is excised, and a small drain is sutured in place to ensure that the distal wound stays open.
- The patency and drainage of the construct is tested by the injection of sterile saline through the proximally placed catheter.
- A variation on this technique is to bring the distal end of the catheter out the distal wound and allow passage of saline in the sheath by two to three openings made in the catheter within the sheath.

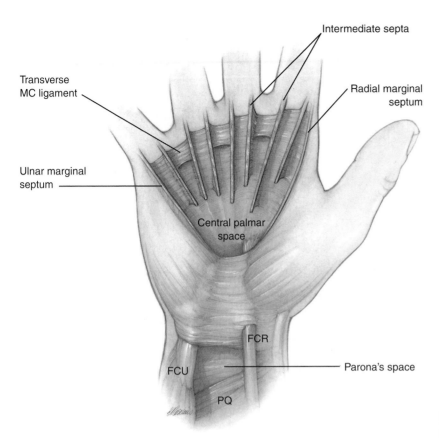

Intermediate septa

Transverse
MC ligament

Radial marginal
septum

Ulnar marginal
septum

Central palmar
space

FCR

FCU

Parona's space

PQ

Figure 5-12   The palmar space and Parona's
space (see text for details).

- The proximal portion of the catheter is brought out through the dressings, and attached to a sterile 50-mL syringe.
- The distal wound is left exposed in the splint and dressings for visual verification of patency of the system.
- The system is flushed with sterile saline every 2 hours for 48 hours, and then the finger is inspected. Comparable end results might be achieved without postoperative irrigation.
- If the infection has abated, the catheter should be removed and gentle range of motion exercises should begin.
- If there is some question about the status of the infection, the irrigation can be continued for another 24 hours.
- General principles in this technique include preservation of the annular pulleys during placement of the catheter, and concomitant intravenous antibiotic therapy.

Central Palmar Space Infections

Pertinent Anatomy
I recommend that the following concept regarding the palmar space, based on the work of Bojsen-Moeller and Schmidt, be accepted as valid.

- The *central palmar space* is bounded radially and ulnarly by marginal septae that begin as an expansion of the sidewalls of the carpal canal.
- The floor is formed by the palmar interosseous fascia, transverse metacarpal ligaments, and adductor fascia.

- The roof is formed by the palmar aponeurosis.
- The radial marginal septum extends distally to the proximal phalanx of the index finger, and forms the radial wall of the lumbrical canal.
- The ulnar margin septum is attached to the shaft of the small finger metacarpal.
- Between these two marginal septae are seven intermediate septae that divide the distal aspect of the central palmar space into four canals for the flexor tendons and four canals to accommodate the lumbrical muscle and neurovascular bundles.
- *Thus, the historical concepts of a thenar and midpalmar or, as later modified, an adductor and deep palmar ulnar space should be abandoned in my opinion* (Figure 5-12).

Clinical Appearance and Diagnosis
- An infection of the central palmar space may result from a penetrating injury to the space or an extension of an infected digital synovial sheath.
- There may be swelling, redness, and tenderness in the central aspect of the palm, and active and passive movement of the fingers may be painful.

Treatment
- Surgical drainage may be performed through an incision in or parallel to the proximal palmar crease or thenar crease to correspond to the site of maximum fluctuance.
- A drain is placed to promote continuous egress, and a splint is applied.

■ Elevation of the extremity, bed rest, and appropriate antibiotics complete the treatment regimen.

SPECIAL SITUATIONS

Several conditions may present as unique situations and may seem somewhat out of the ordinary.

Horseshoe Abscess

■ This term is used to describe an infection that may begin in the thumb or little finger flexor sheath and that may infect the opposing digit.
■ This occurs when sufficient pressure in the respective sheath results in passage of the infected material into Parona's space in the wrist and then into the opposing tendon sheath. (see Figure 5-9 and Figure 5-12)
■ The treatment principles described for flexor tenosynovitis are used, and drainage is required for both of the digits involved and at the wrist (Parona's space).

Collar Button Abscess

■ This term has been used to describe interdigital web-space infections.
■ The infections usually begin in the palm.
■ The palmar fascia attachments to the skin provide resistance to superficial palmar spread, and the infection will spread dorsally in the path of least resistance. Thus, the lesion presents in the shape of a collar button or an hourglass.
■ Patients present with painful swelling in the web space and distal palm.
■ Palmar and dorsal drainage is effective treatment through appropriate incisions such as a zigzag palmar incision and a longitudinal web incision dorsally.

Osteomyelitis

Although osteomyelitis may be seen in the hand by direct extension from an adjacent soft tissue infection, it may also result from direct penetration. It seldom occurs by the hematogenous route. *Staphylococcus aureus* and *S. epidermidis* are the usual organisms involved.

Clinical Appearance and Diagnosis

■ Osteomyelitis should be suspected in any longstanding or deep infection that is adjacent to bone, or in an infection following a deep, penetrating wound.
■ Chronic swelling and infections that fail to resolve with standard treatment may indicate osteomyelitis.
■ Elevation, increased thickness of the periosteum, or an osteolytic lesion in the bone, seen on radiograph, are signs of bone infection.
■ A foreign body with an osteolytic halo is also suggestive of osteomyelitis.
■ C-reactive protein may be elevated.
■ A technetium bone scan may be diagnostic.

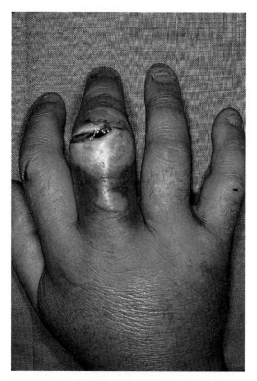

Figure 5-13 This neglected glass laceration resulted in a chronic infection of the middle finger involving soft tissues, bone, and joint. The problem could not be resolved with elevation, rest to the part, and antibiotics. An amputation was performed with resolution of the infection.

Treatment

■ Drainage of the bone is indicated through drill holes in the cortex or a small window.
■ Necrotic bone (sequestrum) is removed if it is present.
■ The wound may be packed open, or the catheter irrigation method may be used.

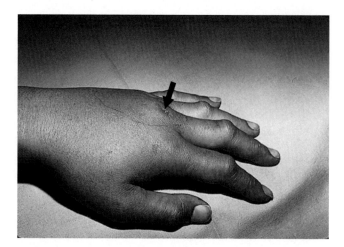

Figure 5-14 Human bite wound. This policeman sustained a penetrating tooth wound (*arrow*) to the MCP joint of the left middle finger, and shortly thereafter noted pain and swelling in the hand. Incision and drainage was required, along with hospitalization and intravenous antibiotics.

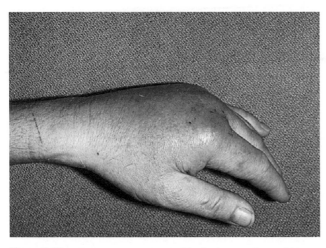

Figure 5-15 This cat owner sustained multiple scratches and bites to the dorsum of her hand that resulted in cellulitis, with swelling, redness, and pain. The infection developed overnight. The organism was *Pasteurella multocida*, and the condition quickly resolved with intravenous penicillin.

- In some cases with severe bone and soft tissue involvement, amputation may be the best treatment (Figure 5-13).

Human Bite Wounds

These wounds are most often seen over the metacarpophalangeal (MCP) joint and are due to a fist blow to an opponent's mouth. The history of injury is not often forthcoming due to embarrassment.

Clinical Appearance and Diagnosis
- These wounds are often small and may initially appear very benign.
- The opponent's tooth penetrates the MCP joint space and inoculates this closed space with a variety of organisms, including *Staphylococcus aureus*, *Streptococcus viridans*, and *Eikenella corrodens*.
- Later on there is swelling, redness, and increasing pain (Figure 5-14).
- A radiograph of the injured hand may reveal a fracture or a piece of the opponent's tooth in the joint.

Treatment
- *These injuries should never be closed primarily.*
- They should be opened and debrided extensively. This includes excision of the initial wound margins and extension of the wound to allow proper exposure, inspection, and irrigation of the joint involved.

- The wound is cultured prior to irrigation and debridement.
- It is left open and the hand is dressed and splinted.
- Appropriate antibiotics are started after cultures have been obtained.
- Patients with bite wounds from humans may not always keep their follow-up appointments, and serious consideration should be given to hospitalization until the condition is resolved.

Animal Bites

Clinical Appearance and Diagnosis
- Domestic animal bites or scratches may result in the rapid onset of cellulitis and lymphangitis.
- The most commonly isolated organisms from dog and cat bites are *Streptococcus viridans*, *Pasteurella multocida*, *S. aureus*, and anaerobes.
- Figure 5-15 represents a case of *P. multocida* (a small gram-negative coccus) cellulitis following a bite from the patient's house cat.
- The condition must be distinguished from *cat scratch disease* or fever, which is usually associated with small red lesions on the hand or wrist, lymphadenopathy, and a history of cat scratch. The organism is *Rochalimaea henselae*, a gram-negative bacillus.
- A skin test may be confirmatory.

Treatment
- Penicillin is the antibiotic of choice for animal bites.
- The treatment for cat scratch disease is said to be controversial because it is a self-limiting disease.
- Ciprofloxacin has been used.

SUGGESTED READING

Bojsen-Moeller F, Schmidt L. The palmar aponeurosis and the central spaces of the hand. J Anat 1974;117:55–68.

Cornwall R, Bednar MS. Infections. In: Trumble TE, ed. Hand surgery update-3, hand, elbow & shoulder. Rosemont, IL: American Society for Surgery of the Hand, 2003:433–457.

Jebson PJL, Louis DS, eds. Hand infections. Hand Clinics 1998;14(4):511–711.

Neviaser RL. Acute infections. In: Green DP, Hotchkiss RN, Pederson WC, eds. Green's operative hand surgery. 4th Ed. New York: Churchhill Livingstone, 1999:1033–1047.

Tosti A, Piraccini BM, Ghetti E, Colombo MD. Topical steroids versus systemic antifungals in the treatment of chronic paronychia: an open, randomized double-blind study and double dummy study. J Am Acad Dermatol 2002;47:73–76.

Wright PE II. Hand infections. In: Canale ST, Dougherty K, Jones L, eds. Campbell's operative orthopedics. vol. IV, 10th Ed. Philadelphia: Mosby, 2003:3809–3825.

TENOSYNOVITIS AND EPICONDYLITIS

This chapter discusses some of the most common clinical entities in the fingers, thumb, and wrist (stenosing tenosynovitis), as well as medial and lateral epicondylitis of the elbow.

Epicondylitis, although anatomically not in the hand or wrist, is commonly seen on a Hand and Upper Extremity Service and is appropriately included in this text on the hand and wrist.

Trigger digits and de Quervain's tenosynovitis may be classified as inflammatory conditions that involve the respective tendon sheaths and retinacular structures.

Stenosing tenosynovitis is an apt term to describe trigger digits and de Quervain's, since *narrowing* of the channel through which the respective tendons travel is the common denominator in these conditions. There may not be agreement as to the relative role of tendon, retinacular, or synovial tissues in causing this narrowing, but perhaps all three play varying roles. The fact that the problem may be relieved by rest, medication, or surgery indicates that stenosis is a valid concept when discussing this disorder.

Epicondylitis, in contrast, may have multiple pathophysiologic factors in its etiology.

TRIGGER DIGIT (ADULT)

Pertinent Anatomy

This condition involves the first annular pulley (A1) of the fingers and thumb. These structures are depicted in Figure 6-1.

The A1 pulley in the finger arises from the metacarpophalangeal (MCP) joint palmar plate and, to a lesser extent, from the base of the proximal phalanx. It is located in the *distal palm* and not the finger. In the thumb, the A1 pulley arises from the MCP joint palmar plate and, to a lesser extent, from the base of the proximal phalanx.

History, Clinical Appearance, and Diagnosis

- This condition is more common in women, with the peak incidence at 40 to 60 years of age.

- The ring finger is most commonly involved, followed by the thumb and middle finger.
- Single or multiple digits may be involved.
- Patients give a history of a "clicking" sensation with motion of the affected finger or thumb.
- Sometimes a "lump" is described in the palm, and anatomically this lump corresponds to the A1 pulley.
- The clicking may progress to "locking" of the digit.
  - This "locking" is in the flexed position. Attempts at extension of the digit are often painful.
  - The locked position in a trigger digit is with both the MCP and proximal interphalangeal (PIP) joint flexed.
  - Sometimes the patient must use the other hand to passively extend, or "unlock," the digit.
- Repetitive use or overuse of the hand may be associated with the onset of the condition.
- Commonly associated conditions are rheumatoid arthritis, diabetes mellitus, and gout.
- Other reported causes of trigger digit include localized enlargement of the flexor digitorum profundus (FDP) in the region of the A3 pulley. In patients with rheumatoid arthritis, the triggering may be due to proliferative synovium about the profundus tendon and subsequent trapping at the flexor digitorum superficialis (FDS) decussation.
- Stenosing tenosynovitis does not usually result in a fixed or permanently locked position.
  - If a "trigger finger" cannot be passively extended, it is probable that true locking of the finger is present due to a cause such as a spur from the metacarpal that is trapped in a small fenestration in the palmar plate.
  - The posture of true locking is with varying degrees of flexion at the MCP joint, whereas the PIP joint is in full extension and actively and passively mobile.
  - The locked trigger finger is in a flexed posture at both the PIP and MCP joints (Figure 6-2).
- In early or mild cases, crepitation with flexion of the digit and tenderness over the region of the A1 pulley may be the most prominent findings.
- As the condition progresses, definite locking and catching may occur. This is usually painful.

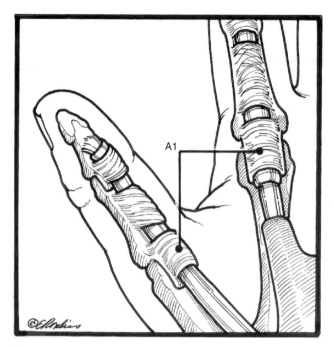

Figure 6-1 The arrangement of the finger and thumb flexor tendon sheath and pulleys.

■ The patient may become apprehensive when asked to flex the finger, because the locking and release of the locked digit are painful.

Treatment

Nonsurgical Treatment
■ Conservative management in the form of rest to the hand, splinting, and anti-inflammatory medication may be of benefit in mild or early cases.

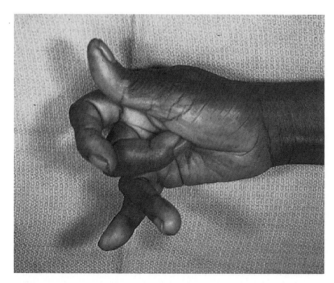

Figure 6-2 The clinical appearance of a typical "locked" trigger finger. Note that flexion is present in the MCP, PIP, and DIP joints.

■ The next level of treatment includes a steroid injection into the flexor sheath.
■ One injection (or a second 2 weeks later) may result in relief.
■ Patients with a discrete palpable nodule, single digit involvement, and a short duration of symptoms appear to have the best response to injections.

Injection Technique
■ The site to be injected is prepped with Betadine or a similar solution, and the skin at the injection site is anesthetized with ethyl chloride spray.
■ A short, 25-gauge needle attached to a 1-mL syringe with 0.5 mL of corticosteroid designed for intrasynovial use (Kenalog-40 or similar agent) is introduced through the skin and into the *proximal* synovial sheath.
■ The ideal injection site is just proximal to the A1 pulley into the synovial sheath.
■ Entering at a slight angle aids in placement of the needle.
  ■ Marked resistance indicates that the needle may be in the substance of the tendon, and the needle should be withdrawn slightly or repositioned.
■ As the steroid is injected into the sheath, the filling of the sheath may be palpated by the injector's finger positioned over the proximal or middle phalanx.
■ Serial injections in the anatomy laboratory by the author have demonstrated that a fluid volume of 0.5 mL is more than sufficient to fill the sheath in most digits.
■ Figure 6-3 shows the injection technique.

Surgical Treatment
■ The goal of surgical treatment is to incise (release) the first annular pulley through a transverse or longitudinal incision.
■ In general, the incisions should not cross a palmar or digital flexion crease at right angles.
■ Some suitable longitudinal incisions for the fingers and the recommended transverse thumb incision are depicted in Figure 6-4.
■ My preference for longitudinal finger incisions is based on the ease of exposure. The line of incision parallels the underlying tendons, nerves, and blood vessels (they are less likely to be injured), and is oriented in a more suitable plane to facilitate postoperative exercises.
■ The proximal part of the incision over the middle finger is angled slightly, to parallel the distal palmar flexion crease.
■ Four digits may be released simultaneously with these incisions without compromise to the skin.
■ The soft tissues are retracted with two vein retractors that protect the neurovascular bundles. The A1 pulley is incised with a no. 15 blade under direct vision.
■ All of the A1 pulley is incised and, if necessary, so are a few millimeters of the proximal portion of the A2 pulley.
■ The flexor tendons may be pulled up into the wound to verify complete release. In the thumb, the radial digital sensory nerve crosses the flexor pollicis longus (FPL) sheath from ulnar to radial at or proximal to the A1 pulley and must be identified and protected.

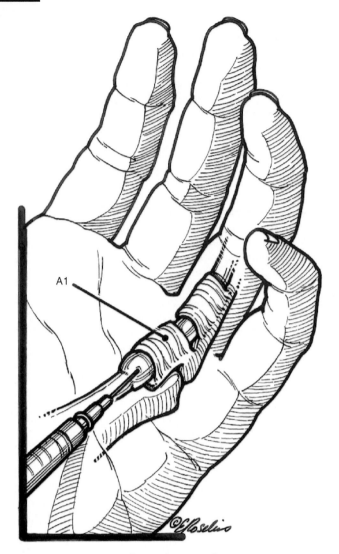

Figure 6-3   Injection technique for trigger fingers.

- The A1 pulley is incised, but the oblique pulley is preserved.
- Percutaneous release has been developed for trigger finger release and, in experienced, operators may be a useful adjunct to the open technique.

CONGENITAL TRIGGER THUMB

Trigger digits in infants and children usually involve the thumb rather than fingers.

History, Clinical Appearance, and Diagnosis

- These children are usually brought to the pediatrician or other caregiver when the family notes that the thumb interphalangeal (IP) joint is in a flexed posture and cannot be passively extended.

- The child presents with a locked IP joint that cannot be actively or passively extended.
- A prominent but nontender nodule is noted in the region of the palmar aspect of the thumb MCP joint. It may be bilateral in 25% to 33% of patients diagnosed.
- The wise practitioner will not attempt to passively extend the IP joint with undue force, because such a maneuver may be painful.
- The diagnosis is usually made by the clinical appearance and physical findings.
- Other diagnoses may be considered, such as congenital clasped thumb, absent extensor tendons, arthrogryposis, or spasticity.
- Figure 6-5 shows the clinical appearance of bilateral congenital trigger thumbs.

Treatment

Nonsurgical Treatment

Spontaneous resolution of this condition has been reported in some series with or without conservative treatment, such as splinting, massage, and passive extension exercises to the IP joint. It is unknown how many of these thumbs spontaneously resolve without ever being diagnosed. Conservative treatment may be tried based on the perceived needs of the family and the age of the child. Little or no harm will result from delaying the trigger thumb release should it be required.

Surgical Treatment

- The first annular pulley is incised through a transverse incision that is centered over the nodule.
- The neurovascular bundles are close by and must be protected.
- In contrast to the adult trigger thumb, the FPL tendon has a prominent nodule (*Notta's node*).
- This nodule is not excised because it will resolve following release of the first annular pulley (Figure 6-6).

CONGENITAL TRIGGER FINGER

- Trigger fingers in children are much less common than trigger thumbs.
- Pathologic findings may include a nodule in the FDP and FDS, and a bunching up or buckling of one or more slips of the FDS.

Treatment

- In contrast to congenital trigger thumb release, release of the first annular pulley in congenital trigger finger may be inadequate.
- The incision should be extensile, because correction, in addition to release of the A1 pulley, may require excision of tendon nodules, one or both slips of the FDS, and release of the A3 pulley.
- A Bruner zigzag incision is useful for this more comprehensive exposure.

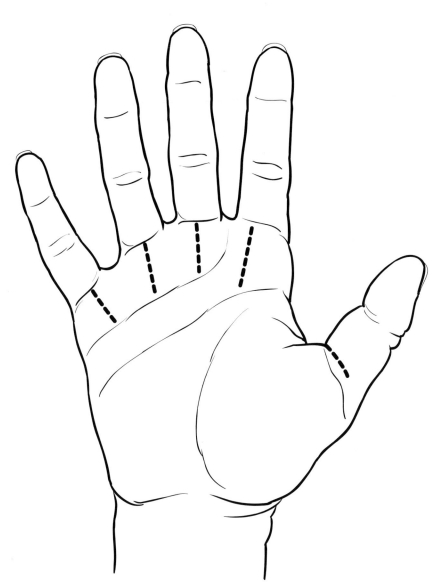

Figure 6-4 Suitable longitudinal incisions for trigger finger release, and the recommended transverse incision for release of the thumb A1 pulley.

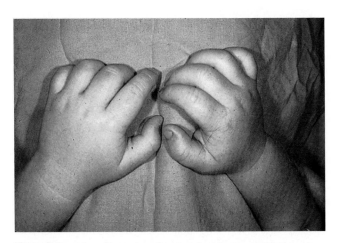

Figure 6-5 Bilateral congenital trigger thumbs in a child. Note the flexed posture of the interphalangeal joints of the thumbs.

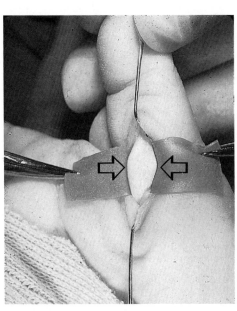

Figure 6-6 Congenital trigger thumb. Intraoperative photo showing release of the first annular pulley, and the prominent nodule (*arrows*) in the FPL called *Notta's node*.

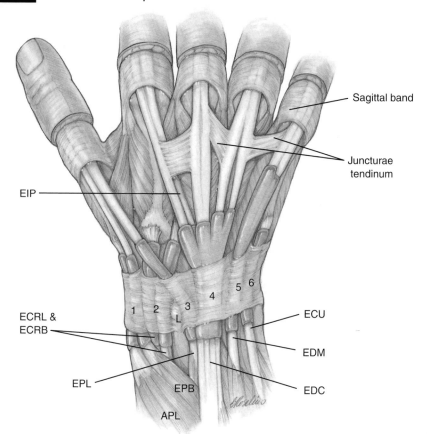

EIP

Sagittal band

Juncturae
tendinum

ECRL &
ECRB

1 2 3 L 4 5 6

ECU

EDM

EPL EPB EDC

APL

Figure 6-7 The six dorsal extensor compartments.

DE QUERVAIN'S TENOSYNOVITIS

Pertinent Anatomy

The first extensor compartment contains the abductor pollicis longus (APL) and the extensor pollicis brevis (EPB) tendons (Figure 6-7). The wrist, thumb, and finger extensor tendons enter the hand beneath a fibrous tissue retinaculum that contains six tunnels. Five of these tunnels are fibroosseous and one (the fifth) is fibrous. This extensor retinaculum (ER) is a wide fibrous tissue band that prevents bowstringing of the tendons and improves their mechanical advantage. At this level, the extensor tendons are covered by a synovial sheath. The ER has two distinct layers: the supratendinous layer and the infratendinous one. The latter is limited to the area deep to the ulnar three compartments.

The tendons in the first extensor compartment are variable in their number of slips and tunnels. The APL may have two, and up to four, tendon slips, whereas the EPB usually has only one and may be absent in 5% to 7% of cases. Anatomic studies have revealed that the first compartment may consist of two distinct compartments in as many as 33% of patients. These two tunnels are an ulnar tunnel for the EPB, and a more radial one for the abductor pollicis longus (APL). Even a third tunnel containing an anomalous tendon has been reported. Failure to recognize these variations may lead to treatment failure (Figure 6-8).

The anatomic relationship of the radial artery and nerve to this region must be recognized to prevent injury to these structures (see Figure 6-8). The radial artery passes obliquely across the anatomical snuff box from the palmar aspect of the wrist *deep* to the APL and the radial wrist extensors (extensor carpi radialis longus [ECRL] and extensor carpi radialis brevis [ECRB]). Two or more sensory branches of the radial nerve are immediately *superficial* to the first extensor compartment.

History, Clinical Appearance, and Diagnosis

- A history of radial-sided wrist pain of variable duration may be identified, in association with overuse of the wrist and thumb. The condition may be associated with diabetes or pregnancy.
- There is tenderness over the first extensor compartment, and there may be swelling and redness over the region of the radial styloid.
- Flexion and extension of the thumb is usually painful, and crepitation may be noted.
- *Finkelstein's* test is pathognomonic and is properly performed as described.
  - The thumb is grasped by the examiner, and the hand is quickly abducted (bent ulnarward).
  - The test is *inappropriately* performed by placing the thumb in the palm before wrist abduction, because this may produce pain even in a normal wrist (Figure 6-9).
  - A positive test is manifested by pain over the radial styloid due to stretching of the inflamed tendons.

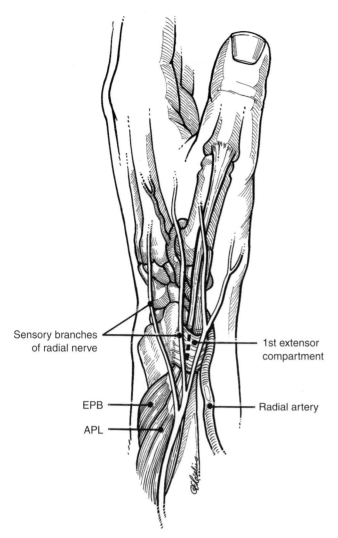

Figure 6-8   Relevant anatomy for de Quervain's tenosynovitis. The APL and EPB ordinarily share a common fibroosseous canal, but in 33% of cases a separate canal may be present that contains the EPB. Failure to recognize and release this second compartment will result in an incomplete release. Note the relationship of the radial artery and radial nerve to the first extensor compartment.

Sensory branches of radial nerve

1st extensor compartment

EPB

Radial artery

APL

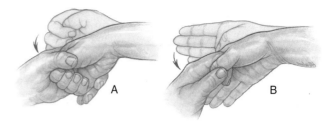

Figure 6-9   Finkelstein's test. (**A**) The incorrect technique. (**B**) The correct technique. The test is appropriately performed by grasping the patient's thumb, and then ulnar deviating the hand. A false-positive test may result if the thumb is flexed into the palm and grasped by the patient's fingers followed by ulnar deviation of the wrist (see text).

- De Quervain's tenosynovitis must be distinguished from arthritis of the trapeziometacarpal joint of the thumb.
  - Tenderness and swelling over this joint, along with pain and crepitation, are signs of arthritis.
  - This arthritic condition may co-exist with de Quervain's tenosynovitis.

Treatment

Nonsurgical Treatment

- Rest to the thumb and wrist by means of a splint that immobilizes both, along with anti-inflammatory medication, may be useful in mild cases.
- If these simple measures are not successful, a steroid injection into the first extensor compartment should be considered.

  - This is performed under sterile techniques and local anesthesia (1% Xylocaine without epinephrine).
  - Ethyl chloride spray is a suitable alternative to temporarily anesthetize the skin.
- An intrasynovial steroid injection is placed into the first compartment using a short 25- or 27-gauge needle.
- The injection site is about 1 cm proximal to the tip of the radial styloid.
- The needle is guided by palpation of the tendons in the first compartment. Needle placement may be verified by noting enlargement of the sheath with instillation of the cortisone.
- The injection may be repeated in 4 to 6 weeks if symptoms are not relieved.
- Water-soluble steroid preparations in volumes of 1 mL or less are preferred. Informed consent prior to the injection includes the possibility of depigmentation of the skin and atrophy of the subcutaneous fat.

Surgical Treatment

- If conservative treatment fails, surgery by release of the first extensor compartment is performed.
- A 2 cm transverse incision is made about 1 cm proximal to the tip of the radial styloid.
- Branches of the radial sensory nerve are identified and carefully retracted.
- The retinaculum is incised longitudinally, all compartments released, and the respective tendons are gently lifted from the wound to verify complete release.
- Traction on one of the unroofed tendons must result in extension of the MCP joint, indicating release of the EPB tendon.
- If this does not occur, then a second compartment must be searched for and released.

INTERSECTION SYNDROME (CROSSOVER TENDONITIS)

Pertinent Anatomy

This condition is a type of tenosynovitis of the second dorsal compartment. The APL and EPB muscle bellies cross over the tendons of the ECRL and ECRB, and this is the

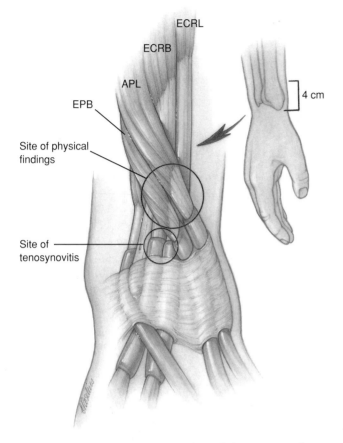

ECRL

ECRB

APL

EPB

Site of physical findings

Site of tenosynovitis

4 cm

Figure 6-10   Intersection syndrome. Although the symptoms of swelling and tenderness present in the crossover area 4 cm proximal to the radial styloid, the true pathology is distal in the second extensor compartment.

site of physical findings. The pathology, however, is located distally in the synovial sheath of the second compartment. The ECRL and ECRB are encased in a tight compartment, and the symptoms and the physical findings of swelling and tenderness do not present at this site. Rather they present about 4 cm proximal to the radial styloid. Surgical release of the second compartment distal to the area of symptoms and findings reveal characteristic synovitis (Figure 6-10).

Clinical Appearance and Diagnosis

- Pain and swelling about the muscle bellies of the APL and EPB at the dorsal and radial aspect of the wrist are characteristic of this syndrome.
- This area is about 4 cm proximal to the radial styloid.
- It may be seen after overuse of the wrist, and is often associated with sports activities such as rowing or weight lifting.

Treatment

- If conservative measures including splinting and/or steroid injections into the second compartment fail, then surgical release of the second dorsal compartment is

performed through an incision centered over the radial wrist extensors (ECRL and ECRB).
- The extensor pollicis longus (EPL) tendon and sensory branches of the radial nerve are in the area and are identified and protected.

EXTENSOR INDICIS PROPRIUS (EIP) SYNDROME

Pertinent Anatomy

The muscle belly of the EIP may extend into the relatively small (8 to 10 mm wide) fourth compartment when the wrist is flexed. This produces relative occlusion or compromise of the already limited space. Hypertrophy of this muscle, or synovitis of the surrounding tendon sheath, may be implicated.

Clinical Appearance and Diagnosis

- This condition may manifest itself as swelling and tenderness in the radial side of the fourth extensor compartment, which is most noticeable in wrist flexion.
- With the wrist in full flexion, the patient is asked to extend the index finger against resistance.
- The production of pain that is adjacent to Lister's tubercle represents a positive test for EIP syndrome.

Treatment

- Partial release of the extensor retinaculum or partial excision of a hypertrophied EIP muscle belly may be indicated if conservative measures fail.

EXTENSOR POLLICIS LONGUS TENOSYNOVITIS

Pertinent Anatomy

The EPL curves around Lister's tubercle in the third extensor compartment. Its movement is through a relatively long osseous groove and Lister's tubercle acts as a "turning fairlead" to change its initial course that is parallel to the long axis of the forearm to an oblique axis to reach the thumb. Any condition that compromises the osseous groove or inflames the surrounding synovial sheath will result in pain, swelling, and tenderness.

History, Clinical Appearance, and Diagnosis

- EPL tenosynovitis is often seen following a Colles fracture, and its tendency to rupture may be related to local ischemia in an unyielding fibro-osseous groove.
- Tenderness, swelling, and crepitation may be noted along the course of the tendon.

Treatment

■ Attritional rupture of the EPL may occur in these circumstances, and steroid injections are not advised.
■ Re-routing of the tendon radial to its anatomic tunnel is recommended.

CALCIFIC TENDONITIS

Etiology, Clinical Appearance, and Diagnosis

■ Release of calcium salts into the synovial and peritendinous space results in acute pain, swelling, redness, and tenderness.
■ The onset is sudden and is not usually associated with a precipitating incident.
■ The redness and swelling may mimic infection.
■ Gouty tenosynovitis may present in a similar fashion and may be diagnosed by history or laboratory studies.
■ A high index of suspicion and a radiograph more often than not lead to the diagnosis of acute calcific tendonitis.
■ The lesions may occur anywhere in the hand or wrist, and the region of the flexor carpi ulnaris (FCU) and pisiform bone is the most common site (Figure 6-11).

Treatment

■ This condition is usually self-limited and may resolve in a matter of days.
■ Symptomatic treatment is indicated in the form of splints, mild anodynes, and anti-inflammatories as needed.

LATERAL EPICONDYLITIS

Pertinent Anatomy and Possible Etiology

Most treaters of lateral epicondylitis have focused on the ECRB muscle and its fibrous tissue origins from the lateral epicondyle. It arises from the common extensor origin from the lateral epicondyle, radial collateral ligament of the elbow joint, and the intermuscular septum. Various entities have been implicated, and include such conditions as an inflamed synovial fringe, fibrositis of the annular ligament around the radial head and neck, periostitis of the ECRB origin, and angiofibroblastic hyperplasia of the ECRB tendon of origin. Most now agree that some form of noninflammatory degeneration of the ECRB tendon is responsible, because acute inflammatory cells are not often present in the specimens removed.

The findings at surgery have identified a grayish and edematous ECRB origin and rupture of portions of the ECRB origin in about one-third of the patients treated. Specialized stains of these abnormal tissues have demonstrated myofibroblast cells that are not normally found in tendons.

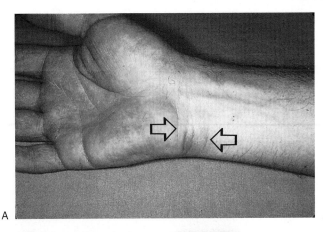

A

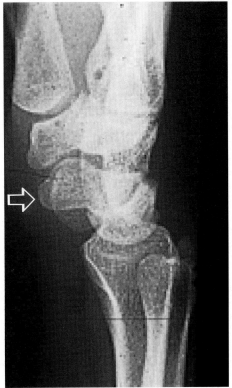

B

Figure 6-11   Acute calcific tendonitis. (**A**) This young reporter noted the sudden onset of pain, swelling, and redness on the flexor aspect of his wrist (*arrows*). (**B**) Radiographs demonstrated a calcium deposit in the region of the FCU tendon and pisiform bone (*arrow*).

History, Clinical Appearance, and Diagnosis

■ Patients with this condition present with the insidious onset of pain on the outer aspect of the elbow that may radiate into the extensor surface of the forearm.
■ Racket sports have been implicated, especially in those that play often or have faulty technique.
■ Repetitive use of the wrist and finger extensor muscles is often noted. Swelling is not a usual feature, but point tenderness over the lateral epicondyle and the tendon of origin of the ECRB is present.
■ Symptoms are reproduced by resisted dorsiflexion of the wrist with the elbow extended.

- Differential diagnosis may include cervical disc disease, radial tunnel syndrome, posterior interosseous nerve syndrome, radiocapitellar arthritis, or osteochondral injury.
- Radiographs should be obtained to rule out bone pathology.

Treatment

Nonsurgical Treatment

- Initial treatment is conservative in the form of activity modification, rehabilitation exercises, ice, and anti-inflammatories.
- Some patients will benefit from a so-called tennis elbow brace that applies pressure to the extensor tendon origin on the proximal forearm.
- Steroid injection, directed to the osseous origin of the ECRB tendon, may be beneficial.

Surgical Treatment

- Surgery is indicated for those patients that have failed to improve after several months of conservative treatment, and who, for a variety of reasons, cannot or chose not to live with the condition.
- Most current surgical approaches to this problem are extra-articular, and consist of debridement of the abnormal tissue on the deep or underside of the ECRB and adjacent tendons.
- In open techniques, the interval between the ECRL and ECRB is exposed through a lateral incision.
- Diseased tissue is removed from the ECRB after detaching it from its epicondylar origin.
- Other sites of diseased tissue are looked for and removed from the ECRL or common extensor origin.
- Reattachment of these tendons is facilitated by roughening of the adjacent bone or by mini-epicondylectomy.
- The collateral ligament is protected during the procedure to avoid the postoperative complication of posterolateral rotatory instability of the elbow (Figure 6-12).
- Arthroscopic debridement of the ECRB has also shown favorable results.

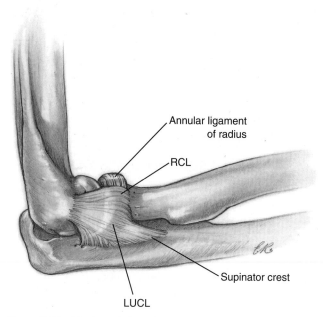

Figure 6-12   The lateral elbow ligaments. LUCL, lateral ulnar collateral ligament; RCL, radial collateral ligament.

History, Physical Examination, and Diagnosis

- Medial epicondylitis is the most common cause of medial elbow pain, but it is much less common than lateral epicondylitis.
- The onset, like lateral epicondylitis, is insidious in the majority of cases.
- The patients often describe activity-related pain associated with repetitive and forceful forearm pronation and/or wrist flexion.
- Many cases are associated with occupational activities.
- Sports-related activities such as throwing and golfing are often associated with this condition.

MEDIAL EPICONDYLITIS

Pertinent Anatomy and Possible Etiology

The flexor-pronator muscle group originates from the medial epicondyle and supracondylar ridge, and include the pronator teres (PT), flexor carpi radialis (FCR), palmaris longus (PL), flexor digitorum superficialis (FDS), and the FCU. The PT (humeral head) and FCR share a common tendon origin from the epicondylar ridge, and are the usual muscles involved. The anterior elements of the medial collateral ligament (A-MCL) are the major ligamentous stabilizers of the medial aspect of the elbow, and must be protected during any surgical releases in this area. The A-MCL originates from the inferior and anterior aspect of the medial epicondyle (Figure 6-13).

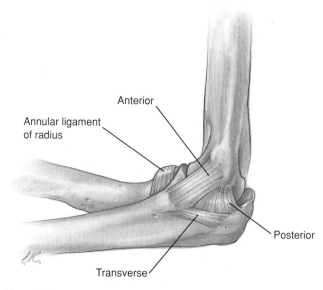

Figure 6-13   The medial elbow ligaments.

- The sites of maximum tenderness are over the medial epicondyle and just distal at the tendinous origin of the flexor-pronator muscles.
- Resisted pronation and wrist flexion often reproduce the symptoms.
- Symptoms of cubital tunnel syndrome may also be present, and are manifested by tenderness and a positive Tinel's sign over the ulnar nerve in the cubital tunnel.
- Additional differential diagnostic entities include ulnar nerve subluxation, subluxing medial head of the triceps, medial collateral ligament insufficiency (especially in throwers), elbow arthritis, and cervical radiculitis.

Treatment

Nonsurgical Treatment
- Conservative treatment is represented by activity modification, ice, and anti-inflammatory medication.
- A steroid injection deep to the site of the origin of the flexor-pronator group may also be tried.
- If symptoms resolve in a timely fashion, flexor-pronator stretching exercises are performed.

Surgical Treatment
- Surgery is indicated for those patients that have failed to improve after several months of conservative treatment, and who, for a variety of reasons, cannot or chose not to live with the condition.
- The commonly recommended treatment is debridement and reattachment of the flexor-pronator origin through an incision just anterior to the medial epicondyle.
- A small cuff of tissue may be left proximally to facilitate reattachment.
- Pathological tissue on the underside of the PT or FCR, or elsewhere in the flexor-pronator origin, is excised.
- Some surgeons perform a limited epicondylectomy to facilitate reattachment of the flexor-pronator muscles.

- The ulnar nerve in the cubital tunnel, and the branches of the medial antebrachial cutaneous nerve, must be identified and preserved during the procedure.

SUGGESTED READING

Baker CL Jr, Murphy KP, Gottlob CA, Curd DT. Arthroscopic classification and treatment of lateral epicondylitis: two-year clinical results. J Shoulder Elbow Surg 2000;9:475–482.

Cardon LJ, Ezaki M, Carter PR. Trigger finger in children. J Hand Surg 1999;24:1156–1161.

Carroll RE, Sinton W, Garcia A. Acute calcium deposits in the hand. JAMA 1950;157:422–426.

Carrozzella J, Stern PJ, Von Kuster LC. Transection of radial digital nerve of the thumb during trigger release. J Hand Surg 1989;14A:198–200.

Doyle JR. The Elbow. In: Doyle JR, Botte MJ, Surgical anatomy of the hand and upper extremity. Philadelphia: Lippincott, Williams & Wilkins: 2002:371–402.

Doyle JR. Palmar Hand. In: Doyle JR, Botte MJ, Surgical anatomy of the hand and upper extremity. Philadelphia: Lippincott, Williams & Wilkins: 2002:532–641.

Dunsmuir RA, Sherlock DA. The outcome of treatment of trigger thumb in children. J Bone Joint Surg 2000;82B:736–738.

Elliott BG. Finkelstein's test: a descriptive error that can produce a false positive. J Hand Surg (Br) 1992;17:481–82.

Finkelstein H. Stenosing tendovaginitis at the radial styloid process. J Bone Joint Surg 1930;12:509–540.

Gabel GT, Morrey BF. Operative treatment of medial epicondylitis: influence of concomitant ulnar neuropathy at the elbow. J Bone Joint Surg 1995;77A:1065.

Grundborg AB, Reagan DS. Pathologic anatomy of the forearm: intersection syndrome. J Hand Surg 1985;10A:299–302.

Morrey BF, An K-N. Functional anatomy of the ligaments of the elbow. Clin Orthop 1985;201:84–90.

Musgrave DS, Sotereanos DG. Tenosynovitis, de Quervain's syndrome and epicondylitis, In: Trumble, TE, ed. Hand surgery update-3, hand, elbow, shoulder. Rosemont, IL: American Society for Surgery of the Hand, 2003:271–284.

Pate MD, Bassini LB. Trigger fingers and thumb: when to splint, inject or operate. J Hand Surg 1992;17A:110–113.

Ritter WA, Inglis AE. The extensor indicis proprius syndrome. J Bone Joint Surg 1969;51-A:1645–1648.

Weiss APC, Akelman E, Tabatabai M. Treatment of de Quervain's disease. J Hand Surg 1994;19A:595–98.

Wolfe S. Tenosynovitis. In: Green DP, Hotchkiss RN, Pederson WC, eds. Green's operative hand surgery. 4th Ed. New York: Churchill Livingstone, 1999:2022–2044.

ENTRAPMENT NEUROPATHIES

Common entrapment neuropathies or nerve compression syndromes of the sensory and motor nerves in the arm, elbow, forearm, and wrist will be presented in this chapter. Compression syndromes that occur in the arm, elbow, and forearm are included because their major manifestations are often in the hand.

The term *compression neuropathy* is an appropriate description of abnormal pressure on a nerve from an adjacent anatomic structure. The underlying pathophysiology, however, is not understood as well, but may be related to mechanical factors and abnormal fluid homeostasis associated with conditions such as diabetes, chronic renal failure, hypothyroidism, or pregnancy. The role of mechanical factors is easily appreciated in those diseases or tumors that result in a space-occupying lesion. Rheumatoid arthritis that produces inflammation, and proliferation of the synovium and ganglion cyst, may be extrinsic mechanical factors that result in nerve compression.

The pertinent anatomy will be presented with each clinical entity. Important features in the history, pertinent physical findings, and treatment options will be given for each condition.

7.1 MEDIAN NERVE

Carpal Tunnel Syndrome (CTS)

Compression of the median nerve in the carpal canal is more often than not seen as a *chronic condition* related to a variety of causes. Some have placed it in the category of repetitive stress syndrome, but it is beyond the scope of this chapter to discuss this issue. This *chronic condition* is appropriately contrasted to *acute median nerve compression* seen most commonly in association with fractures about the wrist.

Pertinent Anatomy

The median nerve enters the hand from the forearm and wrist through a fibroosseous canal or tunnel. The floor and sides of this tunnel are formed by the pronator quadratus muscle and the carpal bones. Figure 7.1-1 shows the roof of this structure, which is formed by the *flexor retinaculum*. The flexor retinaculum is composed of the following:

1. Proximally, the antebrachial fascia and deep investing forearm fascia.
2. The central portion is the transverse carpal ligament that is defined by its attachments to the pisiform and hook process of the hamate ulnarly, and radially to the tuberosity of the scaphoid and ridge of the trapezium.
3. The distal portion is the aponeurosis between the thenar and hypothenar muscles.

Nine flexor tendons accompany the median nerve through this canal. These tendons are covered by a synovial sheath called the ulnar and radial bursa (Figure 7.1-2). The reader is referred to the suggested reading list for details of the complex anatomy of this region.

Pathophysiology

Although the carpal canal is open proximally and distally, it acts as a closed compartment. Chronic median nerve compression results when pressure levels exceed those normally tolerated by the median nerve. Carpal tunnel (CT) pressure levels in normal subjects have been recorded at 2.5 to 10 mm Hg, whereas CTS patients may exhibit levels of approximately 30 mm Hg. It is unclear, and experts have debated, if the underlying cause of nerve dysfunction is the relationship between mechanical factors or ischemia. It has been observed that nerve compression of 20 to 30 mm Hg will block venous blood flow and axonal transport, and compression of 60 to 80 mm Hg will block intraneural blood flow. Nerve conduction block occurs at 130 to 150 mm Hg.

Pressure catheters placed in the CT of both CTS patients and normal subjects have revealed that CT pressures

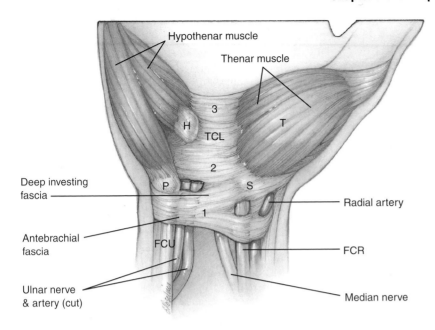

Figure 7.1-1   The anatomy of the flexor retinaculum. 1, antebrachial and deep investing forearm fascia; 2, central portion of the transverse carpal ligament (TCL); 3, distal aponeurosis. H, hook process of hamate; P, pisiform; S, scaphoid; T, thenar eminence.

are affected by finger, wrist, and forearm position, and activities such as pinching and grasping. Carpal tunnel (CT) pressure increases with wrist flexion and with extension. Anatomic studies have noted incursion of the distal muscle bellies of the FDS when the fingers are extended. They have also noted similar incursion of the lumbrical muscles when the fingers are flexed. This may partly explain the pressure changes noted in various finger and wrist positions.

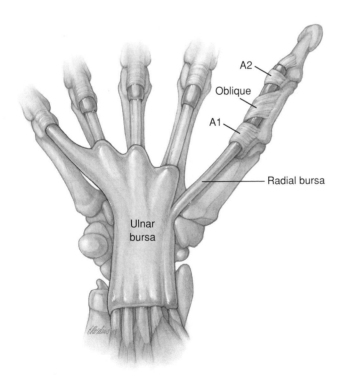

Figure 7.1-2   The synovial tissue that surrounds the nine flexor tendons as they pass through the carpal tunnel is called the ulnar and radial bursa.

Abnormal fluid homeostasis and carpal canal edema are also factors leading to CTS in patients with diabetes, chronic renal failure, hypothyroidism, and pregnancy. Rheumatoid, gouty, or other inflammatory arthritis can cause hyperplasia of the tenosynovium, which can diminish the space available in the carpal canal for the median nerve. This compresses the nerve. Diabetic patients have a predilection to develop CTS because of increased nerve susceptibility to injury, and because of a lower pressure threshold for blockage of fast axonal transport.

Acute Carpal Tunnel Syndrome

Fractures about the wrist, including the distal radius and the carpus, are the most common causes of acute compression of the median nerve. These injuries are often characterized as space-occupying lesions in terms of the carpal canal and the median nerve. A volarly displaced lunate or a fragment of a Colles fracture may significantly compromise the volume of the CT. This may compress the median nerve against the flexor retinaculum. As part of a Colles fracture treatment, a hematoma block and extreme wrist flexion have both been shown to further increase pressure within the canal. Post-traumatic edema associated with these injuries also plays a significant role in the production of acute CTS.

Diagnosis

Patient History
■ Patients with CTS often present with multiple complaints, but the most common is numbness and tingling in the fingers and thumb.
　■ The patient is often unable to tell the examiner which digits tingle.
　■ The numbness may be constant or intermittent, and commonly occurs 2 to 3 hours after retiring for the night. These nocturnal symptoms have been ascribed to the fact that the normal use of the hand during the day promotes the flow of well-oxygenated blood

to the median nerve. At night, however, venous stasis occurs, and oxygen tension in the nerve decreases to a level that promotes or triggers the symptoms. This concept is supported by the fact that patients often relieve the numbness through vigorous massage or by shaking their hands.

- Patients often complain of dropping things, and they sometimes complain of pinch or grip weakness.
- Predisposing or associated conditions should be asked about. Those include occupational and sports activities, as well as associated disorders such as rheumatoid arthritis, diabetes, and thyroid disease. Other peripheral neurological disorders that may produce hand numbness are cervical radiculopathy, brachial plexopathy, thoracic outlet syndrome, apical lung tumor, pronator syndrome, cubital and ulnar tunnel syndrome, and peripheral neuropathy.
- Bilateral CTS in a young male should prompt an investigation for acromegaly.

Physical Examination

Sensory Tests

- Sensory evaluation may be by static or moving two-point discrimination (2PD) and Semmes-Weinstein (SW) monofilaments.
  - The static 2PD evaluates the status of slowly adapting large myelinated fibers, while the moving 2PD evaluates the fast adapting large myelinated fibers.
  - SW monofilaments are threshold tests that evaluate sensory end organ function.
- The SW test is more sensitive in identifying compressive neuropathy than 2PD; when abnormal 2PD is present, the disease is more severe.

Motor Evaluation

- Motor evaluation consists of looking for thenar atrophy and strength testing the abductor pollicis brevis.
- The disease is considered severe and is usually longstanding when there is thenar muscle atrophy.
- Atrophy is seldom, if ever, recovered following CT release.

Provocative Tests

- Commonly used provocative tests for CTS include Phalen's and Tinel's signs, the CT compression test (Durkan's sign), the tourniquet test, and a combined Phalen's maneuver with SW monofilament testing. These and other useful tests are given in Table 7.1-1.

Electrodiagnostic Tests

- Electrodiagnostic studies include nerve conduction velocity (NCV) and electromyography (EMG).
- An abnormal nerve conduction result includes decreased action potential amplitude, increased distal latency, and decreased velocity.
- A distal motor latency of >4.5 ms and a sensory latency of >3.5 ms constitute and abnormal result. These measurements are achieved using an orthodromic stimulus and recording across the wrist.
- Additional diagnostic accuracy has been shown with nerve conduction measurements assessing short nerve segments (such as the inching technique or the comparison of palm-to-digit and wrist-to-digit latencies). In the case of CTS, measurements are made by isolating the wrist segment.
- Electromyography measures insertional activity, resting potential, and muscle activation.
  - Increased insertional activity, fibrillations at rest, positive sharp waves, complex repetitive discharges, and decreased motor unit recruitment are all consistent with nerve compromise.

Diagnostic Reliability.   Szabo and co-workers noted that the accuracy with which a patient can be diagnosed with CTS depends on the population being studied. They observed that a combination of findings in the history and physical exam was more accurate than the same findings in isolation. The CTS was accurately diagnosed 86% of the time when night pain, a positive SW monofilament test, a positive Durkan's test, and a positive Brigham hand diagram were all present; the probability of having CTS was 0.68% when all of these tests were negative. These authors noted that electrodiagnostic studies did not add to the diagnostic power of this combination of tests.

Some believe that electrodiagnostic studies provide the only objective evidence, and equate it to the "gold standard" for diagnosis of CTS. But not all agree. These tests may be positive in asymptomatic individuals, and negative in individuals with classic signs and symptoms. Some observers have noted that a significant number of patients diagnosed with CTS on clinical grounds—but with negative electrodiagnostic studies—have improved following a CTR.

Median Nerve Contusion

It is important to distinguish median nerve contusion from acute CTS, because delayed release of an acute CTS may result in a poor outcome. Contusion may be treated by observation, whereas acute CT syndrome requires immediate release.

- Signs and symptoms of contusion appear *immediately*, in contrast to those of compression that may occur later, as swelling increases. Thus, initial and careful sensory evaluation is mandatory.
- SW or 2PD tests are useful.
- In some cases, direct pressure measurements are indicated. Pressure greater than 40 mm Hg as measured by a wick catheter in the CT indicates the need for immediate CT release.

Treatment

Nonsurgical Treatment.   Conservative or nonoperative treatment is indicated for mild CTS, and is initially indicated for moderate cases. Any associated conditions should be identified and treated as indicated.

- Treatment is aimed at the underlying process, and may include activity modification such as ergonomic studies and corrections, splints that immobilize the wrist in a neutral position, and oral nonsteroidal medication. In some cases, treatment includes a short course of steroidal anti-inflammatory medication.

TABLE 7.1-1 TESTS FOR CARPAL TUNNEL SYNDROME (CTS)

Test	How Performed	Condition Tested	Positive Result	Interpretation of Positive Result
Phalen's test	Elbows on table, forearms vertical, wrists flexed	Paresthesia in response to position	Numbness or tingling on radial digits within 60 seconds	Probable CTS (sens 0.75, spec 0.47)
Percussion test (Tinel sign)	Lightly tap along median nerve from proximal to distal	Site of nerve lesion	"Electric" tingling response in fingers	Probable CTS if positive at the wrist (sens 0.60, spec 0.67)
Carpal tunnel compression test (Durkan)	Direct compression of median nerve at carpal tunnel	Paresthesia in response to compression	Paresthesia within 30 seconds	Probable CTS (sens 0.87, spec 0.90)
Hand diagram	Patient marks site of pain or altered sensation on outlined hand diagram	Patient's perception of symptoms	Markings on palmar side of radial digits, without markings in palm	Probable CTS (sens 0.96, spec 0.73, negative predictive value 0.91)
Hand volume stress test	Hand volume measured by displacement, repeat after 7-minute stress test and a rest of 10 minutes	Hand volume	Hand volume increased by 10 mL or greater	Probable dynamic CTS
Direct measurement of carpal tunnel pressure	Wick or infusion catheter placed in carpal tunnel	Hydrostatic pressure in resting and provocative positioning	Resting pressure 25 mm Hg or more (variable and technique related)	Hydrostatic compression is felt to be probable cause of CTS
Static 2-point discrimination	Determine minimum separation of two distinct points when applied to palmar fingertip	Innervation density of slow-adapting fibers	Failure to determine separation of at least 5 mm	Advanced nerve dysfunction
Moving 2-point discrimination	As above, with movement of the points	Innervation density of fast-adapting fibers	Failure to determine separation of at least 4 mm	Advanced nerve dysfunction
Vibrometry	Vibrometer placed on palmar side of digit, amplitude set to 120 Hz, and increase to threshold of perception; compare median and ulnar bilaterally	Threshold of fast-adapting fibers	Asymmetry compared to contralateral hand or median to ulnar in ipsilateral hand	Probable CTS (sens 0.87)
Semmes-Weinstein monofilaments	Monofilaments of increasing diameter touched to palmar side of digit until patient can determine which digit is touched	Threshold of slowly adapting fibers	Value greater than 2.83	Median nerve impairment (sens 0.83)
Distal sensory latency and conduction velocity	Orthodromic stimulus and recording across wrist	Latency, conduction of sensory fibers	Latency greater than 3.5 msec, or asymmetry of conduction velocity of greater than 0.5 msec versus opposite hand	Probable CTS
Distal motor latency and conduction velocity	Orthodromic stimulus and recording across wrist	Latency, conduction velocity of motor fibers of median nerve	Latency greater than 4.5 msec, or asymmetry of conduction velocity of greater than 1.0 msec	Probable CTS
Electromyography	Needle electrodes placed in muscle	Denervation of thenar muscles	Fibrillation potentials, sharp waves, increased insertional activity	Advanced motor median nerve compression

Sens, sensitivity; spec, specificity. (From Abrams R, Meunier, M. Carpal tunnel syndrome. In: Trumble TE, ed. Hand surgery update 3, hand, elbow, shoulder. Rosemont, IL: American Society for Surgery of the Hand, 2003:299–312.)

- Steroid injection or steroid iontophoresis into the CT, along with splinting, may give short-term benefit. It occasionally gives long-term benefit.
- A positive response affirms the diagnosis, and may be a predictor of a satisfactory surgical outcome, if required.
- Stretching, strengthening, and flexibility exercises may also play a significant role in recovery and avoidance of surgery in selected patients.

Surgical Treatment
Indications

- Surgical treatment of CTS is indicated for patients who have failed conservative treatment, and for patients with thenar muscle weakness, atrophy, or with signs of motor denervation on electrodiagnostic studies.

Open Surgical Technique
INCISION

- The incision for open CT release is a longitudinal incision that begins at the wrist flexion crease and ends about 1 cm proximal to the proximal palmar crease. Its axis is somewhat parallel to the radial border of the ring finger.
  - Others have tried to identify the ideal site of placement, and have noted that the depression between the thenar and hypothenar eminence is the ideal site for the incision.
  - This sought-after zone is the zone in which the *least number* of superficial nerves are present. But there is no true internervous or nerve-free zone for this incision (Figure 7.1-3).
  - The incision just described places the dissection to the ulnar side of the CT, which is considered to be the relatively safe side for entering the canal and releasing the TCL.
- Some surgeons have used smaller, single- or two-portal incisions to accomplish exposure and release of the TCL. Many of these techniques use special blade-guide instruments to facilitate section of the TCL.

DEEP DISSECTION. The goal of this operation is to completely release the ulnar margin of the TCL without injury to vital structures such as the median nerve and its branches—including the recurrent or motor branch—and the superficial palmar arch that is just distal to the distal end of the TCL. The technical details of the various CT release techniques are beyond the scope of this text.

ENDOSCOPIC RELEASE OF THE CARPAL CANAL. A variety of techniques have been developed that utilize the arthroscope to assist in TCL section. Single- and two-portal techniques have been used with success.

OPEN VERSUS ENDOSCOPIC CT RELEASE. Studies comparing these two basic techniques have suggested that there is earlier functional recovery in the endoscopic technique compared to open techniques. However, there is no current evidence available to show that the endoscopic technique is superior in terms of *final outcome* to the open technique.

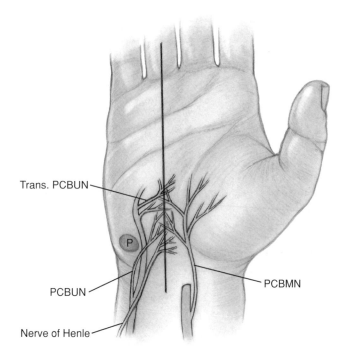

Trans. PCBUN
P
PCBUN
Nerve of Henle
PCBMN

Figure 7.1-3 Cutaneous innervation of the palm as it relates to open carpal tunnel release. Four nerves are at risk (all nerves that may be cut or pass within 2 mm of the incision): the palmar cutaneous branch of the median nerve (PCBMN); the palmar cutaneous branch of the ulnar nerve (PCBUN); the nerve of Henle; and transverse palmar branches (Trans. PCBUN) from the ulnar nerve in Guyon's canal.

Caveat: CT release by any means, including open, limited-open with or without special guide instruments, and endoscopic release, have all been associated with complications.

ANCILLARY PROCEDURES WITH CT RELEASE. Studies have shown that there is no added benefit from tenosynovectomy, epineurotomy, or internal neurolysis in idiopathic CTS.

Pronator Teres Syndrome and Proximal Sites of Median Nerve Compression

Sites of Compression
There are five potential sites of proximal median nerve compression: two are in the distal arm and three are in the proximal forearm (Figure 7.1-4).

The *first distal arm site* is an abnormal proximal origin of the superficial head of the pronator teres from the supracondylar ridge rather than the medial epicondyle. This abnormal muscle position results in lateral displacement of the neurovascular bundle, and has the potential for compression of the underlying median nerve and brachial artery.

The *second distal arm site* is represented by a supracondylar process and a ligament of Struthers, which spans between the supracondylar process and the medial epicondyle, thus creating an arcade that contains the median nerve and brachial artery. The supracondylar process is a hook-shaped projection of bone from the

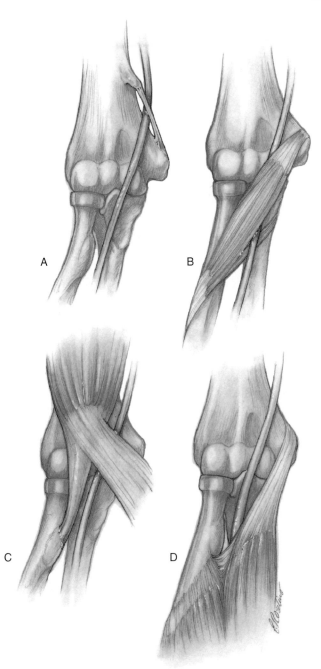

Figure 7.1-4   Sites of compression of the median nerve in the arm/forearm. (**A**) The ligament of Struthers from an anomalous supracondylar process to the medial epicondyle. (**B**) The pronator teres. (**C**) The lacertus fibrosus (the least common cause). (**D**) A fibrous arch in the flexor digitorum superficialis of the middle finger.

anteromedial aspect of the distal humerus. It arises 3 to 5 cm proximal to the medial epicondyle and is 2 to 20 mm in length. Its incidence is approximately 1%, and it is a rare cause of pressure on the under lying median nerve and brachial artery.

In the proximal forearm, the median nerve may be compressed at one of three levels, in the following order of frequency: the pronator teres, the flexor superficialis arch, and the lacertus fibrosus.

Pronator Teres (PT).   Dissections of the proximal forearm have revealed either a fibrous band on the dorsum of the superficial head of the pronator overlying the median nerve, or a fibrous band as a component of the deep ulnar head of the pronator when the latter was present, or, when the deep head was absent, a separate fibrous band attached to the coronoid process of the ulna proximally. In some instances, fibrous bands were noted on both heads, which formed a definite fibrous arcade.

Flexor Superficialis Arch.   A fibrous arcade was observed in approximately one third of the dissections spanning from the proximal margin of the FDS to the middle finger.

Lacertus Fibrosus.   Entrapment of the median nerve beneath the lacertus fibrosus is the least common cause of median nerve entrapment in the proximal forearm. It may be secondary to hypertrophy or enlargement of the lacertus.

Diagnosis
Functional muscle testing may give some indication of the site of compression (Figure 7.1-5).

■ If complaints are produced by flexion of the elbow against resistance between 120 and 135 degrees of elbow flexion, compression may be in the distal arm beneath a ligament of Struthers.

■ Compression by the lacertus fibrosus may be aggravated by active flexion of the elbow against resistance when the arm is pronated.

■ If symptoms are increased by resisted pronation of the forearm (usually combined with wrist flexion to relax the FDS), the nerve may be compressed between the pronator.

■ If the symptoms are aggravated by resisted flexion of the FDS to the middle finger, compression may be at the FDS proximal arch.

Treatment
■ The operative technique for treatment of pronator syndrome includes complete exploration of the median nerve, from the distal arm to the proximal forearm.

■ The median nerve is explored from the region of a possible anomalous supracondylar process and an associated ligament of Struthers to the proximal edge of the FDS, with release of all potentially constricting structures, including the ligament of Struthers and the lacertus fibrosus.

■ At the level of the PT, compression may be because of muscle hypertrophy or constricting muscle fascial bands.

■ Further decompression of the median nerve is achieved by tracing the median nerve into the substance of the PT, and then releasing any areas of constriction.

■ The final site of possible constriction is in the proximal edge of the FDS, which may be exposed by entering the interval between the FCR and the PT.

■ The median nerve may be constricted here beneath a fibrous tissue arch along the leading edge of the FDS.

■ A persistent median artery has also been observed as a cause of pronator syndrome. Reported cases have demonstrated penetration of the median nerve by the median artery, and constriction of the nerve by vascular leashes from the median artery.

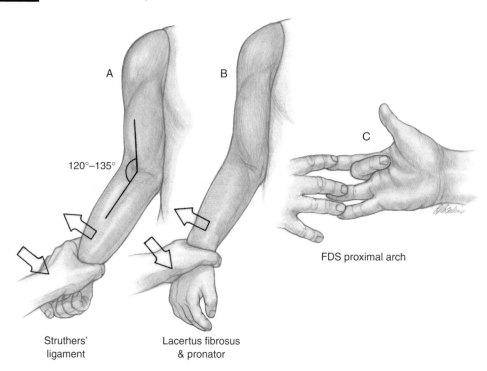

120°–135°

Struthers'
ligament

Lacertus fibrosus
& pronator

FDS proximal arch

Figure 7.1-5   Localizing tests for median nerve compression in the proximal forearm. (**A**) Test for presence of a ligament of Struthers. (**B**) Test for lacertus fibrosus and pronator teres compression. (**C**) Test for median nerve compression by fibrous tissue arch of flexor digitorum superficialis of the middle finger (see text).

Anterior Interosseus Nerve Syndrome

Compression of the anterior interosseus nerve (AIN) characteristically results in complete or partial loss of function of the FPL and the flexor digitorum profundus (FDP) of the index finger and long fingers, as well as of the PQ. This occurs without any sensory deficits. These findings may be associated with vague complaints of discomfort in the proximal forearm. In the complete AIN syndrome (AINS), the affected patient assumes an unusual pinch posture with the distal joint of the index and thumb in extension. Although the FPL and FDP of the index are innervated exclusively by the AIN, the FDP of the long finger is exclusively innervated by the AIN only 50% of the time. In the remaining 50%, the long finger FDP is at least partially innervated by the ulnar nerve. Variations from the classic AINS include isolated paresis or paralysis in either the index profundus or the FPL. In both complete and partial types, there is often an antecedent history of unusual muscular exertion, blunt trauma, or edema in the extremity.

Diagnosis

Differential Diagnosis

- AINS, especially the incomplete type, must be distinguished from flexor tendon rupture, flexor tendon adhesion, and stenosing tenosynovitis.
- If a Martin-Gruber connection is present between the AIN and the ulnar nerve, there may be intrinsic muscle paresis or atrophy.
- The incomplete type of AINS may be distinguished from rupture of the FPL by noting passive flexion of the interphalangeal joint of the thumb with wrist and metacarpophalangeal (MCP) joint hyperextension in AINS, in contrast to absence of thumb interphalangeal joint flexion in rupture of the FPL.

Compression Sites

- The nerve is usually compressed by fibrous bands that run from the deep (most common) or superficial head of the PT to the brachialis fascia (Figure 7.1-6).
- Other sites of compression have been identified, including the fibrous tissue arcade of the FDS, which the AIN passes beneath to sit on the interosseous membrane (IOM).
- Other reported causes of compression include enlarged bursae or tumors, aberrant or thrombosed vessels, a double lacertus fibrosus overlying the nerve, compression of the nerve as it runs deep to both heads of the PT, and fractures of the forearm and distal humerus.
- Three aberrant muscles have been identified in association with AINS, including an accessory head of the FPL called Gantzer's muscle, the palmaris profundus, and the flexor carpi radialis brevis (FCRB).
  - Although an accessory head of the FPL (Gantzer's muscle) has been identified as a cause of AINS, some observers have noted that Gantzer's muscle always is posterior to the median nerve and AIN. However, in dissections of the forearm in which Gantzer's muscle was present, the authors demonstrated the possibility of a pincer-like effect between this abnormal posterior head and the adjacent anterior FDS. This could produce compression of the median nerve, as well as the AIN. The median nerve and AIN passed through the interval between these two muscles, which share a common origin on the medial epicondyle.
- The common denominator in this condition appears to be localized edema, superimposed on an anatomic abnormality that is either congenital or acquired.

Treatment

Nonsurgical Treatment.   Patients who present with paresis may be observed, because most improve spontaneously

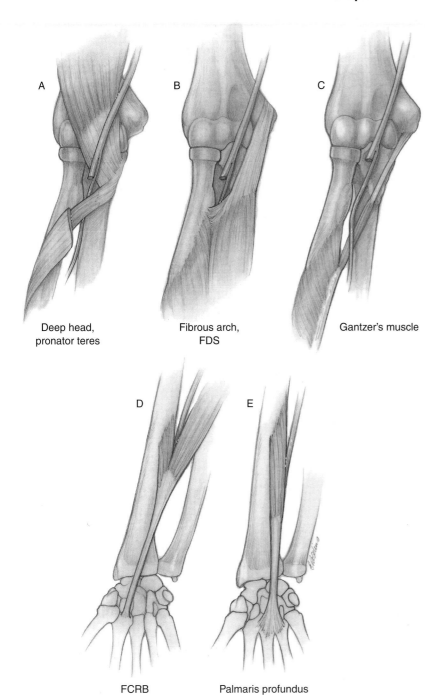

Deep head,
pronator teres

Fibrous arch,
FDS

Gantzer's muscle

FCRB

Palmaris profundus

Figure 7.1-6 Anterior interosseous nerve compression sites. (**A**) Deep head of the pronator teres. (**B**) Fibrous arch of the middle finger flexor digitorum superficialis. (**C**) Gantzer's muscle. (**D**) Abnormal flexor carpi radialis brevis (FCRB). (**E**) Abnormal palmaris profundus muscle. FDS, flexor digitorum superficialis.

without surgery. This is especially true in children with AINS associated with fractures of the forearm and elbow region.

Surgical Treatment

■ Exploration and decompression is advised in patients who present with complete paralysis of either muscle tendon unit and who have shown no improvement, as determined by physical examination or repeat EMG after 12 weeks of observation.

■ The AIN is exposed through a curved incision beginning at the antecubital flexion crease just medial to the biceps tendon.

■ The median nerve is traced distally to its entrance between the two heads of the PT, and the superficial head of the PT is mobilized and retracted to reveal the usual site of origin of the AIN, from the posterior aspect of the median nerve.

■ The site of compression may be identified by noting a pale discoloration in the nerve, with or without a concomitant indentation of the nerve.

■ All potential sites of compression are released; it is not necessary to perform an internal neurolysis.

■ It may be necessary to divide the insertion of the PT, in order to facilitate exposure of the AIN at the superficialis fibrous arcade.

7.2 ULNAR NERVE

Ulnar Nerve Compression (Wrist)

Compression of the ulnar nerve at the wrist is significantly less common than compression at the elbow.

- Subjective complaints include loss of dexterity in the hand, which results in clumsiness, dropping things, or weakness.
- Numbness in the ring and little fingers may be prominent symptoms, and may be verified on physical examination.
- Motor weakness of the intrinsic muscle may be present in early cases, and atrophy of the intrinsic muscles may be present in late cases or severe compression of the motor component of the nerve.
- A characteristic claw deformity of the ring and little fingers may be observed with motor deficit.

Pertinent Anatomy

Ulnar Tunnel (Guyon's Canal). Guyon's canal, or the ulnar tunnel, is the space that the ulnar nerve and artery traverse to gain entrance to the hand from the forearm.

Guyon's canal begins at the proximal edge of the palmar carpal ligament and ends at or beyond the fibrous arch of the hypothenar muscles. Beginning from proximal to distal, the roof of the canal is formed by the palmar carpal ligament, portions of the palmar aponeurosis, and the palmaris brevis muscle. The floor is formed by the TCL, the pisohamate and pisometacarpal ligaments, and the FDM. The ulnar wall is composed of the flexor carpi ulnaris (FCU), the pisiform, and the ADM. The radial wall is formed by the tendons of the extrinsic flexors, the TCL, and the hook process of the hamate. The average length of Guyon's canal is 27 mm, with a range from 20 to 34 mm. The ulnar nerve and artery branches in this region are covered by the palmaris brevis muscle, and are surrounded by a thick fat pad.

Ulnar Nerve in Guyon's Canal.   The ulnar nerve, accompanied by the ulnar artery on its radial side, enters the hand on the radial side of the pisiform bone through Guyon's canal (Figure 7.2-1). The ulnar nerve may divide into motor and sensory components proximal to, at, or in Guyon's canal, but the most common configuration is division in

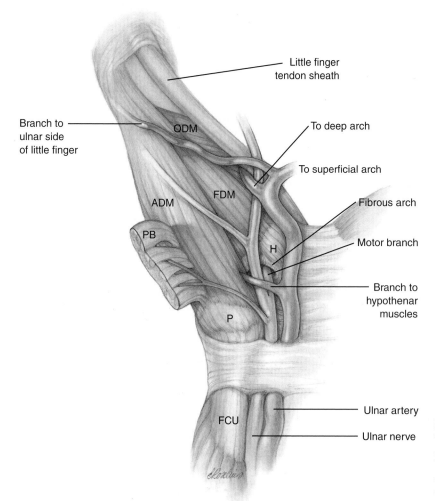

Figure 7.2-1   The ulnar nerve in Guyon's canal. The ulnar nerve may divide into motor and sensory components proximal to, at, or in Guyon's canal, but the most common configuration is division in Guyon's canal an average of 8.6 mm (range, 0–15 mm) from the proximal edge of the pisiform. H, hook process of hamate; P, pisiform.

Guyon's canal at an average of 8.6 mm (with a range of 0 to 15 mm) from the proximal edge of the pisiform.

Ulnar Motor Branches.   The motor component of the nerve at the level of the pisiform is ulnar and dorsal. The motor branch gives off one to three (usually two) branches to the hypothenar muscles before it enters the depths of the palm. Its course into the palm has been variously described as passing between the origin of the FDM and ODM, or beneath the proximal origin of the FDM. It then courses around the ulnar and distal aspect of the base of the hook process of the hamate. The proximal edge of the FDM often demonstrates a fibrous arcade, where the motor branch may become entrapped. It then traverses the hand to innervate the ring and small finger lumbricals, the palmar and dorsal interossei, the adductor pollicis, and the deep head of the FPB (Figure 7.2-2).

Ulnar Sensory Branches.   After division into a sensory trunk and a motor branch in Guyon's canal, the sensory component divides into the sensory branch to the ulnar side of the little finger, and the common sensory nerve to the fourth web space, which subsequently divides into the PDN to the radial side of the little finger and the ulnar side of the ring finger. The motor branch to the palmaris brevis usually arises from the sensory branch to the little finger.

The Zones of Guyon's Canal.   Guyon's canal has been divided into three zones to aid in identification of the most common or likely causes of nerve compression in the ulnar tunnel. Zone 1 is from the proximal edge of the proximal commissural ligament (PCL) to the bifurcation of the ulnar nerve. Zones 2 and 3 are parallel zones that begin at the bifurcation of the nerve and that end at the region just beyond the fibrous tissue arch of the hypothenar muscles. Zone 2 contains the motor branch of the ulnar nerve, and zone 3 contains the sensory branch of the nerve. Zones 2 and 3 are not divided by an anatomic structure, but rather are arbitrary divisions that have useful clinical applications.

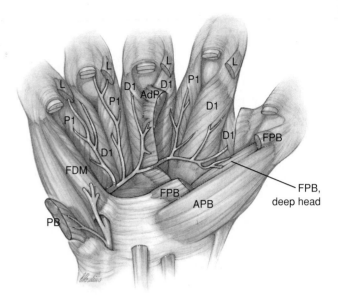

Figure 7.2-2   The deep motor branch of the ulnar nerve in the palm. See text for details.

Diagnosis

The clinical relevance of these zones is apparent in Table 7.2-1. These zones are useful for the localization and correct prediction of the cause of ulnar neuropathy in Guyon's canal. This information, along with a careful history, sensory and motor examination, careful palpation, Allen's test, and radiographs of the wrist, may lead to an accurate prediction of the cause of the ulnar deficit.

Treatment

■ Decompression of the ulnar nerve in Guyon's canal is performed through a longitudinal zigzag incision centered over the interval between the pisiform and the hook process of the hamate (Figure 7.2-3).

■ The roof of the canal is incised to reveal the underlying nerve and artery on the radial side of the FCU tendon.

TABLE 7.2-1 AREAS AND CAUSES OF ULNAR NERVE COMPRESSION IN GUYON'S CANAL

Deficit	Zone 1	Zone 2	Zone 3	Causes	Occurrence (%)
Motor and sensory	42			Ganglions	45
				Fractures	36
				Anomalous muscles	7
Motor alone	1	42		Ganglions	60
				Fractures	12
				Thickened pisohamate ligament	7
Sensory alone	7		10	Thrombosis	30
				Synovitis	24
				Anomalous muscles	12

These represent the most frequent causes of ulnar nerve compression, and do not add up to 100%. Those patients with combined motor and sensory loss without a history of trauma had a ganglion as the cause of the ulnar deficit 45% of the time. Isolated motor deficits occurred most frequently in zone 2 and were due to a ganglion 60% of the time. Isolated sensory deficits occurred most commonly from compression in zone 3, but also may occur in zone 1; thrombosis of the ulnar artery was the most frequent cause. (Taken from Doyle JR, Botte MJ. Palmar hand. In: Surgical anatomy of the hand and upper extremity. Philadelphia: Lippincott Williams & Wilkins, 2002:578.)

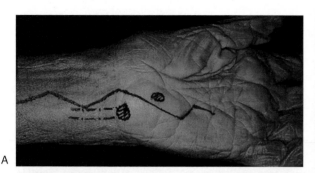

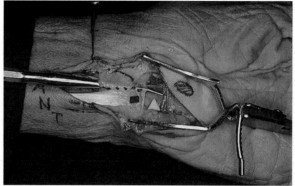

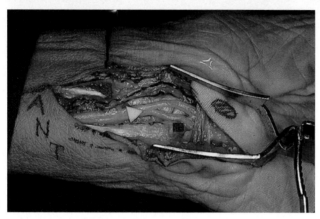

Figure 7.2-3   Surgical approach to Guyon's canal. (**A**) A longitudinal zigzag incision is used in the interval between the pisiform and hook process of the hamate (*dots*) in order to unroof the canal. (**B–C**) Note the arrangement of the artery, nerve, and tendon (ANT) from radial to ulnar, and also note the relationship of the nerve to the FCU tendon, pisiform, and hook process of the hamate bone.

Cubital Tunnel Syndrome (Elbow)

The term cubital tunnel syndrome was proposed in 1958 to identify a specific site of entrapment of the ulnar nerve, and to distinguish it from tardy ulnar palsy that is associated with posttraumatic cubitus valgus.

Pertinent Anatomy

The ulnar nerve enters the posterior aspect of the arm at approximately the midpoint of the arm, and continues distally toward the elbow behind the medial intermuscular septum on the medial head of the triceps muscle. The nerve continues to the elbow, where it enters the fibroosseous cubital tunnel. The tunnel can be divided into three parts. The *first part* of the cubital tunnel is the entrance of the tunnel formed by the ulnar groove in the medial epicondyle. At this level, the ulnar nerve usually provides one or several small articular branches to the elbow joint, and these branches usually are proximal to the branches given off to innervate the FCU.

The *second, and middle, part* of the tunnel consists of a fascial arcade that is a fan shaped ligament covering the tunnel. It attaches to the medial epicondyle and to the olecranon, and connects the ulnar and humeral heads of the origin of the FCU muscle. In this area, the nerve lies on the posterior and oblique portions of the ulnar collateral ligament, and usually gives off two branches to innervate the FCU. One branch usually supplies the humeral head, and one supplies the ulnar head. The first branch exits the main nerve trunk horizontally. The second branch continues dis-

tally for several centimeters before entering the FCU. Up to four motor branches to the FCU may be given off, exiting the main nerve at a point between 4 cm proximal and 10 cm distal to the medial epicondyle. The motor branches enter the FCU on its deep surface. The distance between the medial humeral epicondyle and the olecranon is shortest with elbow extension. This distance increases with elbow flexion. The roof or fascial arcade becomes taut with elbow flexion.

The *third, and most distal, part* of the tunnel consists of the muscle bellies of the FCU. The FCU provides a portion of the roof in this area. The nerve courses through the interval between the humeral and ulnar heads of the FCU, or between the FCU and the FDP muscles. It continues distally in the forearm between the FDP, located dorsally and laterally to the nerve, and the FCU, located anteriorly and medially. The volume of the tunnel decreases with elbow flexion, and the pressure within it increases—even in the normal elbow when the aponeurotic arch or surrounding soft tissues are not thickened.

Pathophysiology

The ulnar nerve at the elbow is subcutaneous throughout much of its course, and also is partially fixed in a fibroosseous canal. Because of its exposed position, and the fact that it wraps around the medial condyle in flexion, prolonged elbow flexion—which stretches the nerve and narrows the tunnel—combined with resting the elbow on a hard surface may result in paresthesias in the ring and little fingers. This occurs even in normal people. When swelling of, or elbow inflammation or congestion of, the flexor-pronator muscles is added to this stretch–compression, the vascular supply of the ulnar nerve may be compromised, and nerve symptoms may result. Sustained elbow flexion combined with vigorous finger and wrist motion—such as that which a musician might perform—can also result in ulnar nerve symptoms. The motions used to throw a ball and for a tennis serve are similar, and can place significant stress on the ulnar nerve. They may be associated with ulnar nerve symptoms. Perioperative ulnar neuropathies are more common in men than in women. Although there is no gross anatomic difference between the sexes regarding the course of the ulnar nerve in the upper extremity, there is a significantly larger (2 to 19 times greater) fat content on the medial aspect of the elbow in women compared to men. Also, the tubercle of the coronoid process on the ulna is 1.5 times larger in men.

Sites of Compression

Surgical treatment of cubital tunnel syndrome is facilitated by knowledge of the potential sites of compression, and of the anatomy specific to each of those areas.

Arcade of Struthers. Although recently contested by some observers as to its name and occurrence, there is a potential site of entrapment of the ulnar nerve that lies 8 cm proximal to the medial epicondyle called the arcade of Struthers. When the arcade is present, both the ulnar nerve and the superior ulnar collateral vessels pass through it. In a study of 25 arms, the arcade of Struthers was present 68% of the time. The arcade has a medial-facing roof, formed by the deep investing fascia of the arm, superficial muscle fibers from the medial head of the triceps, and the internal brachial ligament arising from the coracobrachialis tendon. The floor, which is lateral, is formed by the medial aspect of the humerus, and is covered by the deep muscular fibers of the medial head of the triceps. The anterior border is the medial intermuscular septum (Figure 7.2-4).

Medial Head Triceps. The ulnar nerve may be buried in the medial head of the triceps muscle, and this overlying muscle roof may be a source of compression. When it is, it should be incised.

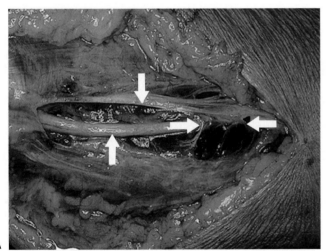

A

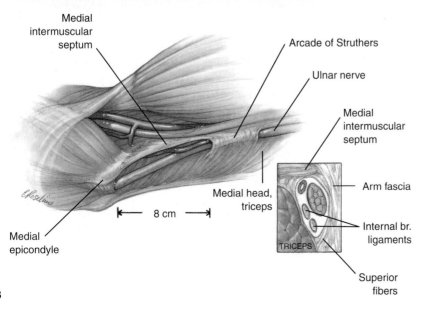

B

Figure 7.2-4 Fresh cadaver dissection of the so-called arcade of Struther's. (**A**) The appearance of the arcade over the ulnar nerve and its relationship to the medial intermuscular septum (MIMS). Here, the upper vertical *arrow* marks the MIMS, the lower vertical *arrow* marks the ulnar nerve, and the opposed horizontal *arrows* mark the arcade. (**B**) Artist's depiction of the relationship of the arcade to the MIMS and the medial epicondyle.

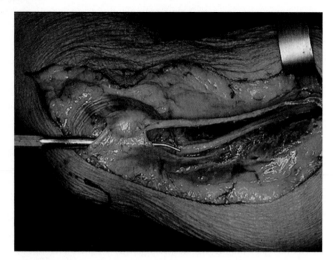

Figure 7.2-5   Fresh cadaver dissection of the medial aspect of the arm and elbow. Note the probe under the cubital tunnel retinaculum.

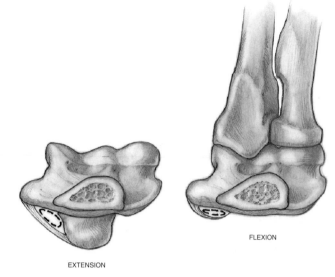

FLEXION

EXTENSION

Figure 7.2-6   Changes in the cubital tunnel with flexion and extension.

Medial Intermuscular Septum.   The ulnar nerve lies posterior to the medial intermuscular septum (MIMS)—and when the ulnar nerve is transposed anteriorly—it can represent a sharp edge that may cause impingement of the nerve. The MIMS should be excised as part of ulnar transposition, as discussed under the treatment section (see Figure 7.2-4).

Elbow (Cubital Tunnel).   The ulnar nerve in its passage from the arm to the forearm transits the cubital tunnel, which is an osseous canal formed by the medial epicondyle and the proximal ulna. It is covered by a retinaculum formed by the deep investing fascia of the arm that is attached to the medial epicondyle and the olecranon. This cubital tunnel retinaculum (CTR) is 2 to 3 cm wide from proximal to distal, and 0.5 to 0.75 mm thick—and its distal margin blends with the investing fascia of both the humeral and ulnar heads of the FCU. Osborne's band and the arcuate ligament are other names often used to describe this fibrous tissue roof of the ulnar tunnel (Figure 7.2-5). Because of the somewhat eccentric origin of this fascial roof, the cubital tunnel changes contour and volume during elbow flexion and extension. In flexion, the cross-sectional contour changes from slightly ovoid to elliptical (Figure 7.2-6). Any swelling in the canal—or inflammation or thickening of the fascial roof—may compress the nerve or its vasculature.

Forearm.   At the distal end of the cubital tunnel the ulnar nerve enters the forearm through the flexor pronator group of muscles, usually between the humeral and ulnar heads of the FCU. The flexor-pronator muscles are arranged in two groups. The superficial group is formed by five muscles (the PT, FCR, PL, FDS, and FCU) that originate from a common origin created by the fusion of several fibrous septae. Those septae arise from the anterior surface of the medial humeral epicondyle, the ulnar collateral ligament, and medial surface of the coronoid process. They form well-defined fascial compartments for the muscles, as well as a common aponeurosis from which adjacent muscles originate. These septae fuse, beginning approximately 3.5 to 4 cm distal to the epicondyle. This fused structure is commonly known as

the flexor-pronator origin, or the flexor-pronator aponeurosis. An additional aponeurosis in this area is present between the FDS to the ring finger and the humeral head of the FCU that did not fuse with the previously described common flexor pronator origin but rather arose from the medial surface of the coronoid process 0.3 to 0.5 cm medial to it. If present, it may not be possible to transpose the ulnar nerve adjacent to the median nerve in a relatively straight course unless this septum is detached along with the radial two-thirds of the flexor-pronator group. Others have identified a structure deep to the FDS, and superficial to both the FDP and the FCU, that provided a point of origin for all of these muscles. That structure extended approximately 5 cm distal to the epicondyle. This deep aponeurosis of the FCU, which bridges and forms a common origin for muscle fibers of the FCU, FDS, and FDP, should be released by separating the two heads of the FCU and exploring the deep surface of the muscle for at least 5 cm distal to the epicondyle.

Diagnosis

- Clinical findings include complaints of medial elbow pain, numbness and tingling—or burning—in the ring and little fingers, hand clumsiness, and weakness of pinch.
- Physical findings may include tenderness behind the medial condyle over the course of the ulnar nerve, as well as a positive Tinel's sign over the nerve 2 cm proximal and distal to the cubital tunnel.
- Other physical findings include decreased sensibility in the ring and little fingers, as well as decreased pinch and grip strength.
- Claw deformity of the ring and little fingers, as well as intrinsic muscle atrophy, are seen in severe and prolonged cases.
- Physical findings that aid in the diagnosis are tenderness over the ulnar nerve at the elbow, reproduction of the patient's symptoms with elbow flexion, and positive findings with sensory evaluation.

- Electrodiagnostic studies have a high rate of false negatives.
- Other causes of symptoms that mimic cubital tunnel syndrome (such as thoracic outlet syndrome) should be eliminated by appropriate tests.
- Weakness of the FDS to the little finger may be present in cubital tunnel syndrome, but not in ulnar nerve compression at the wrist. This finding may be helpful in distinguishing these two conditions.

Treatment

Nonsurgical Treatment
- Conservative treatment is appropriate for mild and early cases of cubital tunnel that present without motor deficit.
- Avoidance of elbow flexion and pressure over the point—or medial aspect—of the elbow, along with oral anti-inflammatories, may be beneficial.

Surgical Treatment
- Common to all ulnar nerve transpositions is elimination of compression or traction problems by removing the nerve from the fibroosseous tunnel and permanently transposing it to an anterior location.
- Permanent transposition has been achieved by subcutaneous transposition, subcutaneous transposition with some form of tether to prevent the nerve from assuming its original position, or submuscular or intramuscular transposition.
- The *sine qua non* of ulnar nerve transposition is permanent realignment of the ulnar nerve in an anterior position, without entrapment (absence of compression) or fixation (traction). Such complications would prevent the nerve from gliding.
- It also must be recognized that the ulnar nerve remains subcutaneous throughout most of its new course, and that even submuscular or intramuscular transposition eliminates only a portion of this subcutaneous position.
- The effectiveness of transposition is based on decompression of the nerve and on elimination of any potential for traction injury.
- A factor in the avoidance of secondary entrapment following transposition might be early and protected mobilization of the elbow joint.

The debate concerning the best technique for ulnar nerve transposition and the role of *in situ* ulnar nerve neurolysis without transposition (with or without medial epicondylectomy) is not addressed in this text. Rather, the reader is referred to the suggested reading list at the end of this chapter.

7.3 RADIAL NERVE

Although this is a text on the hand and wrist, radial nerve palsy originating in the arm will be encountered on an upper extremity service and it is appropriate to discuss it in the context of this book.

Radial Nerve Palsy with Fracture of the Humerus

Radial nerve palsy in the arm is associated most often with fractures of the humerus in the middle third or at the junction of the middle and distal thirds. Radial nerve palsy at this location is distinguished from the more proximal "Saturday night palsy" and "crutch palsy" seen in the upper arm and axilla, respectively. These more proximal lesions usually recover spontaneously in 60 to 90 days and are not the topic of discussion here.

Pertinent Anatomy
At the level in the humerus under discussion, the radial nerve is subject to injury based on at least two anatomic factors:

1. The proximity of the radial nerve to bone in the spiral groove.
2. The relative fixation of the radial nerve in the spiral groove and at the site of penetration of the nerve through the lateral intermuscular septum on its way from the posterior to the anterior aspect of the arm.

Based on these anatomic findings, it is appropriate to postulate the etiology of the neurapraxia based on traction, contusion, or hematoma.

Surgical Exploration
Although much discussion has been generated around the issue of early versus late exploration of radial nerve palsy associated with humeral fracture, most palsies recover spontaneously, and early surgical exploration is recommended in only three circumstances: (1) open fractures, (2) fractures that require open reduction and or fixation, and (3) fractures with associated vascular injuries. The onset of radial nerve palsy after fracture manipulation is not an indication for early nerve exploration.

Holstein-Lewis Fracture
In 1963, Holstein and Lewis described a spiral oblique fracture of the distal humerus in seven patients, five with radial nerve paralysis and two with paresis. They noted radial angulation and overriding at the fracture site. As the radial nerve courses anteriorly through the lateral intermuscular septum, it is less mobile and subject to being injured by the movement of the distal fracture fragment. Because of the high incidence of radial nerve dysfunction, early operative intervention was advised.

In a larger and more recent study of this fracture associated with radial nerve palsy, 11 of 15 patients were treated without exploration of the radial nerve and had complete recovery; in the 4 patients who were explored, the nerve was in continuity. They also demonstrated complete recovery.

Radial Nerve Entrapment in the Arm

Pathophysiology
Radial nerve entrapment in the arm is rare compared with trauma-related palsy. A fibrous arch and accessory part of the lateral head of the triceps has been associated with nerve compression secondary to swelling of the muscle after muscular effort. Some cases of radial nerve entrapment in this region of the lateral head of the triceps have been reported as spontaneous in onset and some following strenuous muscular activity. What appears to be a familial radial nerve entrapment syndrome has been reported in a 15-year-old girl with a total and spontaneous radial nerve palsy. Her sister had recently sustained an identical lesion that improved spontaneously, and her father also suffered from intermittent radial nerve palsy. These cases appear to represent a genetically determined defect in Schwann cell myelin metabolism.

Treatment
■ Although a patient with entrapment neuropathy with an acute onset after overactivity sometimes recovers spontaneously, entrapment in the advanced stage should be surgically decompressed because prolonged compression might result in intraneural fibrotic changes secondary to long-term compression.
■ The surgical approach of choice is posterior between the long and lateral heads of the triceps.

Radial Sensory Nerve Entrapment at the Wrist

Wartenberg in 1932 described an isolated neuritis of the superficial radial nerve at the wrist that he called cheiralgia paresthetica. The condition is characterized by pain, burning, or numbness on the dorsal and radial aspect of the distal forearm and wrist that radiates into the thumb, index, and middle fingers. The symptoms are often associated with a history of a variety of traumatic and iatrogenic causes, including a direct blow to the nerve, a tight wristwatch band or bracelet, handcuffs, or an injury due to laceration or compression from retraction during surgery. Although Wartenberg classified it as "neuritis," it is a form of nerve entrapment.

Pertinent Anatomy
The sensory branch of the radial nerve (SBRN) is positioned beneath the BR muscle as it travels towards the wrist, where it exits from beneath the BR tendon and between the ECRL tendon to pierce the antebrachial fascia. In 10% of specimens, the nerve may pierce the tendon of the BR. It becomes subcutaneous at a mean of 9 cm (with a range of 7 to 10.8 cm) proximal to the radial styloid. In supination the SBRN lies beneath the fascia, but without compression. In pronation, the ECRL crosses over the BR and may create a scissoring or pinching effect on the SBRN.

Diagnosis
■ A useful provocative test is to ask the patient to fully pronate the forearm. A positive test is manifested by paresthesia or dysesthesia on the dorsoradial aspect of the hand.
■ In addition to this provocative test, a positive Tinel's sign may be noted over the nerve distal to the BR muscle belly as well as altered moving touch and vibratory sense.

Treatment
■ Treatment is based on the particular cause, and is usually conservative in the form of splinting, altered physical activities, and physical therapy including stretching and tissue gliding exercises.
■ In patients who require surgery, release of the deep fascia and the fascia joining the BR and ECRL, as well as neurolysis of the SBRN, may be utilized in selected cases.

Radial Tunnel Syndrome

Pertinent Anatomy
In the mid-portion of the arm, the radial nerve passes through the spiral groove to enter the anterolateral aspect of the distal third of the arm on its way to the forearm, where it lies between the brachioradialis laterally and the brachialis medially. The ECRL covers it anterolaterally, and the capitellum of the humerus is posterior. The radial tunnel begins at the level of the radiohumeral joint and extends through the arcade of Frohse to end at the distal end of the supinator. Division of the radial nerve into motor (posterior interosseous) and sensory (superficial radial) components may occur at any level within a 5.5-cm segment, from 2.5 cm above to 3 cm below Hueter's or the interepicondylar line (a line drawn through the tips of the epicondyles of the humerus). The superficial radial nerve remains on the underside of the brachioradialis until it reaches the mid-portion of the forearm and is not subject to compression in the radial tunnel.

Sites of Compression
The five structures in the radial tunnel that represent potential sites of compression may be recalled by a useful mnemonic *FREAS* (Figure 7.3-1). The structures, from proximal to distal, are Fibrous bands, Recurrent radial vessels (the leash of Henry), Extensor carpi radialis brevis, Arcade of Frohse, and Supinator (the distal border). The fibrous bands are anterior to the radial head at the beginning of the radial tunnel, and are the least likely cause of compression. The radial recurrent vessels cross the PIN to supply the adjacent brachioradialis and ECR muscles, and it is postulated that engorgement of these vessels with exercise may compress the nerve. The tendinous proximal margin of the ECRB also may compress the PIN, and may be mistakenly identified as the arcade of Frohse, which lies deep to the proximal margin of the ECRB muscle. The arcade of Frohse is the fibrous proximal border of the superficial portion of the supinator. It is the most common site of compression of the PIN, and is located from 3 to 5 cm below Hueter's line (Figure 7.3-2). Sometimes the tendinous margin of the ECRB and the arcade of Frohse may overlap and form a scissors-like pincer effect on the radial

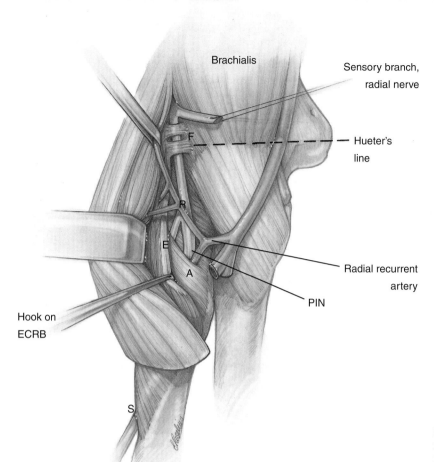

Brachialis

Sensory branch, radial nerve

F

Hueter's line

R

E

A

Hook on ECRB

PIN

Radial recurrent artery

S

Figure 7.3-1 Potential sites of compression of the radial nerve in radial tunnel syndrome (RTS). F, fibrous tissue bands; R, radial recurrent vessels; E, fibrous edge of ECRB; A, arcade of Frohse; S, supinator (see text).

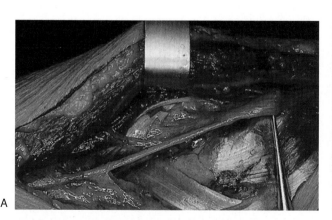

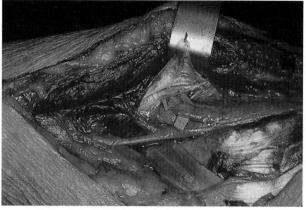

A   B

Figure 7.3-2 Fresh cadaver dissection of the ECRB and supinator. (A) The fibrous tissue edges of the ECRB and the supinator are in close proximity to the PIN as it enters the supinator. (B) The ECRB has been reflected superiorly. Fat has been removed from around the supinator to reveal its two heads and to reveal the fibrous tissue edge of the superficial head that forms the arcade of Frohse.

nerve in this area. It is appropriate to continue the exploration to the distal border of the supinator, although it is a rare site of compression. More often, a mass, such as a ganglion, may be found beneath the superficial portion of the supinator.

Diagnosis

Differential Diagnosis
- The radial tunnel syndrome (RTS) must be distinguished from PIN syndrome (PINS).
  - RTS is a subjective symptom complex without motor deficit, which involves a motor nerve. This is in contrast to PINS, which is an objective complex with motor deficit affecting a motor nerve.
  - The symptoms in RTS are similar to lateral epicondylitis, with complaints of pain over the lateral aspect of the elbow that sometimes radiates to the wrist. Because compression of a motor nerve is believed to cause the pain, the description of the pain as a deep ache is not surprising.
  - A dynamic state may exist in which pronation, elbow extension, and wrist flexion are combined with contraction of the wrist and finger extensors to produce compression of the PIN.

Physical Examination
- Physical findings may include point tenderness 5 cm distal to the lateral epicondyle.
- The absence of sensory or motor disturbances in RTS is characteristic.
- To a limited extent, provocative tests may give some indication of the anatomic location of the compression, but are not always reliable.
- The so-called middle finger test involves extension of the middle finger with the elbow in extension and the wrist in neutral. The test is considered to be positive if pain is produced in the region of the proximal portion of the ECRB. Sanders has modified this test as follows:
  - With the elbow in full extension, the forearm in full pronation, and the wrist held in flexion by the examiner, the patient is asked to actively extend the long and ring fingers against resistance.
  - According to Sanders, these positional modifications produce maximum compression on the PIN, and represent a more reliable form of the test.
  - If symptoms are reproduced with the elbow in full flexion, the forearm in supination, and the wrist in neutral, then fibrous bands are suspected.
  - Reproduction of symptoms by passive pronation of the forearm—with the elbow in 45 to 90 degrees of flexion and the wrist in full flexion—indicates entrapment by the ECRB.
  - Compression at the arcade of Frohse is suspected if the symptoms are reproduced by isometric supination of the forearm in the fully pronated position.
- The most reliable test is the injection of 2 to 3 mL of 1% lidocaine without epinephrine into the radial tunnel. Relief of pain and a PIN palsy confirms the diagnosis.
- A prior injection into the lateral epicondylar region that did not relieve pain also supports the diagnosis.

- Electrodiagnostic studies to date have not been useful in the diagnosis because there are no motor deficits, and studies of conduction velocity through the radial tunnel are unreliable.

Treatment
- Treatment may be nonoperative, in the form of rest to the extremity and avoidance of the activities that aggravate the condition.
- The judicious injection of steroids about the site or sites of possible compression may result in some relief.
- Surgical intervention is in the form of release of all possible points of compression of the nerve.

Posterior Interosseus Nerve Syndrome

In contrast to RTS, PINS is characterized by objective motor signs of entrapment of the PIN manifested by weakness or complete palsy of the finger and thumb extensors. There usually is no history of antecedent trauma.

Diagnosis

Physical Examination
- In complete PINS, active extension of the wrist occurs with radial deviation owing to loss of the ECRB, whereas the more proximally innervated ECRL remains intact.
- There is associated loss of finger and thumb extension.
- Partial loss of function is more common, with lack of extension of one or more fingers or isolated loss of thumb extension.
- Sensation always is intact.

Diagnostic Tests
- In contrast to RTS, EMG is positive in the muscles innervated by the PIN.
- Computed tomography scans or magnetic resonance imaging may show a mass in the radial tunnel.

Treatment
The reader is referred to the sections on RTS, since the approaches and principles of decompression are very similar.

- The nerve should be explored from the arm to the distal aspect of the supinator, based upon the clinical findings and the findings at surgery.

Bowler's Thumb and Cherry Pitter's Thumb

Bowler's thumb is a neuroma in continuity of the ulnar digital nerve of the thumb. It results from external pressure from the margin of the thumb hole in a bowling ball. It usually involves the ulnar nerve, and is characterized by pain, paresthesias, and a tender mass on the ulnar aspect of the proximal phalanx of the thumb. A variation known as cherry pitter's thumb has been described by Viegas.

Treatment
- Both conditions may be treated by activity modification, and, in the case of bowler's thumb, by enlarging the thumb hole in the bowling ball.

SUGGESTED READING

Abrams R, Meunier M. Chapter 21. Carpal tunnel syndrome. In: Trumble, TE, ed. Hand surgery update 3, hand, elbow & shoulder. Rosemont, IL: American Society for Surgery of the Hand, 2003:299–312.

Cobb TK, Dalley BK, Posteraro RH, et al. Anatomy of the flexor retinaculum. J Hand Surg 1993;18:91–99.

Dellon AL, Chiu DTW. Chapter 22. Cubital and radial tunnel syndromes. In: Trumble, TE, ed. Hand surgery update 3, hand, elbow & shoulder. Rosemont, IL: American Society for Surgery of the Hand, 2003:313–323.

Dellon AL. Diagnosis and treatment of ulnar nerve compression of the elbow. Techniques in Hand and Upper Extremity Surgery 2000;4:127–136.

Dellon AL, Mackinnon SE. Radial sensory entrapment in the forearm. J Hand Surg 1986;11A:199–205.

Dobyns JH, O'Brien ET, Linscheid RL, et al. Bowler's thumb: diagnosis and treatment. A review of seventeen cases. J Bone Joint Surg 1972;54:751.

Doyle JR, Botte MJ. Elbow. In: Surgical anatomy of the hand and upper extremity. Philadelphia: Lippincott Williams & Williams, 2002:365–406.

Doyle JR, Botte MJ. Forearm. In: Surgical anatomy of the hand and upper extremity. Philadelphia: Lippincott Williams & Williams, 2002:407–485.

Doyle JR, Botte MJ. Palmar hand. In: Surgical anatomy of the hand and upper extremity. Philadelphia: Lippincott Williams & Williams, 2002:532–641.

Ehrlich W, Dellon AL, Mackinnon SE. Cheiralgia paresthetica (entrapment of the radial sensory nerve). J Hand Surg 1986;11:196–199.

Gelberman RH, Eaton R, Urbaniak JR. Peripheral nerve compression. J Bone Joint Surg 1993;75:1854–78.

Gross NS, Gelberman RH. The anatomy of the distal ulnar tunnel. Clin Orthop 1984;196:238–247.

Sanders WE. Letter. J Bone and Joint Surg 1992;309–310.

Szabo RM. Acute carpal tunnel syndrome. Hand Clinics 1998;14:419–429.

Szabo RM, Slater RR, Farver TB, et al. The value of diagnostic testing in CT syndrome. J Hand Surg 1999;24A:704–714.

Szalay EA, Rockwood CA Jr. The Holstein-Lewis fracture revisited. Orthop Trans 1983;7:516.

8 ANESTHESIA

CHARLES L. MCDOWELL
KEVIN CUNNINGHAM

Relief from pain delivered with a minimum of discomfort and a high degree of safety is a building block of patient reassurance and a hallmark of modern outpatient surgery. The methods to be described are effective and safe in emergency rooms, outpatient settings, as well as in more formalized operating theaters. Emphasis upon outpatient surgery has dramatically increased the desirability of effective regional and local anesthesia methods that can be used by operating surgeons and anesthesiologists. In many of the settings where surgery is performed today, there is not an anesthesiologist available—or even necessary. This is an additional stimulus to the operating surgeon to become proficient in the administration of local and regional anesthesia.

GUIDELINES

1. Determine the patient's allergy status to the drugs.
   - Despite the fact that genuine allergies to local anesthetics are exceedingly rare, if the patient describes an allergy to a local anesthetic, the surgeon should not use it, even if the history is inconclusive or vague.
     - If the patient is right, and a reaction occurs, the physical and legal consequences can be serious.
   - If a local anesthetic agent is necessary for medical or other reasons, the surgeon should consider using an alternative drug or skin testing.
   - Of the two types of local anesthetics, esters, being derived from para-aminobenzoic acid (PABA), are far more likely to produce an allergic reaction than amide-type agents are.
   - Symptoms of allergic reactions include itching, burning, tingling, hives, erythema, angioedema, dyspnea, chest discomfort, wheezing, coughing, sneezing, shock, and tachycardia.
   - Much more commonly, the patient will not have had a true allergic reaction to the local anesthetic, but rather symptoms associated with one of the following:
     - Inadvertent direct intravenous or arterial injection of the agent or a drug overdose. These symptoms can include convulsions, disordered speech, tachycardia, or bradycardia.
     - Reaction to local agents containing epinephrine (palpitations, severe anxiety, tachycardia).
     - A vasovagal reaction.
     - An anxiety-hyperventilation event.
   - One can choose another type and perform a skin test.
   - Otherwise, consult an anesthesiologist and proceed with another method.
2. Ensure the site of injection is sterile.
3. Do not inject directly into a wound. This increases the risk of implanting and spreading bacteria.
4. Inject more proximally to avoid multiple needle sticks and the resulting multiple punctures and patient discomfort.
   - Block a peripheral nerve well proximal to the site of surgery.
   - This will result in less needle sticks and a larger area of anesthesia.
5. Know the anatomy.
   - Knowing the location of peripheral nerves is necessary to accomplish a successful regional nerve block.
   - The sensory distribution of peripheral nerves is reasonably consistent.
   - Figure 8-1 represents the distribution of the three major peripheral nerves in the upper extremity.
   - It is important to know this anatomy so as to be able to perform a neurologic examination prior to inducing anesthesia for the purpose of making a proper diagnosis.
   - A patient's injury may have resulted in damage to a nerve, and that fact should be known before surgery so that one can select a proper treatment plan and choose the appropriate peripheral nerve, or nerves, to block.
6. Take care in choosing the needle bore and type.
   - One has to balance the issues of pain versus effectiveness and safety.
   - We tend to assume that needles of small diameter cause less pain. However, the disposable needles we use are so sharp that patients cannot tell the difference between one with a gauge of 25 or 22.
   - There are several advantages to using a larger-bore needle.

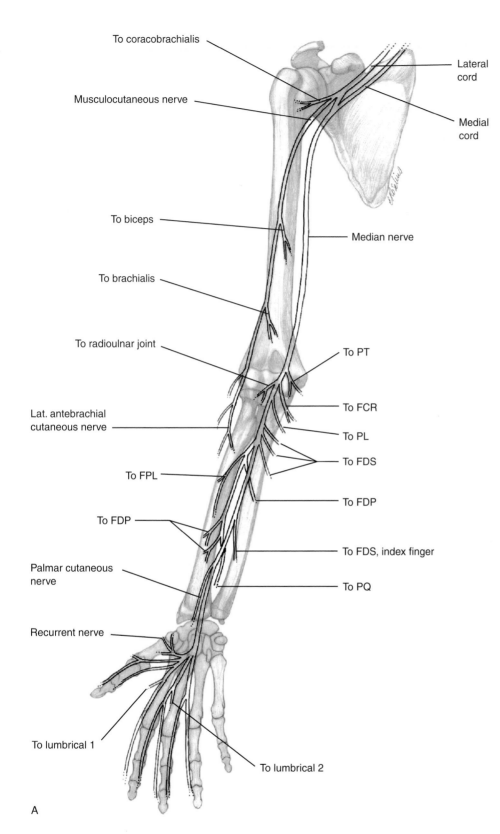

To coracobrachialis

Musculocutaneous nerve

Lateral cord

Medial cord

To biceps

Median nerve

To brachialis

To radioulnar joint

To PT

To FCR

Lat. antebrachial cutaneous nerve

To PL

To FDS

To FPL

To FDP

To FDP

To FDS, index finger

Palmar cutaneous nerve

To PQ

Recurrent nerve

To lumbrical 1

To lumbrical 2

A

Figure 8-1 The anatomy of the major nerves of the upper extremity, showing their sensory and motor components. (**A**) Median nerve. *Figure continues.*

- Increased stiffness of the needle allows the surgeon to direct it more effectively.
- There is less chance of breaking it or having to deal with retrieving a broken needle.
- One obtains useful information feedback from rate of flow.

☐ Because there is greater resistance to flow in a small-bore than in a large-bore needle, one has to push harder on the plunger.
☐ If the surgeon inadvertently places the needle into the substance of a tendon or ligament, it would be more difficult to push the plunger

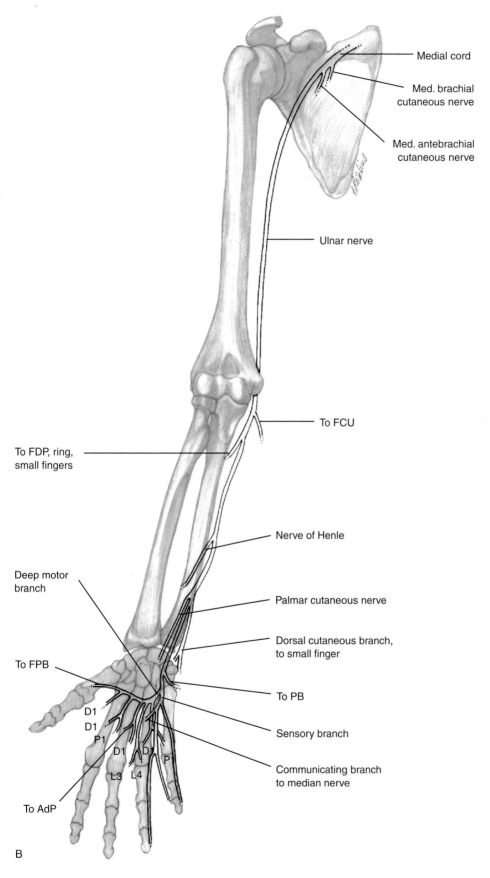

Medial cord

Med. brachial
cutaneous nerve

Med. antebrachial
cutaneous nerve

Ulnar nerve

To FCU

To FDP, ring,
small fingers

Nerve of Henle

Deep motor
branch

Palmar cutaneous nerve

Dorsal cutaneous branch,
to small finger

To FPB

To PB

D1
D1
P1
D1 D1 P1
L3 L4

Sensory branch

Communicating branch
to median nerve

To AdP

B

Figure 8-1 (*continued*) (**B**) Ulnar
nerve.

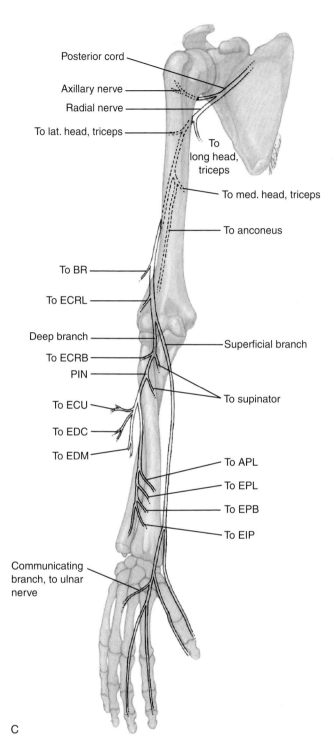

Posterior cord

Axillary nerve

Radial nerve

To lat. head, triceps

To long head, triceps

To med. head, triceps

To anconeus

To BR

To ECRL

Deep branch

To ECRB

PIN

To ECU

To EDC

To EDM

Superficial branch

To supinator

To APL

To EPL

To EPB

To EIP

Communicating branch, to ulnar nerve

C

Figure 8-1 (*continued*) (**C**) Radial nerve.

■ Smaller diameter needles will penetrate the substance of a peripheral nerve more easily than larger diameter needles.
  ☐ Axons will be damaged if a needle is inserted into the substance of a peripheral nerve.
  ☐ Also, the patient will usually have severe pain upon penetration.

When the surgeon and the patient both move violently because of pain or surprise, additional damage can be done to the nerve.

■ For all peripheral nerve blocks, one should use needles designated "blunt tip," when available.
  ▪ *This is especially important when doing infraclavicular and axillary blocks.*
  ▪ The angle of the bevel is 30 to 45 degrees instead of the usual "sharp tip" needles, which are beveled at 12 to 15 degrees.
  ▪ Using a blunt-tip needle further reduces the chance of penetrating the epineurium and injecting into the substance of the nerve.
  ▪ Experience has shown that the blunt-tip needle is more likely to push or roll the nerve out of the way, rather than perforating or impaling it.
  ▪ Injecting into the substance of a peripheral nerve may cause significant mechanical injury.

7. Inject the local anesthetic slowly and steadily.
  ■ Avoid fast and forceful injections, especially with larger volume blocks.
  ■ Remember, nerves can usually recover from mechanical trauma from needle contact, but needle insertion plus deposition of local anesthetic injected under high pressure can significantly damage nerve fascicle architecture and compromise its microvasculature, *with devastating permanent results.*
  ■ Always inject smaller volumes of local anesthetic (3 to 5 mL) at a time, with intermittent aspiration to rule out a direct intravascular injection.
  ■ When aspirating on a syringe for blood, some smaller veins may collapse, even with the tip of the needle in the lumen of the vessel.
  ■ Patient response is the key to diagnosis of intravascular injection of local anesthetic agent.
  ■ Never inject local anesthetic when high resistance to the injection is encountered.
    ▪ Withdraw the needle, reassess surface landmarks, reinsert the needle, and try again.
    ▪ Painful paresthesias and resistance to injection strongly suggest an intraneural injection.

8. Do not inject into a vein or artery.
  ■ Many peripheral nerves are in close association with veins and arteries.
  ■ In some locations, such as the axillary sheath, the median nerve at the elbow, and the ulnar nerve at the wrist, the relationships are intimate.
  ■ The old and true admonition to withdraw the plunger of a syringe before injecting applies yet again.

9. Consider the time it takes for local or regional anesthesia to become effective, and use this period to further your relationship with the patient.

than if the needle had been placed in a space such as the ulnar bursa, which contains the median nerve.
  ☐ If the surgeon uses a small-bore needle, he or she may not be able to distinguish between being in a tendon or the space around a peripheral nerve.
  ☐ A large-bore needle will give the surgeon important information about the location of the end of the needle.

- Because anesthetic materials take a few minutes to become fully effective, there is a potential time gap in the operating room schedule.
  - Anesthesia should preferably be administered in an anteroom to the operating room.
  - Nurses in this setting can prepare the patient so that the surgeon can administer the anesthetic immediately after the preceding operation.
  - The anesthetic will be acting while the paperwork and room preparation is proceeding.
  - If one assumes a 20-minute turnover time, there will be adequate time for the anesthetic to become effective.
- This is an important time to establish a doctor-patient relationship in the surgical environment, before the patient is separated from the operating team by a wall of draping cloth.
  - Giving the anesthetic well before the operation gives the surgeon time to reassure the patient and to discuss the process.
  - When administering the anesthetic, the surgeon has time to chat, describe the process, and answer questions that all patients have.
  - The patient may remember the surgeon only in a white coat in an office. Often, patients will not even recognize the surgeon in a scrub suit.
  - Preoperative contact with the operating surgeon is in itself reassuring to patients, even though an anesthetic agent is being injected.
  - The patient will be reassured by knowing that anesthesia is complete before being rolled into the operating room.
  - If the surgeon has to administer additional injections after the patient has been blinded to the process by drapes and other items, the patient may lose confidence and become anxious.
  - Making the patient as comfortable as possible in the operating room can enhance the feeling of reassurance.
    - Keeping the environment warm and quiet is helpful.
    - A pillow for the head and behind the knees adds comfort.
    - The arm board should be placed so that the arm is not abducted more than perpendicular to the trunk, in order to reduce shoulder stiffness or pain.
10. Confirm that anesthesia is accomplished by using light touch.
    - Pinching or sticking skin merely produces more pain and unnecessary anxiety in the patient.
    - If the patient feels light touch, the anesthetic is not adequate. If the patient does not feel light touch, anesthesia is complete.
    - This method must be used in children, or the additional pain or threat thereof will bar any possibility of cooperation. Adults appreciate the same consideration.
    - The examiner has to be careful to not stimulate a proprioceptive response from the patient by moving skin or joints in an area not anesthetized. Many

patients will respond if they feel anything, including a proprioceptive sensation.
11. Remember that managing anesthesia for children is different from that for adults.
    - Children have minimal tolerance for pain and threatening surgeons. And one is wise to assume that they have food in their stomachs.
    - In many emergency situations, local anesthesia is the safest method for obtaining anesthesia for children, but successful administration requires the surgeon to be skilled at management of the psychological and technical issues.
    - In the more controlled operating room environment, anesthesiologists, equipment, and premedication are available. Adults appreciate efficient, minimally painful, and effective anesthesia, too.
12. Consider use of a pneumatic tourniquet when more distal blocks (wrist and digits) are used.
    - Most patients can tolerate a tourniquet without parenteral drugs for up to 20 minutes.
    - The pressure should not exceed 225 to 250 mm Hg.
    - If the systolic pressure is so high that bleeding occurs in spite of the tourniquet pressure set as described, one should probably not be doing surgery except in an emergency situation.
    - The tourniquet can be deflated and reinflated 5 to 10 minutes later if necessary, but one should carefully choose operations that can be performed with confidence within the 10 to 20 minute time limit.
    - Planning approaches, reviewing radiographs, and other such procedures should be done before inflating the tourniquet, and wound irrigation, bleeding control, and closure can be done after the tourniquet has been deflated.

COMMONLY AVAILABLE AGENTS AND THEIR USES

Lidocaine

Lidocaine (Xylocaine) without epinephrine produces rapid onset of anesthesia but is short acting. Using epinephrine can increase the time of effective anesthesia. The latter drug may produce some unpleasant side effects to deal with in an outpatient setting, including drowsiness, lightheadedness, and vertigo. If blood concentration continues to rise, one sees agitation and excitement, and then, seizures. Fortunately, these symptoms are not common, but one must be prepared. One complication reported from the use of epinephrine with local anesthetic agents when used for digital nerve blocks is ischemia of the digit caused by vasoconstriction of the digital arteries. Most of these unfortunate effects can be avoided by using mepivacaine, which has a longer effect without using epinephrine.

Mepivacaine

Mepivacaine (Polocaine/Carbocaine) is ideal for an outpatient setting. Its time of effectiveness is adequate for most upper extremity operations, and it doesn't act so long that it interferes with postoperative evaluation of pain symptoms. The safety record for this drug is excellent.

Marcaine

Marcaine (Bupivicaine) can produce anesthesia for up to 12 hours. During that time, the patient will be relieved of pain from the injury or operation. However, the surgeon will have placed the patient at risk. Consider, for example, if the operation were performed successfully and a dressing or cast applied after wound closure—and then the patient developed a compartment syndrome. By the time the patient and surgeon were aware that there was a problem, it would be too late to prevent necrosis of soft tissue. Surgeons depend on careful observations to warn of an impending compartment syndrome. Usually, the first warnings come from the patient who complains of inordinate pain. If that information is not available because of the anesthetic, the first indication that a problem exists will come too late to reverse the course of the injury. A better choice of agent is mepivacaine. It will provide adequate anesthesia for an operation and recovery up to 3 to 4 hours. Then the patient will be able to alert the surgeon if the pain is so severe that it cannot be adequately controlled by 30 to 60 mg of codeine, or its equivalent. There will be sufficient time to relieve pressure from the cast or dressing, or to do a fasciotomy if needed, to prevent soft tissue necrosis.

INDICATIONS AND OPERATIVE SITES

When the site or sites are in the same upper extremity, and if the sites to be operated upon are located within the digits or palm, a wrist block would suffice. However, the surgeon must be aware of the tourniquet time. An axillary or infraclavicular block is usually more comfortable for the patient, and provides better flexibility for the surgeon if the tourniquet time will extend beyond 10 to 20 minutes.

When the procedure requires an additional surgical site in addition to the operated extremity for skin, bone, vessel, or tendon graft material or distant skin flap, one could still use regional anesthesia if the patient and anesthesia services are prepared to use a general anesthetic when needed, or if the other site can be anesthetized with regional or local anesthesia. Otherwise, proceed with general anesthesia from the outset.

When one is doing a procedure where the patient's cooperation is required or useful, such as tenolysis of adhesions to tendons or tendon balancing, as in quadregia, a combination of regional anesthesia (wrist block) and sedation/pain relief to control tourniquet pain (ischemia) is used. This requires coordination with anesthesiology. The tourniquet time must be monitored so that the extremity is not paralyzed at the time one needs the patient to contract muscles. Paralysis occurs about 30 minutes after a tourniquet is applied. If the tourniquet is deflated for 5 minutes, patients can respond to commands to contract muscles. For example, if you were doing a tenolysis of a profundus tendon in a digital flexor sheath, you should ask the patient to slowly make a fist. If the regional anesthesia is adequate and

sufficient analgesia has been supplied by the anesthesiologist to block pain from the tourniquet, then the patient should be able to contract the muscles and move the tendon being tenolysed. The procedure described is exceptionally useful when orchestrated properly.

METHODS

Intravenous Regional Anesthesia

This method is mentioned here only to discourage its use. There are four reasons why the procedure should be abandoned. Any procedure that places the patient at unnecessary risk, places the surgeon in the disadvantageous position of restricting options unnecessarily, or favors the person giving the anesthesia over the patient and the surgeon, should not remain in use. The person administering the anesthetic is assured of rapid and easily obtained success, but if an error is made, it can be fatal to the patient. The surgeon cannot consider deflating the tourniquet to evaluate bleeding potential, or for any other reason, before the operation is completed, as anesthesia will be lost as soon as the tourniquet is deflated. Bleeding control, wound closure, and other end-of-operation procedures will have to be done with supplemental anesthetic injected locally, and with attendant discomfort and anxiety for the patient. These are sufficient reasons to discourage the use of intravenous regional anesthesia. Let's add a fourth and more important reason: there are other methods that are safer for the patient and can be performed quickly and easily if the surgeon takes the time to become proficient and efficient using them.

Supraclavicular Blocks of the Brachial Plexus

These should be performed only in an operating room environment because of the risk of pneumothorax (reported up to 6%)—and the resulting need for assistance, positive pressure breathing, and the possibility that a chest tube may have to be inserted. These methods can be used effectively for shoulder operations, as well as for upper extremity operations when experienced personnel and proper facilities are available.

Infraclavicular Blocks of the Brachial Plexus

Blockade of the brachial plexus at the level of the cords can be obtained by an infraclavicular approach.

Anatomy and Technique
- The length of the clavicle is palpated from its manubrial attachment to the coracoid process, and bisected in half.
- The axillary artery pulsation is palpated in the apex of the axilla.
- The surgeon stands on the patient's side opposite the side to be blocked, with the patient's head turned laterally away from that side, with his or her arm abducted 90 degrees at the shoulder, and with the forearm supine.
- The infraclavicular area is prepped and draped.
- A skin wheal is raised 2 to 3 cm below the inferior border of the midpoint of the clavicle.

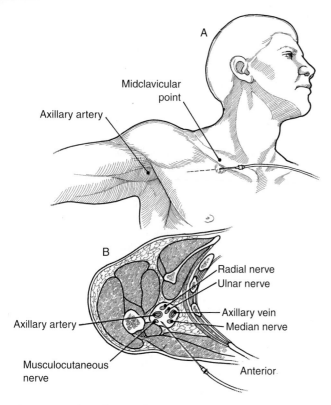

Figure 8-2 The technique of a brachial plexus block, by the infraclavicular approach.

- A nerve stimulator is used to more precisely localize the plexus, usually at a depth of 6 to 8 cm.
- A 10 cm insulated nerve-stimulating needle is then advanced through the skin wheal oriented laterally at a 45 degree angle. It enters tangentially, and away from the rib cage (to reduce the risk of a pneumothorax), and is inserted in the direction of the axillary artery pulsation (Figure 8-2).
  - Initial muscle twitches elicited will be from the pectoralis major/minor.
  - Once the needle has traversed the pectoralis muscles, stimulation of the brachial plexus cords will produce characteristic muscle contractions at the wrist, and will indicate entry of the needle into the sheath.
  - Stimulation of median nerve twitches in particular seems to yield consistently higher success rates.
- The surgeon stabilizes the needle, aspirates carefully for blood, and injects an appropriate volume and concentration of local anesthetic.

Preferred Agent and Volume
- Mepivacaine 1.25% to 1.5% (35 to 45 mL) will provide 3 to 4 hours of anesthesia.

Axillary Block

Axillary block can be undertaken either with or without electrical stimulation. Safety, effectiveness, and ease of performance make this the method of choice in an outpatient setting and in the emergency room. If electrical stimulation is not available, one should use the axillary approach instead of the infraclavicular approach. (Compare with other methods: simplicity, repeatability, effectiveness, risks, effect of obesity on the process, etc.) Also, the axillary approach to the brachial plexus can be used more safely than the supraclavicular and infraclavicular approaches in an outpatient setting.

- All effective proximal nerve blocks are produced by placing the anesthetic agent within the perivascular space (axillary sheath).
- It does not matter where one enters the space. If the volume is sufficient, the anesthetic agent will infiltrate to all four nerves in the sheath.
- The T2 nerve is not located within the axillary sheath. Since it supplies sensibility to the medial arm, one should consider placing a weal of anesthetic material transversely across the proximal arm on the medial surface to relieve pain that could be caused by tourniquet pressure.
- Confirmation of proper needle placement within the axillary sheath can be achieved by any of the following methods:
  - Eliciting paresthesias in the distribution of the median, ulnar, and radial nerves
  - Using a nerve stimulator
  - Dividing the neurovascular bundle into four quadrants, and depositing four aliquots of local anesthetic in each sector around the artery after "fascial clicks" have been obtained. Such clicks are the feedback resistance felt on perforating the axillary sheath, which is more noticeable if one uses a "blunt" needle.

Anatomy and Techniques
No matter which technique is used, one must always withdraw the plunger to be certain that there is no blood returning through the needle.

- The patient lies supine with the upper extremity abducted 90 degrees with or without elbow flexion.
- The axillary artery pulse is palpated as far proximal as possible in the apex of the axilla. Overzealous digital pressure, or having the patient rest the hand behind the head, can obscure the pulse.
- The axillary fold is prepped with Betadine or chlorhexidine solution, and the area is draped with sterile towels.
- The two-finger fixation technique (using the tips of the non-dominant index and long fingers) is used to identify the margins of the pulse, retract the overlying skin and soft tissue, and help immobilize the needle prior to and during the injection.
- A skin wheal is raised over the most prominent area of the axillary artery pulse.
- With the two fingertips gently applied over the pulse, a 22-gauge, 3-to-5-cm conventional needle connected to an intravenous extension set tubing (or alternatively, a 21-gauge butterfly needle with such tubing already attached) is advanced either perpendicular to, or at a more oblique angle with, the needle tip oriented toward the axilla. The needle should intentionally puncture the anterior wall of the axillary artery until bright red blood with a pulsatile pressure head can be seen entering the extension tubing or can be readily aspirated into the syringe.

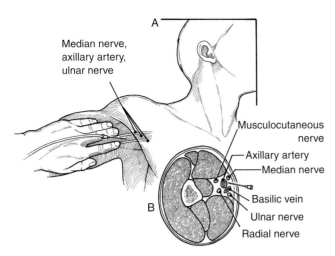

Median nerve,
axillary artery,
ulnar nerve

Musculocutaneous
nerve

Axillary artery

Median nerve

Basilic vein

Ulnar nerve

Radial nerve

Figure 8-3   Technique of a brachial plexus block, by the axillary approach.

- The needle is then slowly advanced 1 cm or more to deliberately puncture the posterior wall of the artery until no more blood flows into the tubing or syringe (Figure 8-3). The needle tip can then be assumed to be residing in the posterior part of the neurovascular sheath.
- Because the axillary sheath is believed to have discontinuous connective tissue septae that compartmentalize or impede the free diffusion of local anesthetic, one should inject half of the total dose of local anesthetic at this location. Do so after careful confirmation that the needle tip is not inside the axillary artery lumen.
- One slowly withdraws the needle through the artery while aspirating for blood into the syringe. The reappearance of blood in the tubing or syringe confirms that the needle tip is back in the lumen of the axillary artery.
- The surgeon continues withdrawing the needle until it exits the artery. At this location one should inject the remaining one-half of the dose of local anesthetic agent.
- After the needle is withdrawn completely, the patient's arm is adducted to the side, and continuous digital pressure is applied to the injection site to promote spread of the anesthetic agent.
- A *single needle* puncture into the axillary sheath often results in an adequate axillary block, but it is not as frequently effective as either the transarterial or the two-needle methods.
    - To use the single needle method, it is only necessary to place the needle into the axillary sheath and then inject 35 to 45 mL of mepivacaine slowly.
    - In the process of inserting the needle into the sheath, one may inadvertently puncture the axillary artery. In case this happens, merely adjust the technique to a transarterial method.
- When performing a *transarterial* axillary block, one deliberately pushes the needle toward the axillary artery, passes through it, and, after withdrawing the plunger to be certain that the tip of the needle is not in either artery or vein, injects the sheath as described above.
    - This method yields a high degree of success. Experience with it suggests that there are not often compli-

cations unless one injects the agent into the artery. If this happens, seizures and other complications can occur.
- A technique that is preferred to either of the above is the *two-needle* method. It is especially useful in urgent and outpatient settings where there may not be expert help available to help deal with the complications from other techniques. The advantage of the two-needle method is that one can avoid the need to search for landmarks after the first injection, which would hide and distort the anatomy because of tissue inflation.
    - A short 22-gauge blunt-tip needle is attached to a syringe to use as a handle, and, for aspiration, to be sure that the needle tip is not in a vessel.
    - The two needles are directed into the axillary sheath, one above and one below the artery. A "click" is often felt when penetrating the axillary sheath.
    - The axillary artery is superficial and should be identified as far proximal in the axilla as possible. This is the best site for injection. All four major nerves are located within the axillary sheath at this level. Recall from our previous discussion that there is a need for a block of T2 nerve root.

Preferred Agent and Volume
- 1% or 1.5% mepivacaine (Polocaine/Carbocaine), 30 to 40 mL.
- When injecting, one can apply digital pressure distal to the site of injection to force more of the fluid into the proximal portion of the perivascular space.
- It takes about 20 to 30 minutes for the anesthetic to become effective, so one should arrange to use the time efficiently.
- If the anesthesia department is planning to perform the block, the patient should be sent for in plenty of time for the anesthesiologist to prepare for and perform the block.
- If the surgeon is doing the block, he should do it immediately following the proceeding case, and then do other paper work, surgical preparations, and other things afterward.

Expected Outcome
A successful outcome will produce complete anesthesia in the upper extremity high enough to prevent pain from a tourniquet. It will also give the surgeon the flexibility to inflate and deflate the tourniquet as needed, do surgery for 2 to 3 hours, and still have sufficient pain relief to last for an additional hour after surgery. Complications from infraclavicular and axillary blocks are rare and are related to intravascular injection of the anesthetic agent.

Blocking Major Nerves in the Arm

There are very few indications for blocking only one or two major nerves in the *arm*. It would be a rare event that would call for such blocks to be used instead of an axillary or other more proximal block. The median and radial nerves in the arm and forearm are deep within the tissue, and lack easily identifiable landmarks. Multiple punctures and an electrical

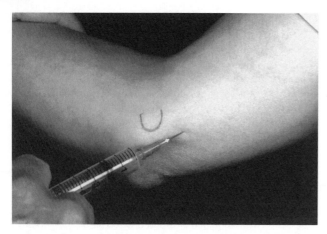

Figure 8-4   Ulnar nerve block at the elbow. The mark on the skin is over the medial epicondyle.

stimulator would be needed to be successful. It is more comfortable for the patient if the axillary block method is used. Also, the success rate is higher.

- The ulnar nerve proximal to the medial epicondyle of the elbow is an exception because it is accessible. In this situation, the nerve is easily palpated just proximal to the medial epicondyle.
- Inserting the needle about 2 to 3 cm proximal to the medial epicondyle and parallel to the nerve, and injecting the agent along side of the nerve at this site, will block it successfully.
- One should not inject posterior to the epicondyle because the nerve is often fixed in the cubital tunnel. Injecting into the cubital tunnel increases the risk that the needle might penetrate the substance of the nerve and cause permanent damage. Also, the hydraulic pressure that is produced by injecting into the partially closed space of the cubital tunnel may cause permanent damage to the ulnar nerve by acute severe compression.

Anatomy and Techniques

The anesthetic agent is injected proximal to the cubital tunnel, and the needle tip is located adjacent to the easily palpated ulnar nerve at this site (Figure 8-4).

Preferred Agent and Volume

- Mepivacaine, 1%, 5 to 7 mL.

Wrist Block

One may wish to use a tourniquet on the arm to control bleeding during a procedure on the hand when some type of peripheral block has been performed. It is possible for the surgeon to inflate a tourniquet to 25 to 50 mm Hg above systolic pressure for about 20 minutes. If more time is required, one will have to deflate the tourniquet, wait about 5 minutes to restore comfort, and begin again. This can be repeated, but the surgeon is likely to push the patient beyond his or her tolerance of pain caused by ischemia. One should reserve this method for operations that can be

performed safely within the 20-minute time limit. The surgeon should not let overconfidence dictate his choice to use this method. If one anticipates that more than 20 minutes will be required to perform an operation with care within the time limit, an axillary block should be undertaken instead. It is a very unhappy scene in the operating room when the surgeon is trying to complete an operation while the patient is complaining of pain, moving around on the table, and threatening to get off the table and leave.

Technique

- The first step is to raise a subcutaneous wheal across the flexor surface of the distal forearm about 2 cm proximal to the wrist flexion crease (Figure 8-5A).
- At this location, the anesthetic material will block the last branch of the lateral antibrachial cutaneous nerve and the palmar sensory branch of the median nerve, producing a numb area for the subsequent injection to block the median and ulnar nerves.
- A second wheal should be raised over the radial styloid to block the sensory branches of the radial nerve (Figure 8-5B).
- One can return to the volar site and inject through the first wheal to block the median and ulnar nerves.
- The median nerve block is accomplished by inserting a 22-gauge needle tip at a location 1.5 to 2 cm proximal to the wrist flexion crease and 1 cm ulnar to the palmaris longus.
- The needle tip is inserted perpendicular to the skin about 1.5 cm and is located within the ulnar bursa. Thus, the median nerve is bathed by the agent and not put at risk of perforation (Figure 8-5C).
- About 5 to 7 mL of mepivacaine is injected.
- The ulnar nerve is blocked by inserting the needle at the same distance proximal to the wrist flexion crease as the median nerve block.
- The insertion should be at the radial edge of the flexor carpi ulnaris (FCU) tendon, to a depth of about 1.5 cm (Figure 8-5D).
- Aspiration is especially important before injecting the agent because the ulnar artery and veins are very close to the nerve.
- About 5 to 7 mL of mepivacaine will be sufficient.
- A complete wrist block using this method will ensue within about 20 minutes.
- A wrist block will, of course, paralyze all of the intrinsic muscles. There may be occasions when preserving function of the small muscles is useful, as in reconstructive operations on the extensor hood mechanism.
    - In such cases, digital blocks and use of an arm tourniquet for a short time will be a better choice.
    - Also, one can coordinate the anesthetic with anesthesiologist as mentioned above, so that the tourniquet can be kept in place for longer than 20 minutes.

Preferred Agent and Volume

- Five to 7 mL of 1% mepivacaine is used at the median and ulnar nerve sites, and 3 to 4 mL is administered in a weal raised over the radial sensory nerve and the dorsal sensory nerve from the ulnar nerve (Figure 8-5B and E).

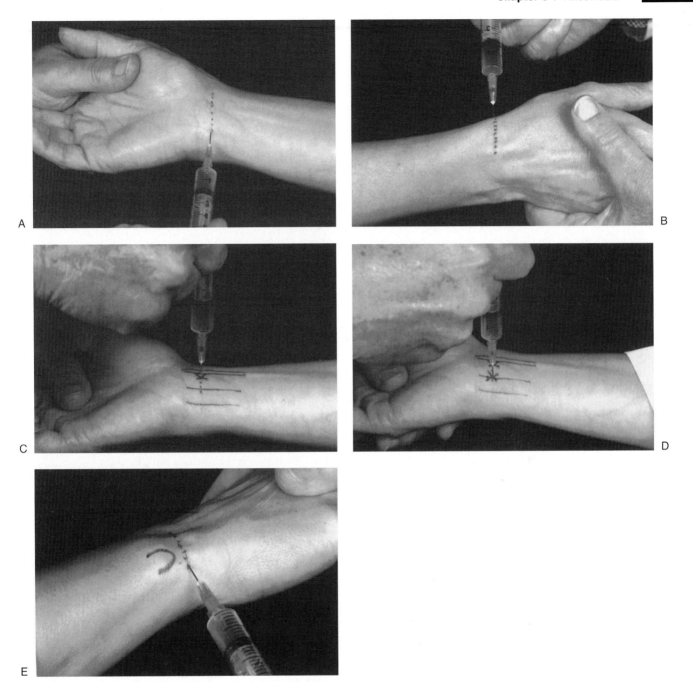

Figure 8-5   Wrist block. (**A**) A wheal is raised to block the sensory branch of the median nerve and produce a numb area for subsequent injection of the median and ulnar nerves. (**B**) Technique to block the sensory branch of the radial nerve. (**C**) Block of the median nerve (**X**). (**D**) Block of ulnar nerve (second **X**). (**E**) Block of the dorsal sensory branch of the ulnar nerve (⊃ mark on skin indicates distal ulna). See text for details of injection techniques.

Expected Outcome

The wrist block described will anesthetize all of the hand except for a small quarter-size area at the base of the thumb on the volar side of the thenar eminence supplied by the branches of the lateral antebrachial cutaneous nerve. A weal placed proximal to this site just proximal to the wrist flexion crease will complete the block if needed. The purpose of this subcutaneous injection of 3 to 5 mL is to block the branches of the medial antebrachial cutaneous nerves and the sensory branch of the median nerve that supply sensation to the base of the thumb and palm, and to anesthetize the sites of injection for the median and ulnar nerve blocks. Some examples of operations that lend themselves to this type of anesthesia are carpal tunnel release and trigger finger release. Longer operations where patient cooperation is necessary, such as tenolysis in digits and palm, should be performed using a wrist block, with sedation and pain control by anesthesia, so that the tourniquet can be used as

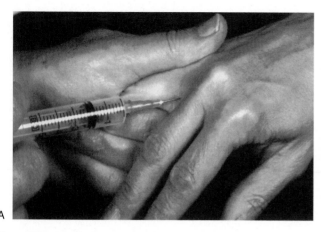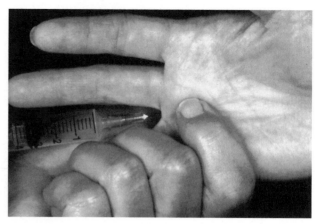

A   B

Figure 8-6 (**A**) Technique for finger nerve block. (**B**) Palmar view of the finger nerve block, showing technique for palpating the flow of the anesthetic material into the web space and lumbrical canal.

needed and the patient can move the tendons undergoing tenolysis at the surgeon's request.

Finger Nerve Blocks

Web space injections are easy to perform, and give a wide area of anesthesia. This approach avoids "circumferential" digital block, with its implied risk of arterial spasm and necrosis of the digit. *Epinephrine is not used in any type of finger or thumb nerve block because of its potential for vasoconstriction and circulatory compromise.* Polocaine/Carbocaine may be injected with a 22-gauge needle.

Technique

■ Assuming the person administering the anesthetic is right handed, he or she should grasp the finger or fingers on the left side of the web space to be injected, place the pulp of his or her index finger in the patient's palm between the metacarpal heads (over the lumbrical canal), insert the 22-gauge needle parallel to the metacarpals and into the lumbrical canal, and inject about 3 mL of Polocaine/Carbocaine into the lumbrical canal (Figure 8-6A).
■ With the index finger, the surgeon should feel the lumbrical canal inflate (Figure 8-6B), confirming that the agent is in the correct space volar to the transverse metacarpal ligament.
■ The next web space is injected in the same manner.
■ Thus, there is a block of both digital nerves to the digit, as well as numbness on the contiguous sides of the adjacent digits. This reduces the sensory feedback that the patient has to tolerate.
■ Additional anesthesia to the digit is produced by raising a weal transversely across the base of the digit about 1 cm proximal to the MCP joint as described elsewhere.
■ The radial digital nerve to the index finger is also superficial enough to be easily palpated over the first lumbrical muscle belly.
■ Two or 3 mL of anesthetic agent placed in a transversely

oriented wheal located about 1 to 2 cm proximal to the metacarpal head will accomplish the block.
■ The situation is a bit different in the case of the ulnar digital nerve to the little finger, as it is under fat resting upon the short flexor muscles of the hypothenar group.
  ■ One cannot palpate the nerve, so the injection should be done from the ulnar side of the palm with the needle directed volar to the hypothenar muscles and into the fat between the muscles and the skin.
  ■ Two to 3 mL of anesthetic agent will produce a successful block.

Thumb Nerve Blocks

Technique

■ In the case of the thumb, the weal can be placed at the level of the mid shaft of the metacarpal or more proximal. This includes doing so at the wrist in order to completely block the radial sensory nerve at the level of the radial styloid.
■ The digital nerves to the thumb are so superficial that they are easily palpated beneath the skin on either side of the flexor pollicis longus.
■ Raising a weal transversely across the flexor surface of the thumb at or just proximal to the MCP joint flexion crease easily blocks them (Figure 8-7).

Preferred Agent and Volume

■ Three mL of mepivacaine is used at each site, and a weal is placed on the dorsum of the palm about 1 cm proximal to the metacarpal head.

Expected Outcome

A satisfactory digital block using mepivacaine will produce pain relief for about 3 hours. Some examples of operations that lend themselves to this type of anesthesia are any operation at or distal to the PIP joint (so there is space for a tourniquet at the base of the digit). A surgeon could use a

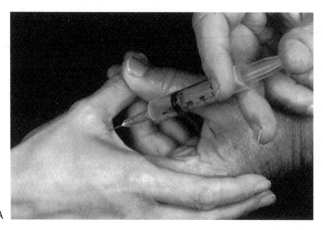
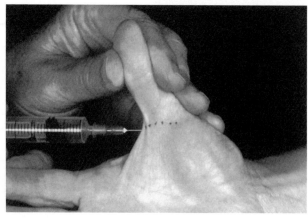

A   B

Figure 8-7   Technique for thumb nerve block. (**A**) Note the convenient and less painful site of injection for a digital nerve block of the thumb. (**B**) The digital nerves of the thumb are located in the subcutaneous tissue, and are easily anesthetized by injecting a wheal of anesthetic across the flexor surface of the thumb at the MCP joint flexion crease.

tourniquet applied more proximally if he or she was very confident that the procedure would take no longer than 20 minutes.

Use of Digital Tourniquets

Murphy's Law is always in force. Only those who either have not heard of the law or think they are above the law would use rubber bands for a temporary tourniquet for bleeding control during operation on a digit. The rest of us know that there is a considerable risk that we could put a dressing over the bands and forget them—and if this happens, when the anesthetic has worn off, the patient will complain of inordinate pain because the digit has been rendered necrotic by prolonged ischemia. We reduce our risk of this happening by using a wider Penrose drain clamped with a hemostat, which will remind us to remove it before applying a dressing. The hemostat is too large to fit inside of most dressings. There is a device being marketed that looks like a finger cot. The device will exsanguinate the digit as it is rolled into place on the digit and provide ischemia during the operation. It has the same inherent drawback that a rubber band has. It can be hidden by dressings, and is not recommended.

CONCLUSION

Both surgeon and patient gain confidence when anesthesia is appropriate, relatively painless, and complete. One must arrange the sequencing of care so that the process is efficient, unhurried, and sufficient time is allowed for the anesthetic agent to become effective.

SUGGESTED READING

Barash P, Cullen B, Stoelting R, eds. Clinical anesthesia. 5th Ed. Philadelphia: Lippincott Williams & Wilkins, 2005.

Hahn MB, McQuillan PM. Regional anesthesia, an atlas of anatomy and techniques. St. Louis: Mosby, 1996.

Kirby RR, et al., eds. Clinical anesthesia practice. 2nd Ed. Philadelphia: W.B. Saunders, 2002.

Miller RD, ed. Miller's anesthesia. 6th Ed. Philadelphia: Elsevier Churchill Livingstone, 2004.

Raj, PP. Pain medicine: a comprehensive review. St. Louis: Mosby, 1996.

Winnie, AP. Perivascular techniques of brachial plexus block. In: Plexus anesthesia. vol I. Philadelphia: W.B. Saunders, 1993.

HAND FRACTURES AND FRACTURE-DISLOCATIONS

This chapter will discuss the general principles of treating fractures of the phalanges and metacarpals and of treating fracture-dislocations in the hand. Fractures of the hand are relatively common, and are second in incidence to lacerations of the hand.

Treatment goals include restoring the bony anatomy, and leaving it with acceptable alignment, length, and rotation. Dislocations and ligament injuries in the hand are presented in Chapter 10.

GENERAL PRINCIPLES

Although restoration of the original anatomic configuration is the goal of treatment, it should not be obtained at the risk of soft-tissue scarring and joint stiffness, or at the risk of altering the blood supply to the bone. This may result in non-union.

Fractures in the hand are considered to be *stable* or *unstable*. Stable fractures may require minimal immobilization, whereas unstable fractures may require special immobilization techniques and or internal fixation. Unstable fractures of the metacarpal diaphysis most often angulate with the apex dorsal whereas fractures of the midaspect of the proximal phalanx angulate with the apex volar. The action of the wrist extensors that insert proximally extend the proximal portion of the metacarpal, and the interosseous muscles and the long-finger flexors flex the distal segment. Unstable fractures of the proximal phalanx are deformed by the extensor mechanism and the intrinsic muscles (Figure 9-1).

The classic fracture deformities described above are not representative of all fracture deformities that may be seen, but they do serve to introduce the concept that unstable fractures angulate and deform.

DIAGNOSIS

Patient History

■ The *history of injury* with a hand fracture is usually straightforward, but fractures associated with a laceration over the metacarpophalangeal (MCP) or proximal interphalangeal (PIP) joints should raise the question of a human bite wound that requires a different treatment approach.

■ To treat a human bite wound, refer to the section of Chapter 5 that deals with human bite wounds.

Physical Examination

■ Physical signs of fracture include swelling, tenderness, ecchymosis, skin abrasions, and deformity—including malrotation.

■ Fractures may be associated with collateral ligament injuries, tendon avulsion, and nerve or vascular injury. These structures should be evaluated by physical examination.

Radiologic Examination

■ Posterior-anterior, lateral, and oblique x-ray views are obtained, along with accurate lateral profile views of the phalanges.

■ Comparison views of the uninjured hand or digit are obtained as needed.

TREATMENT

Closed Treatment

■ Closed treatment and external forms of immobilization are best used in *stable* rather than *unstable* fractures.

■ Stability is defined in this context as the maintenance of reduction following manipulation and external immobilization.

This concept is amplified by noting that a *transverse* fracture is intrinsically more stable than an *oblique* fracture.

Techniques of Closed Reduction

■ The following comments about closed reduction are most appropriately applied to stable fractures of the diaphysis of the middle and proximal phalanges, and the diaphysis

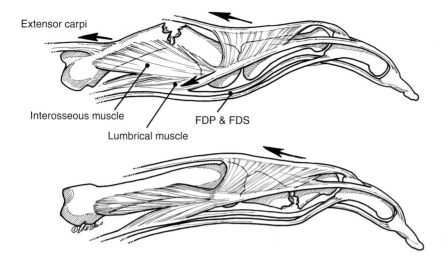

Extensor carpi

Interosseous muscle

Lumbrical muscle

FDP & FDS

Figure 9-1   Classic fracture deformity in unstable fractures of the metacarpals and phalanges (see text for details).

of the metacarpals. They apply to fractures that are stable (usually transverse fractures) and reducible.

■ Specific fractures of a more problematic nature that require operative intervention or special techniques will be discussed later.

Proximal and Middle Phalanges

■ Anesthesia prior to fracture reduction in the hand may be achieved by appropriate nerve blocks. Refer to Chapter 8.

■ Following suitable anesthesia, longitudinal traction is performed, followed by correction of the deformity.

■ This axial traction may be aided by the use of finger traps, and the entire procedure is performed most comfortably for the patient and surgeon by having the patient lay supine with the elbow flexed to 90 degrees.

■ In digital fractures, the potentially deforming forces of the intrinsics are relaxed by flexion of the MCP joints.

■ Wrist extension facilitates flexion of the MCP joints *and* longitudinal traction of the finger or fingers.

■ After reduction, stability of the reduction is determined along with rotational alignment.

■ Rotational alignment is evaluated by "sighting" down the plane of the finger nails (from distal to proximal) to note the relative tilt of the nail plate of the injured finger in comparison to the adjacent fingers and using the uninjured hand for comparison as needed.

■ Rotation may also be checked by noting *absence* of "crossing over" of the digit during flexion, and by noting its normal parallel alignment with the adjacent fingers.

■ Post reduction radiographs are made in sufficient number and detail to verify and document the reduction.

■ Depending on the digits fractured, a radial or ulnar gutter splint is used to immobilize the injured digits.

■ The so-called *intrinsic plus* position is utilized with the wrist in extension, the MCP joints in 90 degrees of flexion, and the PIP joints in extension.

■ Ninety degrees of flexion at the MCP joints may not always be achieved. It has been noted that 60 degrees of flexion of the MCP joint may be adequate.

■ This position results in relaxation of the potential deforming force of the intrinsic muscles, and avoids contracture of the collateral ligaments of the MCP and PIP joints.

■ An alternative to the radial or ulnar gutter splint is to immobilize the wrist and hand in extension, and place the reduced digit on an outrigger splint with the MCP joint flexed to 90 degrees and the PIP joint in extension.

■ This method allows visual evaluation of the alignment; this may be confirmed as indicated by radiograph (Figure 9-2).

■ Protected motion of the fractured digit may begin at 3 to 4 weeks after reduction, with continued splinting as needed and based on the experience of the surgeon.

■ In selected patients, some minimally displaced, stable, and suitably aligned fractures of the proximal and middle phalanges may be treated by strapping the injured digit to an adjacent finger and allowing early protected motion.

■ Appropriate x-ray views should be obtained 1 week or less after reduction, and weekly or biweekly thereafter based on the fracture and the experience of the surgeon.

Metacarpal Fractures

■ The same comments about patient positioning and anesthesia apply as noted for phalangeal fractures.

■ The wrist is extended, and longitudinal traction achieved by grasping the flexed proximal phalanx as a lever for distal traction and aligning and rotating the distal segment of the metacarpal.

■ A "cobra" splint or cast may be used to immobilize these fractures with the wrist in extension and the MCP joints flexed 80 to 90 degrees (Figure 9-3).

■ The PIP joints are left free for flexion; if malrotation is a potential problem, the injured digit may be taped to an adjacent uninjured digit.

■ Splinting may be performed for 3 to 4 weeks based upon the nature of the fracture and the experience of the surgeon.

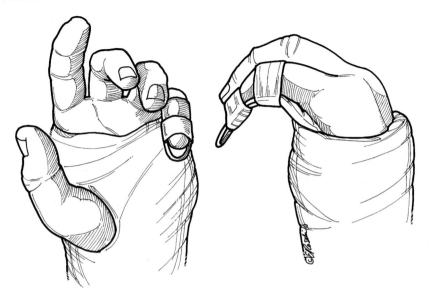

Figure 9-2   Artist's depiction of a Bohler-type outrigger splint used for postreduction immobilization of fractures of the proximal and middle phalanges.

Early Motion in Hand Fractures

- Fractures that are secondary to high-energy trauma, such as crush injuries or those associated with joint injuries, are more likely to develop residual stiffness and loss of function.
- Early mobilization and measures to reduce edema (elevation of the injured part) may be useful adjuncts to avoid this complication.
  - Think of edema and swelling as internal glue that is associated with stiffness.
- True elevation of the hand requires it to be 30 cm or higher than the level of the heart. This is best achieved by lying down and elevating the hand on some form of support.
- Maintaining the hand in an arm sling (although better than letting the hand hang at the side) is *not* elevation.

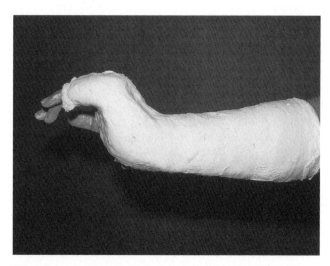

Figure 9-3   An example of a "cobra cast" used to immobilize a fracture of the metacarpal. The carefully padded cast is molded to the contours of the hand and the position of the wrist and MCP joints neutralize the deforming force of the interosseous muscles.

- Early motion is believed to lessen harmful adhesions of the soft tissues, including the extensor and flexor tendon systems and joint capsules.
- Early motion along with proper joint positioning may lessen these complications.
- Some surgeons have noted that immobilization of fingers beyond 4 weeks will lead to long-term stiffness due to tendon adhesions and joint contracture.
  - Thus, fractures treated with closed reduction and splinting are usually mobilized after 3 to 4 weeks, even in the absence of osseous union by radiograph.
- Stability of the fracture at this stage is due to fibrous union that most often proceeds to osseous union.
- In general, only splint the joints that are absolutely needed, in order to allow early motion of uninjured joints.
- The PIP joint does not need to be immobilized in fractures of the distal phalanx or distal interphalangeal (DIP) joint.

Open Treatment

- The indication for closed versus open reduction may depend on many factors, including the special needs of the patient and the experience and preferences of the surgeon.
- Fractures with articular step-off, open fractures (especially in those with bone loss and significant soft-tissue injury), fractures with significant shortening or bone loss, and fractures that fail closed reduction are indications for surgical treatment.
- Other surgical indications include multiple fractures, fractures that are intrinsically unstable, fractures with rotational malalignment as seen in spiral and oblique fractures, and fractures associated with joint subluxation or dislocation.
- Internal fixation should be achieved with minimal soft-tissue disruption in order to limit scarring and disruption of the blood supply of the fractured bone.
- Ideally, the fixation should be rigid enough to allow immediate active motion.

- If this is not possible, protected motion should begin as soon as possible based upon the nature of the fracture and the surgeon's experience.
- Surgical intervention may be associated with stiffness unless early mobilization is used.
- Minimum surgical dissection will favor recovery of motion.
- Many fractures that require reduction and fixation can be treated with percutaneous fixation techniques.
- Phalangeal fractures treated with plates and screws (most likely because of wider surgical dissection) have a higher incidence of stiffness.
- Percutaneous fixation can be performed with Kirschner wires.
- Screws may be placed in selected cases through limited incisions.
- Oblique fractures are prone to rotational malalignment, and stabilization is achieved by compression screws or 0.045-inch Kirschner wires placed perpendicular to the fracture line.
- The fixation devices are positioned to avoid compromise to the tendons, so that early motion is not compromised.
- Figure 9-4 demonstrates an unstable spiral-oblique fracture of the proximal phalanx fixed with two mini-screws.
- The fracture was exposed through a longitudinal incision in the extensor tendon, which gave excellent exposure; this stable construct allowed protected motion early.
- The aftercare and supervised rehabilitation program is very important to achieve maximum recovery and function.
- Dynamic external fixation methods have been developed for treatment of difficult articular fractures, especially about the PIP joint.
- These methods are technically challenging but may be used based on the surgeon's experience and preference.
- Operating room fluoroscopy units are useful aids in reduction and placement of fixation devices.

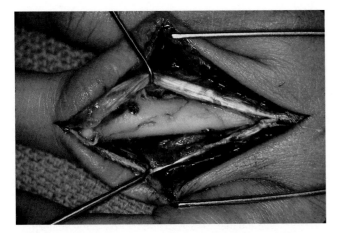

Figure 9-4 An unstable, spiral-oblique fracture of the proximal phalanx exposed through an extensor tendon splitting approach and fixed with two mini screws.

- Arthroscopic evaluation of joint surfaces has allowed some surgeons to more accurately reduce and fix certain intra-articular fractures.

Some Caveats about Kirschner Wires
- Kirschner wires should be placed with understanding that they will be removed at some point in the future.
- They may be cut off beneath the skin, or left protruding from the skin for ease of removal.
- Infection may be avoided by keeping the exit sites of the K-wires clean and dry.
- Inappropriately placed K-wires may damage vital structures such as nerve, blood vessel, or tendon.
- They should be placed so that *soft-tissue gliding* may occur during rehabilitation, without any impingement or compromise to the soft tissues.
- K-wires that cross joints may *break,* and their broken ends may erode and damage articular cartilage.
  - When broken in this manner they are difficult to remove without causing additional joint damage.
- *Transarticular K-wires should be protected with a splint or cast until their timely removal.*
- Making a right-angle bend on the exposed end of the K-wire and cutting it off about 2 to 3 mm beyond the bend may prevent excessive migration. In some instances, this facilitates removal.
- Threaded K-wires are prone to "wrap-up" adjacent soft tissues; for that reason, smooth wires are preferred.

Specific Fractures of the Phalanges and Metacarpals

DISTAL PHALANX
Fractures of the Tuft
- Fractures of the distal phalanx are the most common hand fracture.
- Tuft fractures are usually due to a crush injury, and are often associated with a subungual hematoma and sometimes a nail bed laceration.
- Initial treatment consists of drainage of the subungual hematoma, if present.
- In patients with a disrupted nail and significant laceration or disruption of the nail bed, consider repairing the underlying nail bed with fine absorbable sutures.
- If a suitable nail plate is present, it may be replaced as a biologic stent.
- Splinting of the DIP joint for 2 to 3 weeks may protect the soft-tissue injury and give symptomatic relief for the fracture. Nonunion of one or more fracture fragments is common, and requires no particular treatment.

Fractures of the Shaft
- Fractures of the diaphysis may be transverse or longitudinal.

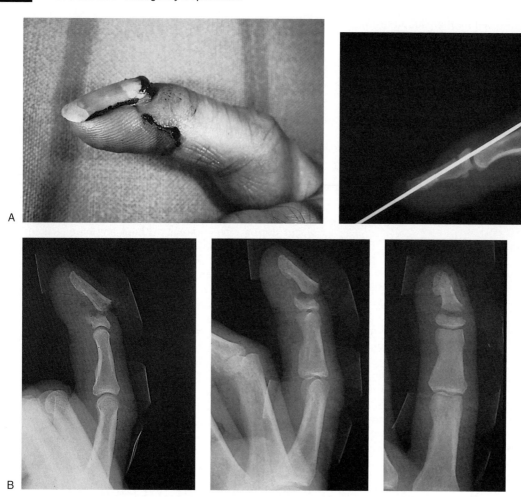

Figure 9-5   Clinical and x-ray appearance of a displaced fracture of the proximal metaphysis of the distal phalanx with K-wire fixation. **A.** Note the displaced fingernail. **B.** Radiographs showing displacement of the fracture. **C.** Longitudinal K-wire fixation.

■ Most are minimally displaced and respond well to 2 to 3 weeks of DIP joint splinting. Fractures from high-energy injuries may damage the germinal matrix.

Fractures of the Proximal Metaphysis

■ These injuries often displace the proximal nail from its bed, and the nail should be anatomically reduced and held in place with sutures. A transfracture K-wire may be used to stabilize the fracture, and is often more advantageous in maintaining the reduction (Figure 9-5).

Fractures of the Base of the Distal Phalanx

■ Three types of these fractures exist. See Table 9-1.

Type I
■ The extensor mechanism is attached to the basal epiphysis, and closed reduction of the fracture results in correction of the deformity.
■ Continuous external splinting of the distal joint in full extension for 3 to 4 weeks results in union of the fracture and correction of the deformity.

Type II
■ This fracture is not to be confused with the more common small bone fragment associated with a tendon avulsion and mallet-finger deformity that is treated as a soft-tissue injury.
■ Operative treatment has been recommended for fracture fragments involving more than one-third of the articular surface.

TABLE 9-1 TYPES OF FRACTURES OF THE BASE OF THE DISTAL PHALANX

Type	Description
I.	*Transepiphyseal fracture* as seen in children.
II.	*Hyperflexion injury* that usually results in a fracture of the articular surface that involves 20–50% of the articular surface (the so-called mallet fracture).
III.	*Hyperextension injury* with fracture of the articular surface that usually involves >50% of the articular surface and is sometimes associated with late volar subluxation of the distal phalanx.

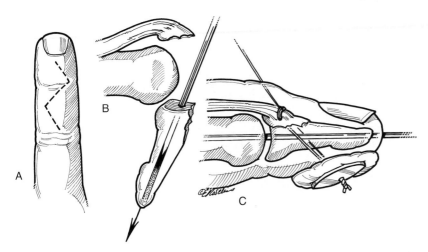

Figure 9-6 Artist's depiction of a method to reduce and fix a mallet fracture. **A.** A zigzag dorsal incision is used to expose the fracture. **B.** A 0.035-inch, double-ended K-wire is drilled longitudinally through the distal phalanx. **C.** The joint is reduced, the K-wire is driven proximally across the joint, and the fracture fragment is reduced. If the fracture fragment cannot be maintained in position, a loop of 4-0 wire is passed through the fragment and distal phalanx and is tied over a padded button. Intraoperative radiographs are made to determine anatomic reduction. The transarticular K-wire is protected with a splint for 6 weeks. The pullout wire may be removed in 3 or 4 weeks.

- An accurate reduction is advocated to prevent joint deformity with secondary arthritis and stiffness.
- This fracture may be treated as depicted in Figure 9-6.
- The reader should note that this is a technically challenging operation, and not all surgeons recommend its use.
- Many surgeons advise closed splinting for this injury.
- Operative repair of a mallet fracture is a technically difficult operation.
- Attempted fixation of the fracture fragment by K-wire or wire loop may result in comminution of the fragment and loss of attachment of the extensor mechanism.

Type III
- Figure 9-7 shows a radiograph of a type III hyperextension injury.
- Treatment for this fracture is the same as for type II fractures.
- Both type I and II injuries have been treated successfully by closed means, and the reader is advised to note the following caveats regarding this fracture.

Caveats
- Wehbe and Schneider recommended nonoperative treatment by extension splinting of all mallet fractures, including the hyperextension type with *subluxation* of the distal phalanx.

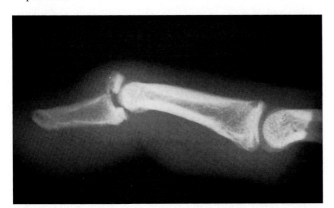

Figure 9-7 Lateral x-ray view of a type III mallet finger fracture (see text for details).

- They believe that restoring joint congruity does not influence the end result, because remodeling of the articular surface is reported to lead to a near-normal painless joint in spite of persistent joint subluxation.
- A further caveat about hyperextension mallet fractures with volar subluxation is that splinting of the deformity in *hyperextension* at the DIP joint should be avoided to prevent volar subluxation of the distal phalanx.

MIDDLE PHALANX

Nondisplaced and Extra-Articular Fractures
- Most nondisplaced extra-articular fractures can be treated with buddy taping for 3 to 4 weeks.
- Spiral fractures or others with potential for instability may be splinted for 3 to 4 weeks, with timely follow-up including radiographs.
- If displacement occurs, the fractures should be treated as noted for unstable displaced fractures (see discussion that follows).

Displaced and Articular Fractures
- Displaced fractures should be considered to be intrinsically unstable, and even when anatomically reduced they may redisplace. This is especially true in oblique or comminuted fractures.

Dorsal Fracture Subluxation of the PIP Joint
- This fracture involves the volar aspect of the articular surface of the base of the middle phalanx, and is one of the most disabling injuries to the finger.
- Diagnosis and treatment are often delayed.
- Figure 9-8 demonstrates the x-ray appearance of such an injury.
- These *comminuted* and *unstable* fractures may be treated by some form of *dynamic traction* that maintains reduction and allows simultaneous movement of the injured joint.
- Another treatment option is that of *dorsal block splinting*, in which the PIP joint is reduced and held in the degree

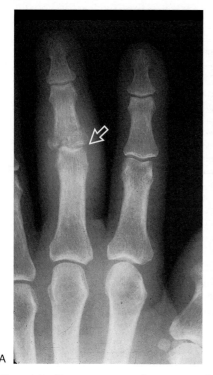 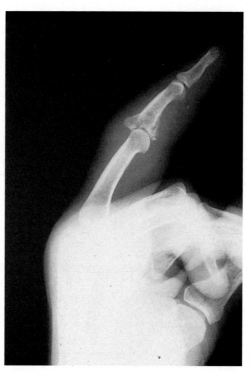

A   B

Figure 9-8   X-ray appearance of a comminuted and displaced fracture subluxation of the base of the middle phalanx.

of flexion that results in and maintains a concentric reduction.

- Active flexion of the joint is performed and the dorsal blocking splint gradually extended over a 4 to 5 week period.
- When seen late, these injuries may be salvaged by a volar plate arthroplasty.
- An example of a similar injury in the proximal phalanx of the thumb demonstrates the use of balanced dynamic traction to treat such an injury (Figure 9-9).
  - This method requires careful monitoring and balancing of the forces involved.
- Some surgeons may elect to treat this injury by a thumb spica cast or splint, and others may choose an open reduction and fixation with K-wires, plates and/or screws.
- These first two examples are contrasted to an unstable fracture-dislocation of the PIP joint with a relative *large and non-comminuted fragment* that can be reduced and fixed.
- Such an anatomic reduction is stable and with early protected motion, an excellent outcome may be anticipated (Figure 9-10).

PROXIMAL PHALANX

Peri-Articular Fractures

At the PIP Joint

- Fractures that involve the articular surface of the proximal phalanx at the PIP joint are intrinsically unstable. If they are not reduced and internally stabilized, deformity and arthrosis will result.

- Figure 9-11 demonstrates a neglected oblique fracture of the proximal phalanx that healed with an *articular offset* and subsequent deformity. A realignment osteotomy corrected the deformity.

At the MCP Joint

- Fractures of the articular surface of the proximal phalanx at the MCP joint are best treated by internal fixation followed by protected early motion. Figure 9-12 demonstrates such a case.

Diaphyseal Fractures of the Proximal Phalanx

- Injuries at this level are prone to angulate with the apex volar due to the action of the intrinsic muscles and extensor mechanism.
- Treatment by closed means, or internal fixation with K-wires or screws, is based on the anticipated stability of the fracture and the preferences of the surgeon.
- Reduction of phalangeal fractures is performed by flexing the MCP joint to relax the intrinsic muscles, followed by axial traction, digital pressure, and accentuation of the deformity to disengage the fracture fragments as needed.

METACARPAL

Fractures of the Neck

- These injuries are relatively common, and most often involve the little finger metacarpal.
- They often occur from punching various things with a tightly clenched fist, and the eponym *boxer's fracture* is often used to describe these injuries.

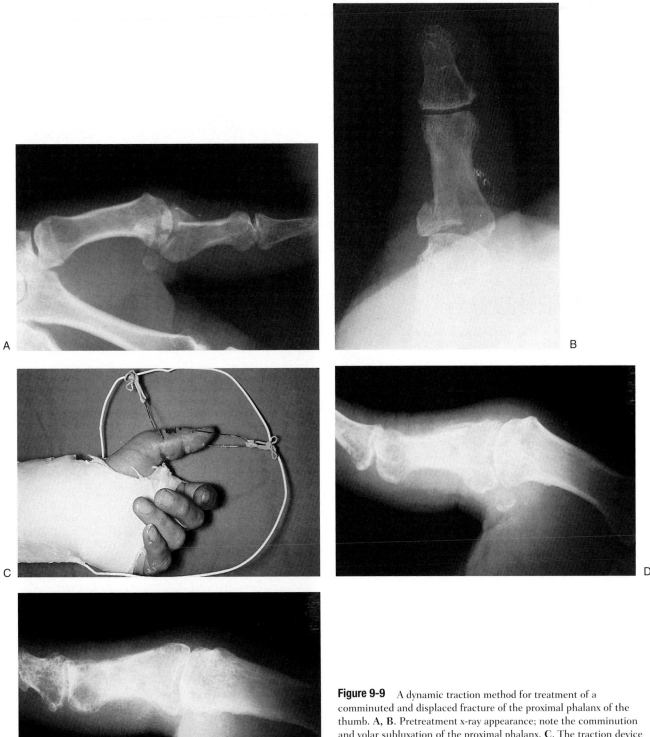

Figure 9-9 A dynamic traction method for treatment of a comminuted and displaced fracture of the proximal phalanx of the thumb. **A, B.** Pretreatment x-ray appearance; note the comminution and volar subluxation of the proximal phalanx. **C.** The traction device in place demonstrating a "dorsal lifting" K-wire in the base of the proximal phalanx, and a longitudinal traction K-wire in the distal phalanx. Traction was achieved by rubber bands between the outrigger device and the K-wires. The device was left in place for 6 weeks. (**D–E**) The x-ray appearance of the fracture at 3 months.

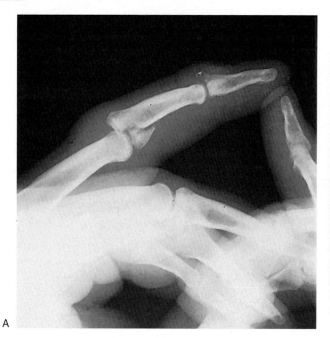
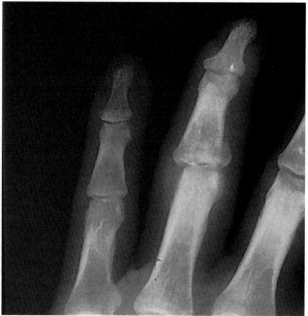

A   B

Figure 9-10 A noncomminuted but *unstable* volar lip fracture-dislocation of the base of the proximal phalanx that is amenable to fixation.

- Some surgeons consider all of these fractures as *stable* and *impacted* ones that are not easily reduced.
- Patients do not always present in a timely fashion, and if seen even after 7 to 10 days, these fractures may be impossible to move even under appropriate anesthesia and vigorous manipulation.
- The most controversial aspect of these injuries is determining which require treatment.
- The basis of treatment for surgeons who treat these more aggressively is determined by the degree of angulation of the fracture as noted on a radiograph. The published acceptable ranges of deformity vary with the finger involved.
  - The little finger appears to tolerate a flexion deformity at the metacarpal neck better than the other fingers due to its hypermobility.
  - Thirty degrees of flexion seems to have no appreciable effect on function in biomechanical studies.
  - Some authors will allow up to 50 degrees of angulation, while others allow up to 70 degrees.
- It has been argued that laborers and athletes that grip bats or racquets may be candidates for more aggressive management.
- Treatment of these fractures is based on the surgeon's experience and the perceived needs of the patient. Most single-bone fractures are treated by closed reduction and some level of immobilization.
- Figure 9-13 demonstrates a useful technique for reduction.
  - It is performed by using the cup or proximal articular surface of the proximal phalanx as a "pusher" to reduce the volar flexed aspect of the head and neck of the metacarpal.

- Multiple displaced fractures may indicate more aggressive treatment.
- In single bone fractures, two parallel percutaneous pins that pass through the reduced distal aspect of the fracture into the adjacent metacarpal keep the fracture in alignment, are minimally invasive, and are easily removed.
- Figure 9-14 shows a patient with significant displacement of fractures of the neck of the metacarpals of the little and ring fingers.
  - Some surgeons would suggest that open reduction and internal fixation is indicated.
  - Closed reduction would no doubt be difficult, if not impossible.

Fractures of the Diaphysis

- Although the ring and little fingers may tolerate up to 40 degrees of angulation of a fractured metacarpal shaft due to carpometacarpal (CMC) motion at the hamate articulation, this amount of angulation leaves a prominent bump on the back of the hand—which most patients find unacceptable.
- Angulation beyond acceptable tolerances requires reduction and some form of fixation or immobilization based upon the patient's needs and the surgeon's preferences.
- Current thinking about the acceptable amount of shortening in metacarpal fractures is said to have decreased from 1 cm to less than 5 mm.
- Extensor lag associated with shortening of the metacarpal may be accommodated by MCP hyperextension in the absence of musculotendinous shortening.
- Although some shortening is acceptable, *rotation* is not.

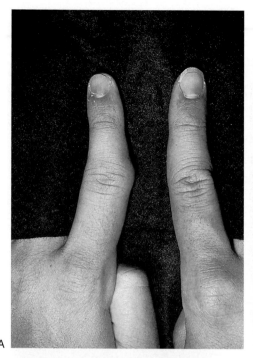

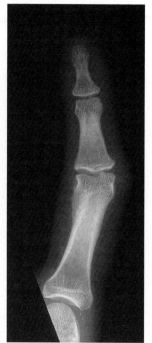

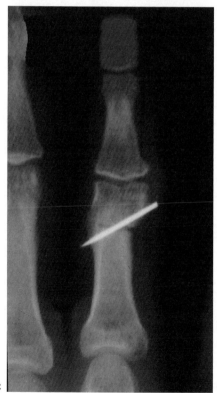

Figure 9-11   A neglected oblique fracture of the articular surface of the neck of the proximal phalanx. **A, B.** Note the clinical and x-ray deformity. **C.** Realignment was obtained by osteotomy.

■ Figure 9-15 demonstrates the clinical appearance of a malrotated index finger following an open reduction and internal fixation.

■ *Caveat*: It does not take much rotation or malalignment at the fracture site to yield a malrotated finger.

■ Treatment of metacarpal shaft fractures may vary from a closed reduction, a well-applied cobra cast (see Figure 9-3), and a careful follow-up including radiographs,

to various forms of fixation, including K-wires, screws, screws and plates, and external fixation devices.

■ Minimum profile plates may be used in certain cases. Figure 9-16 shows such a plate in place.

■ Soft-tissue dissection should be kept to a minimum, and although such techniques allow early protected motion, they should be used in carefully selected patients.

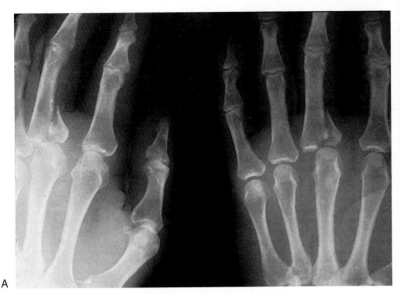

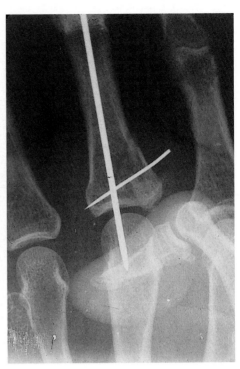

A   B

Figure 9-12   An unstable fracture at the base of the proximal phalanx. **A.** Note the displaced and slightly comminuted fracture at the base of the proximal phalanx. **B.** A single K-wire was used to fix the fragment to the phalanx, and a longitudinal K-wire was used to stabilize the joint. The longitudinal K-wire was removed at 3 weeks, and protected motion was started by strapping the middle finger to the index finger.

- Compression screws placed at right angles to oblique fractures may also be used.
- K-wires may be used in selected cases, either in crossed or parallel configuration.
- Bi-cortical passage of the K-wires promotes better fixation and prevent rotation.
- Stabilization of metacarpal fractures with external fixators, as well as transversely oriented K-wires from an intact metacarpal to one with a fracture or bone loss defect, may be especially useful when severe soft-tissue injuries are present.

Fracture of the Finger Metacarpal Base

- Injuries to the finger metacarpal base most often involve the ring and little fingers.
- They are often associated with fractures of the adjacent carpal bones.
- These fractures may be missed on routine radiographs, and the diagnosis may be aided by an oblique supination view.
- Open reduction and internal fixation is required to restore the normal alignment of the articular surfaces of the CMC joints.
- Figure 9-17 shows such an injury to the base of the little finger metacarpal and an associated fracture of the ring finger metacarpal.
  - Treatment was by open reduction and K-wire fixation of the CMC dislocation, with parallel K-wires across the ring finger metacarpal fracture.

THUMB METACARPAL

Fractures of the Diaphysis

- Fractures of the diaphysis are relatively uncommon, and fractures about the thumb metacarpal usually involve the base.
- The thumb has significant CMC motion, and dorsal angulation of fractures of the diaphysis of the metacarpal may be better tolerated than angulatory deformity in the fingers (especially the index and middle).

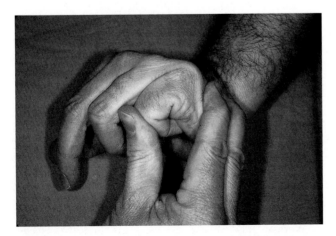

Figure 9-13   Closed reduction technique for boxer's fracture.

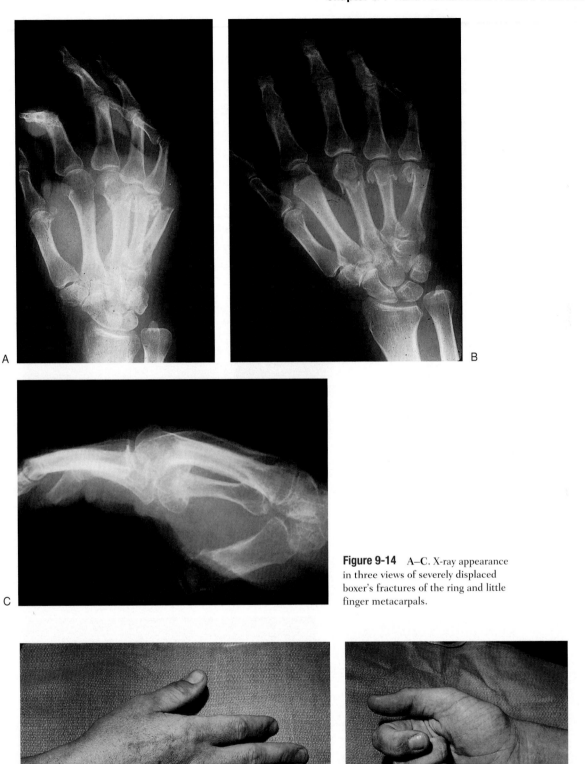

Figure 9-14 **A–C**. X-ray appearance in three views of severely displaced boxer's fractures of the ring and little finger metacarpals.

Figure 9-15 Malrotation deformity of an internally fixed index metacarpal fracture. **A**. Note the scar over the dorsal aspect of the index finger, and the subtle supination deformity seen in the index fingernail. **B**. The deformity is most pronounced during flexion. A corrective derotational osteotomy was performed.

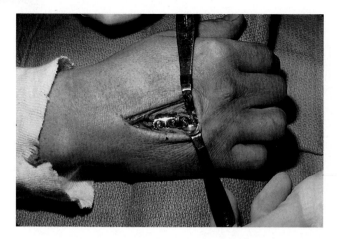

Figure 9-16   Intraoperative view of a miniplate and screws for treatment of a metacarpal fracture.

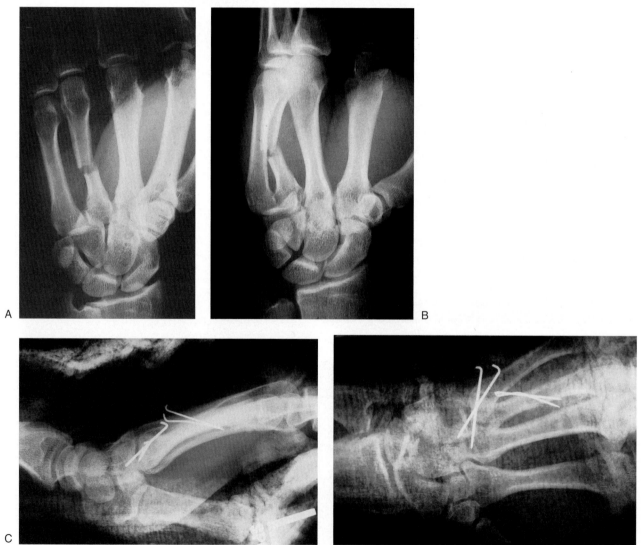

A

B

C

D

Figure 9-17   CMC joint dislocation of the little finger and fracture of the ring finger metacarpal. **A, B**. X-ray appearance of the injury. Note the CMC dorsal dislocation of the little finger metacarpal and fracture of the ring finger metacarpal. Note also that the oblique view is more revealing than the AP view. **C, D**. Postoperative appearance showing anatomic reduction and fixation with K-wires. Note the bent ends of the K-wires (see text).

- Although dorsal angulation of some degree may be functionally acceptable (some surgeons accept up to 30 degrees), it may not always be acceptable from the patient's perspective.
- Both closed and operative methods may be used for reduction and fixation of diaphyseal fractures, as previously described.
- The most suitable position for immobilization of the thumb is abduction and extension of the CMC joint, with minimal flexion of the MCP joint and extension of the IP joint.
- This position may be demonstrated on your own hand by noting the posture of the thumb when it lightly touches the tip of the semi-flexed index finger.

Fractures of the Base

- *Extra-articular* fractures of the base of the thumb metacarpal are treated like fractures of the diaphysis, and most can be managed by closed means.
- It is the *intra-articular* fractures—classified as Bennett's or Rolando's fractures—that are most problematic and challenging for the surgeon.

Bennett's Fracture

Pertinent Anatomy and Pathomechanics
- The volar projection of the base of the thumb metacarpal is firmly held to the adjacent trapezium by the superficial anterior oblique ligament (SOAL) and the deep anterior oblique ligament (DOAL).
  - The latter is also known as the "beak ligament."
- These ligaments firmly hold the volar projection of the thumb metacarpal in place, and in the presence of axial loading, a fracture occurs rather than a dislocation of the CMC joint.
- The resultant fracture is oblique and is displaced by the proximal and dorsal pull of the abductor pollicis longus (APL) tendon that inserts on the dorsal base of the thumb metacarpal.
- In addition, the adductor pollicis (AP) places a radially deforming force on the metacarpal.

Diagnosis
- This injury is most accurately diagnosed by a *true lateral* radiograph of the CMC joint.
- A true lateral is obtained by placing the radial border of the thumb flat on the x-ray plate with the wrist and forearm pronated 15 to 35 degrees.
- Placing the wrist and hand in this position naturally extends the wrist and hand. This position is maintained with a foam wedge placed under the ulnar border of the hand.
- The x-ray beam is centered over the CMC joint and directed at a 15-degree angle from distal to proximal.

Treatment
- An anatomical reduction and maintenance of that reduction is required.
- This is an *unstable fracture,* and it is highly unlikely that a closed reduction can be maintained by a cast or a splint.

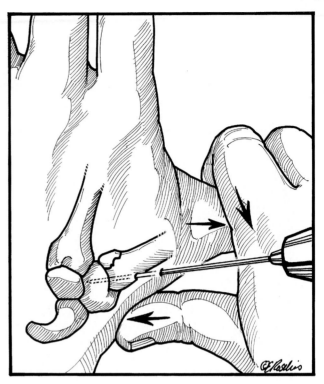

Figure 9-18   Technique for percutaneous fixation of a Bennett's fracture of the thumb (see text for details).

- Some surgeons, however, recommend closed reduction and casting provided a stable reduction can be maintained and provided there is less than 1 mm displacement or articular step-off.
- Maintenance of the reduction is best achieved by some form of fixation, either by closed percutaneous pinning or by open reduction and fixation.

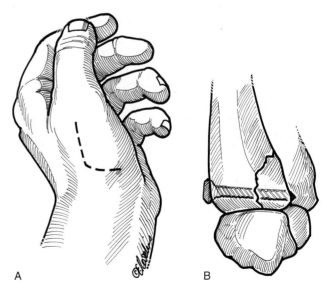

A   B

Figure 9-19   Technique for screw fixation of Bennett's fracture. **A.** The incision. **B.** Reduction and screw fixation.

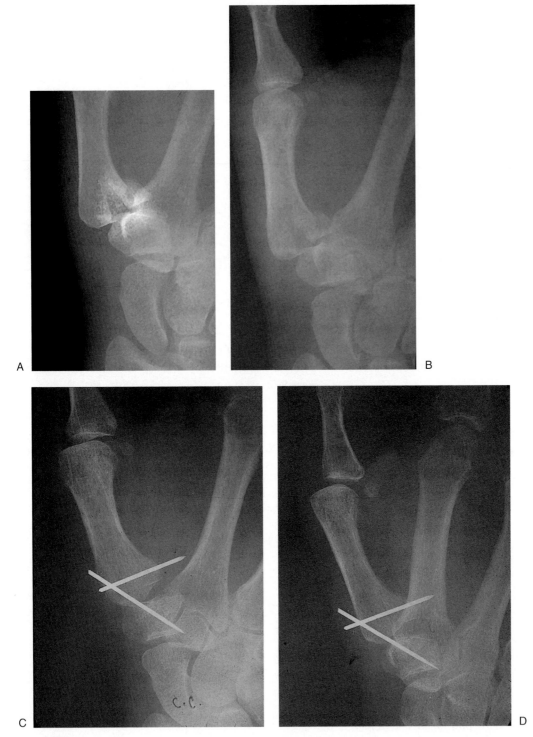

Figure 9-20   X-ray appearance of Bennett's fracture with K-wire fixation. **A, B**. Prereduction appearance. **C, D**. Note the anatomic reduction and K-wire fixation of the fracture fragment, and a second transarticular K-wire across the CMC joint. *Question to the reader: What would you have done differently in terms of the cut off ends of the K-wires? Answer: A 90-degree bend prior to cutting off the K-wires would have prevented migration of the ends of the pins beneath the dorsal cortex of the metacarpal and made pin removal at 6 weeks a less complex procedure.*

- Some surgeons base their decision for closed versus open methods based on the size of the volar lip (articular) fragment.
- If the fragment is less than 15% to 20% of the articular surface, closed reduction and percutaneous pinning is elected.
- If the articular fragment is greater than 25% to 30%, open reduction is performed.
- Management of this fracture by *percutaneous fixation* is performed by longitudinal traction on the thumb, simultaneous pressure over the dorsal aspect of the base of the thumb metacarpal, and pronation of the thumb followed by insertion of a transarticular K-wire across the dorsal base of the metacarpal into the trapezium (Figure 9-18).
  - This construct is protected by a secure cast or splint, the pin is removed at 5 weeks, and motion starts based on the clinical and x-ray findings.
- *Open reduction* is performed through a J-shaped incision that reflects the base of the thenar muscles away from the CMC joint.
  - This approach allows a profile view of the fracture and CMC joint.
  - The fracture fragment is reduced anatomically and fixed to the main body of the metacarpal by one or two K-wires or screws, based on the surgeon's choice and experience.
  - This construct is protected with a cast or splint, and motion is started based on the nature and stability of the fixation (Figure 9-19).
  - Figure 9-20 demonstrates the x-ray appearance of a Bennett's fracture and its reduction and fixation with K-wires.

Rolando's Fracture

- This fracture was originally described as a fracture of the base of the thumb metacarpal with a Y- or T-shaped *intra-articular* component.
- The term has now come to include any comminuted intra-articular fracture of the base of the thumb metacarpal.

Treatment

- In those fractures that meet Rolando's original description, treatment is by open reduction and internal fixation with K-wires, plates, and screws.
- In those more comminuted fractures, treatment techniques have included skeletal traction and mini-external fixators.
- The goals of treatment for these comminuted fractures is to maintain thumb length and as much congruity of the articular surface as possible.

SUGGESTED READING

Doyle JR, Botte MJ. Surgical anatomy of the hand and upper extremity. Philadelphia: Lippincott Williams & Wilkins, 2002.

Eaton RG, Malerich MW. Volar plate arthroplasty of the proximal interphalangeal joint: a review of thirty years experience. J Hand Surg 1980;5:260–268.

Glickel SZ, Barron OA, Eaton RG. Dislocations and ligament injuries in the digits. In: Green DP, Hotchkiss RN, Pederson WC, eds. Green's operative hand surgery. 4th Ed. New York: Churchill Livingstone, 1999:772–808.

Gutow AP, Slade JF, Mahoney JD. Phalangeal injuries. In Trumble T, ed. Hand surgery update 3, hand, elbow and shoulder. Rosemont, IL: American Society for Surgery of the Hand, 2003:1–27.

Markiewitz AD. Metacarpal fractures. In Trumble T, ed. Hand surgery update 3, hand, elbow and shoulder. Rosemont, IL: Amer. Soc Surg Hand, 2003:29–35.

Stern PJ: Fractures of the metacarpals and phalanges. In: Green DP, Hotchkiss RN, Pederson WC, eds. Green's operative hand surgery. 4th Ed. New York: Churchill Livingstone, 1999:711–771.

Wehbe MA, Schneider LH. Mallet fractures. J Bone Joint Surg 1984; 66A:658–669.

DISLOCATION AND LIGAMENT INJURIES

The ligaments of the hand, in conjunction with the configuration of the bone components of the joints, provide for stable yet mobile joints that allow the digits to perform precise movements. These stabilizing ligaments, however, are subject to stresses that sometimes exceed their tolerance. When this happens, they fail. The end result is loss of stability and function due to mechanical factors and pain. Timely recognition and appropriate treatment of these injuries is mandatory in the management of hand injuries. Certain patterns of injury have been identified, and the most common and clinically significant forms of ligament injuries based on their respective joints will be discussed. By definition, the discussion of ligament injuries in this chapter includes joint instability, subluxation, and dislocation. Dislocations may occur without *destabilizing injury or chronic instability* to the respective ligaments involved. However, it is mandatory that the examiner clearly distinguishes those dislocations and subluxations that will inevitably result in instability, and those that are intrinsically stable after reduction.

Our discussion in this chapter will be directed at ligament injuries rather than fracture dislocations. However, some ligament injuries may be associated with an avulsion-type fracture, but the main focus is on the ligament injury and not the fracture. Chapter 9, which focuses on fractures and fracture dislocations, discussed these injuries, and the reader may recognize that some arbitrary divisions have been made in these two chapters for the sake of convenience.

FINGER DISTAL INTERPHALANGEAL JOINT AND THUMB INTERPHALANGEAL JOINT

Incidence and Treatment

- Dislocations of the distal joints of the fingers and thumb are relatively uncommon.
  - The distal phalanx of these joints has a shorter lever arm, and additional stability is present due to the adjacent insertions of the flexor and extensor tendons.

- When dislocations do occur they are most likely to be dorsal or lateral and may be open due to the comparatively diminished skin coverage over this joint (Figure 10-1A).
- Reduction is achieved by longitudinal traction and manipulation of the base of the phalanx into its anatomical bed.
- As in all reductions, joint stability is evaluated by gentle passive and active motion.
- Postreduction radiographs are taken to verify the reduction.
- The joint is splinted in a few degrees of flexion, and motion may be started in 7 to 10 days (Figure 10-1B).
- These dislocations are usually reducible, and reported causes for failed reduction are interposed soft tissue, such as the palmar plate or the flexor tendon.
- Surgery is indicated for those dislocations that cannot be reduced.

PROXIMAL INTERPHALANGEAL JOINT

Pertinent Anatomy

In terms of bony architecture, the PIP joint may be likened to two coffee cups in their respective saucers that have been placed side-by-side, with both cups and saucers firmly attached together. This analogy serves to illustrate the fact that the bicondylar end of the proximal phalanx (the "coffee cups") articulates with a saucer-like component at the base of the middle phalanx, and thus has a certain element of stability or resistance against radial or ulnar deviation. Figure 10-2 depicts the anatomic arrangement of the PIP joint. Add to this fact that the radial and ulnar collateral ligaments are substantial cord-like structures that are firmly attached to the neck of the proximal phalanx and the base of the middle phalanx. It is not surprising to recognize that the majority of dislocations of the PIP joint occur in the dorsal (most common) or palmar plane. Additional stability is added to the PIP joint by the palmar plate and its proximal and distal attachments, and the accessory collateral ligament. Figure 10-3 depicts the soft tissue anatomy of the PIP joint.

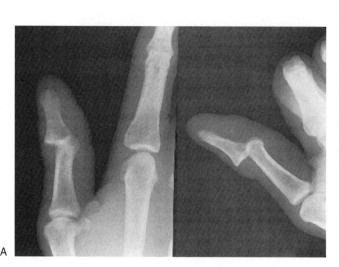

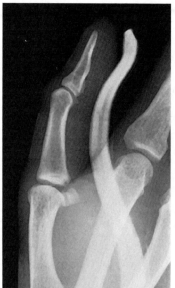

Figure 10-1   (**A**) X-ray appearance of a dorsal dislocation of the IP joint of the thumb. (**B**) X-ray appearance after reduction and splinting.

Dorsal Dislocation

Mechanism of Injury and Pathologic Anatomy

This injury is most commonly associated with a blow to the end of the digit that results in an obvious deformity. The attachments of the palmar plate are disrupted (usually distally). There are also longitudinal but *nondestabilizing tears* of the collateral ligaments in the zone between the proper (cord-like) and accessory (fan-like) region of the collateral ligament complex.

Diagnosis

■ These sports injuries are often reduced shortly after the injury by the patient, a teammate, or coach, and the patient usually presents to the examining physician with a swollen but reduced PIP joint.

■ Profile radiographs in the anterior-posterior (AP) and true lateral planes are obtained to note any fractures.

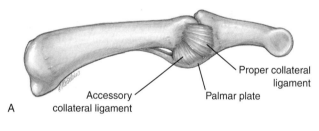

A

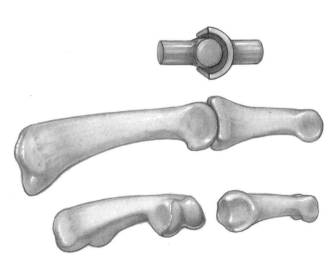

Figure 10-2   The bicondylar arrangement of the PIP joint accounts for its intrinsic bony stability.

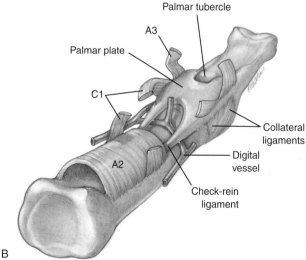

B

Figure 10-3   Artist's depiction of the arrangement of the palmar plate and its proximal and distal attachments, along with the proper and accessory collateral ligaments.

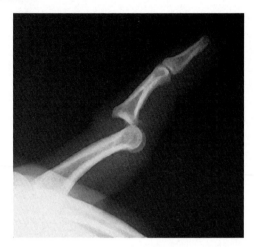

Figure 10-4 X-ray appearance of a dorsal PIP joint dislocation.

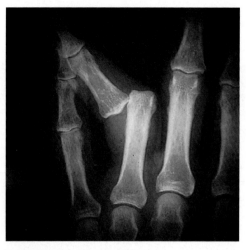

Figure 10-5 X-ray appearance of a lateral dislocation of the PIP joint.

- In the unreduced state, these radiographs most often reveal that the base of the middle phalanx is resting on the dorsal neck of the proximal phalanx (Figure 10-4).
- Sometimes a small fragment of bone is avulsed from the palmar base of the middle phalanx, which indicates that the plane of disruption was through the base of the middle phalanx rather than at the attachment of the palmar plate. This fragment remains attached to the palmar plate volarly.

Treatment
- Closed reduction of the dislocation is performed under digital block anesthesia, followed by longitudinal traction and "pushing" the base of the middle phalanx distally.
- After reduction, stability of the joint is determined by *active* and *passive* movements of the joint.
- Satisfactory active movement without redislocation or deformity indicates that sufficient soft tissue stability remains to allow early protected movement.
- Passive stability is confirmed by stress testing of the collateral ligaments with the PIP joint in full extension and at 30 degrees of flexion, and comparing this to an uninjured but otherwise comparable digit.
- Increased mobility in the AP plane is tested by gentle shear testing, by stabilizing the proximal phalanx and moving the middle phalanx.
- This injury is seldom associated with a *destabilizing* collateral ligament or other soft tissue injury, and the reduced digit may be "buddy taped" to an adjacent digit for protected exercise.
- A large fracture fragment noted on radiograph (usually 40% or more of the articular base of the middle phalanx) indicates a fracture-dislocation and represents a *destabilizing* injury. These injuries are often treated by open reduction and fixation, or other forms of stabilization.
- Instability results due to the fact that the majority, if not all, of the stabilizing collateral ligaments are attached to this fragment and no longer act as stabilizers to the middle phalanx. This topic is discussed in the chapter on *Fractures and Fracture–Dislocations.*

Lateral Dislocation

Mechanism of Injury and Pathologic Anatomy
A mechanism of injury is a direct lateral force on the PIP joint that exceeds the tolerance of the collateral ligament complex (Figure 10-5).

This injury is less common than dorsal PIP joint dislocation. It involves disruption of the origin or insertion of the collateral ligament, disruption of the interval between the proper collateral ligament and the accessory collateral ligament, and partial disruption of the palmar plate attachment.

Diagnosis
- Complete lateral dislocations are clinically apparent, but subluxations may not be as obvious because of swelling.
- Stress testing of the collateral ligament and accessory stabilizers is performed with the PIP joint in full extension.
  - An angular deformity of 20 degrees or more on the stress test is diagnostic of significant instability.

Treatment
- If stability is present with active and passive flexion, and extension of the PIP joint and radiographs demonstrate joint congruity, treatment is through protected motion by "buddy taping" the injured digit to an adjacent digit. Surgery is indicated for soft tissue interposition or a displaced fracture.

Palmar Dislocations

Three types of palmar PIP dislocation have been identified. All are rare.

Rotatory Palmar Subluxation

Mechanism of Injury and Pathologic Anatomy
This condition represents a longitudinal rent in the extensor mechanism between the lateral band and the central slip of the extensor tendon, which allows the head of the proximal phalanx to enter the separation and be trapped. The

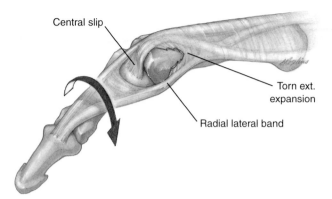

Figure 10-6 Rotatory subluxation of the proximal interphalangeal joint. This lesion occurs due to a longitudinal rent in the extensor mechanism between the lateral band and the central slip of the extensor tendon. This allows the head of the proximal phalanx to enter the separation and be trapped and rotated between the displaced lateral band and the central slip.

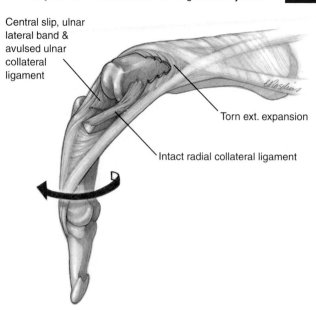

Figure 10-7 Irreducible rotatory palmar dislocation of the PIP joint. The clinical appearance is characterized by almost 90 degrees of flexion at the PIP joint, supination of the distal aspect of the finger, and inability to reduce the deformity.

displaced lateral band is trapped behind the palmar aspect of the condyle, resulting in a rotatory deformity of the middle and distal segment of the finger (Figure 10-6).

The mechanism of injury is due to a combination of forces, including rotation, flexion, and lateral deviation. The PIP joint is most susceptible to torsional force at 55 degrees of flexion, when the lateral bands shift palmar to the mid-axis of the proximal phalanx. Thus, the injury probably is sustained with the PIP joint in moderate flexion. The term subluxation seems appropriate because the PIP joint is not widely separated.

Diagnosis
■ The PIP joint is in moderate flexion, the middle and distal phalanges are rotated, and there is swelling about the PIP joint.
■ A true lateral radiograph of the proximal phalanx demonstrates partial separation of the PIP joint and obliquity of the middle phalanx due to the rotatory component of this injury.

Treatment
■ Although this condition has been reported to be irreducible, closed reduction under appropriate anesthesia may be attempted by simultaneous flexion of the metacarpophalangeal (MCP) and PIP joints to relax the lateral band, followed by gradual extension accompanied by rotation of the middle phalanx that is opposite to the deformity.
■ If this maneuver is not successful, open reduction is performed.

Irreducible Rotatory Palmar Dislocation

Mechanism of Injury and Pathologic Anatomy
This condition is the more complete or severe form of rotatory palmar subluxation.

Irreducibility is due to soft tissue interposition of the central slip, which, along with the ulnar lateral band, is displaced palmar to the neck of the proximal phalanx (Figure 10-7). Findings at surgery reveal the head of the proximal phalanx projecting through an oblique tear in the extensor expansion between the central slip and the radial lateral band. Findings also reveal the central slip and ulnar lateral band displaced to lie together in front of the neck of the proximal phalanx, where they act as a block to reduction. The UCL is avulsed and the RCL is intact. As in rotatory palmar subluxation, the mechanism of injury is a predominantly rotational force. A common cause of injury is a full-spin clothes dryer that catches a finger while it is still moving; the finger most often involved is the index.

Diagnosis
■ The clinical appearance is characterized by almost 90 degrees of flexion at the PIP joint, supination of the distal aspect of the finger, and inability to reduce the deformity.

Treatment
■ The PIP joint is exposed through a dorsal approach. Reduction is achieved by replacement of the displaced central slip and lateral band, followed by repair of the rent in the extensor mechanism.

Reducible Palmar Dislocation

Mechanism of Injury and Pathologic Anatomy
Based on clinical studies and cadaver experiments, the reducible type of palmar dislocation is associated with injury to one collateral ligament, the palmar plate, and the extensor mechanism (usually the central slip insertion of the extensor tendon). Although usually reducible, it is unstable because of loss of dorsal support from the central slip. More

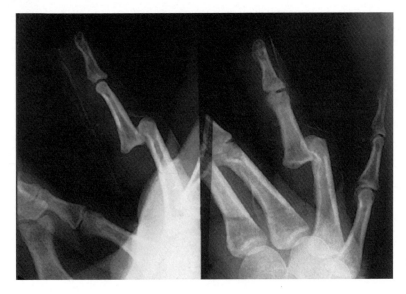

Figure 10-8 X-ray appearance of a palmar dislocation of the PIP joint.

importantly, if not recognized and treated properly, this results in a boutonniere deformity because of the central slip disruption. Unilateral injury to the collateral ligament results in a rotatory deformity because of the suspensory effect of the intact collateral ligament. The mechanism of injury is a varus or valgus stress followed by a palmar force that dislocates the middle phalanx palmarly. Cadaver experiments that used only an anterior force without varus or valgus force resulted in avulsion of the central slip, usually with a fracture fragment and a lesser incidence of collateral ligament rupture. Figure 10-8 depicts the x-ray appearance of reducible palmar dislocation.

Clinical Caveats

- If an anterior dislocation can be reduced, it is important to recognize that an injury to the central slip has occurred and requires appropriate treatment.
- It has been noted that palmar dislocations of the PIP joint always injured the extensor mechanism (most often a tear of the central slip), a collateral ligament, and the palmar plate.
- The associated ligament and tendon injury, if not treated, will result in loss of both static and dynamic PIP joint support, which is manifested by palmar subluxation, malrotation, boutonniere deformity, and fixed flexion contracture.
  - Figure 10-9 demonstrates the clinical and x-ray appearance of such a neglected case involving the PIP joint of the ring finger.
  - Although the joint was reduced and soft tissue reconstruction was performed, the end result was a stiff finger.
- Irreducible palmar dislocations are not usually associated with central slip disruption, and may have a more favorable prognosis.
- Inability to reduce an anterior dislocation is most likely due to interposition of a part of the extensor mechanism, which can be corrected by surgery.
- There are two forms or stages of progression in rotatory injuries.
  - The first, or stage I, is a subluxation injury; the second, or stage II, is an irreducible dislocation.
  - Closed reduction of stage I injuries may be attempted in acute cases.
  - In stage II or complete dislocations, closed reduction is not advised.

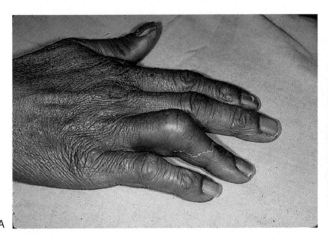

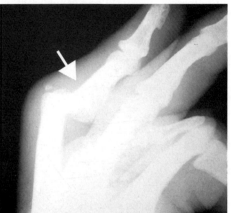

A   B

Figure 10-9 Clinical and x-ray appearance of a neglected palmar dislocation of the ring finger PIP joint.

FINGER METACARPOPHALANGEAL JOINT AND COLLATERAL LIGAMENTS

Pertinent Anatomy

In contrast to the PIP joint architecture, the MCP joints of the fingers may be described as a single coffee cup that is loosely placed in its saucer. The rounded coffee cup (the metacarpal head) sits in its flat saucer (the base of the proximal phalanx) and although the two joint surfaces are joined together, their shape and ligamentous constraints permit mutiplanar movements including flexion, extension, abduction, adduction, and limited pronation and supination (Figure 10-10). Like the PIP joints, they are supported by primary and accessory collateral ligaments. The MCP joint palmar plate is less rigidly fixed proximally, and although a type of checkrein ligament exists, it is less substantial than the one found at the PIP joint. This may explain the normal ability of the MCP joint to hyperextend, whereas the PIP joint is less prone to do so. One collateral ligament injury and two dislocations have been recognized at the MCP joint finger joints.

Finger Metacarpophalangeal Ligament Injuries

Mechanism of Injury and Pathologic Anatomy

The overall incidence of rupture of the collateral ligaments of the fingers is much lower than the incidence of rupture of

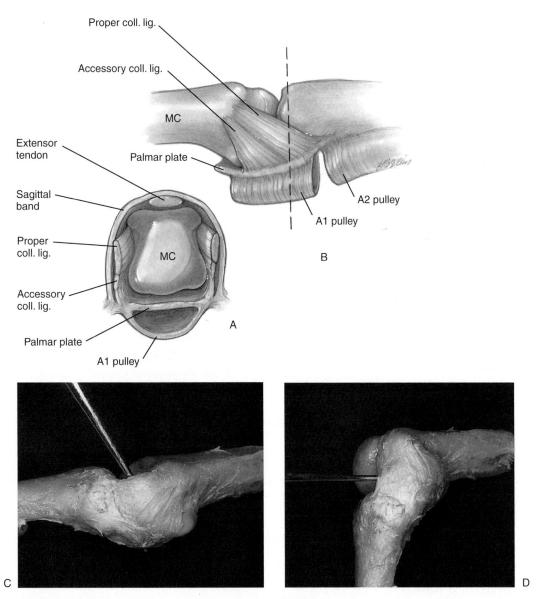

Figure 10-10 Anatomy of the finger MCP joint collateral ligaments. (**A**) A cross section of the MCP joint showing the various stabilizing structures of the joint. (**B**) Lateral view of the finger MCP joint. (**C**) Fresh cadaver dissection of the MCP collateral ligaments showing their comparatively relaxed tension in MCP joint extension. (**D**) Note the increased tension of the collateral ligaments in flexion.

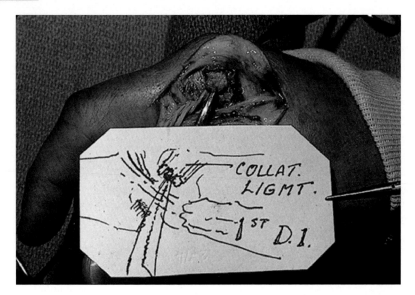

Figure 10-11 Intraoperative appearance of a complete tear of the RCL of the index MCP joint. The curved clamp is on the proximal end of the RCL. The first dorsal interosseous muscle (1st DI) expansion was retracted, and the two ends of the ligament reapproximated with a Bunnell-type pullout suture. Excellent healing and stability was achieved.

either the UCL or RCL of the thumb. Ruptures most often occur in the little and index fingers, and involve the RCL. These fingers are most commonly involved because of their position as border digits, but finger MCP joint RCL ruptures have been reported in all the fingers. The usual mechanism of injury is forced ulnar deviation with the fingers flexed.

Diagnosis
■ There is usually tenderness along the radial side of the joint, and pain on ulnar stress of the joint.
■ An arthrogram may aid in diagnosis.

Treatment
■ Treatment should be based on functional need, and may include primary reattachment, repair, or reconstruction by tendon graft as needed (Figure 10-11).

Dorsal Dislocation of the Finger Metacarpophalangeal Joint

Dorsal dislocation of the finger MCP joints is unusual. The most common digit to be involved is the index, followed by the small finger.

Mechanism of Injury and Pathologic Anatomy
The usual mechanism of injury is hyperextension of the finger, often due to a fall on the outstretched hand. The proximal attachment of the palmar plate is torn, and the suspensory effect of the collateral ligaments allows the hyperextension force to thrust the proximal phalanx and palmar plate dorsally to rest on the dorsal aspect of the metacarpal.

Kaplan identified a four-sided complex of structures that played a role in trapping the metacarpal head in the palm (Figure 10-12). These structures are as follows:

1. Radially, the lumbrical
2. Proximally, the transverse fibers of the palmar aponeurosis

3. Ulnarly, the flexor tendons
4. Distally, the natatory ligaments and the palmar plate

Diagnosis
Physical Examination
■ It is important to distinguish between complete irreducible dislocations and reducible subluxations, because a subluxation can be converted to a complete and irreducible lesion by inappropriate reduction maneuvers.
■ In *complete dislocation* (the irreducible lesion), the MCP joint is held in slight to moderate extension; MCP joint flexion is impossible and the finger is ulnarly deviated.
   ■ A prominence may be palpated in the palm that corresponds to the metacarpal head, and the skin may be puckered. Figure 10-13 demonstrates the clinical appearance of complete dislocation of the MCP joint of the index finger.
■ In *subluxation* (the reducible lesion), the findings are similar except that the proximal phalanx is usually more hyperextended—often 60 to 80 degrees.

Radiographic Findings
■ In complete dislocations, the radiographic findings may be minimal in the anteroposterior view.
■ The oblique view usually demonstrates widening of the joint space, and the lateral view may show the complete dislocation.
■ Lateral or dorsal displacement of the sesamoid in the oblique and lateral views also is an important finding.
■ A tangential or Brewerton view of the metacarpal head may aid in the detection of an avulsion or other fractures in the region of the metacarpal head (Figure 10-14).

Treatment
■ Distinction must be made between subluxation and complete dislocation because the former is reducible by closed means and the latter is not.

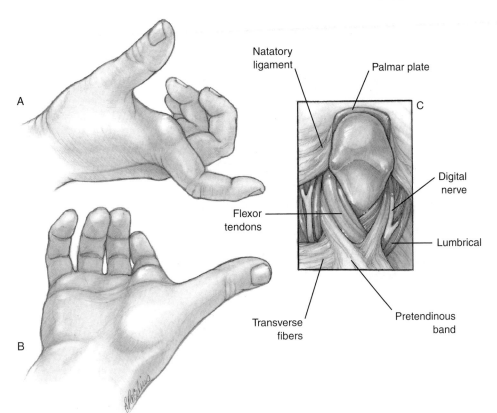

Figure 10-12 labels: Natatory ligament, Palmar plate, A, C, Digital nerve, Flexor tendons, Lumbrical, Transverse fibers, Pretendinous band, B

Figure 10-12 Complete dorsal dislocation of the index finger joint. (**A–B**) Extended and ulnar-deviated index finger. (**C**) The head and neck of the dislocated metacarpal is trapped by the transverse fibers of the palmar fascia, the flexor tendons, natatory ligaments, and the palmar plate, and the lumbrical.

■ In subluxation, the proximal edge of the palmar plate remains palmar to the metacarpal head.
  ■ If either hyperextension or traction is used as part of the reduction technique, the palmar plate may be drawn dorsally and result in a complete and irreducible dislocation.
  ■ The proper reduction maneuver is performed by flexion of the wrist, and distal and palmar force on the base of the proximal phalanx that slides the phalanx over the metacarpal head.
■ Irreducible dislocations are treated by open reduction.

■ Kaplan described a palmar approach for this condition, and others have described a dorsal approach.

THUMB METACARPOPHALANGEAL JOINT AND COLLATERAL LIGAMENTS

Joint Dislocations

Most dorsal dislocations of the thumb MCP joint are reducible; irreducible dislocations are due to a variety of

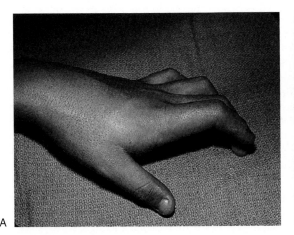
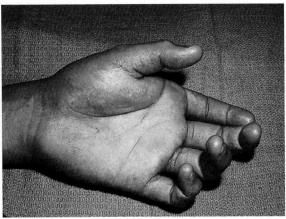

Figure 10-13 (**A**) Clinical appearance of a complete and locked dorsal dislocation of the MCP joint of the index finger. (**B**) Hyperextension at the MCP joint, and ulnar deviation of the index finger.

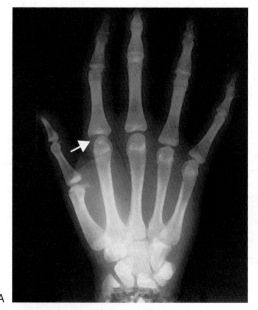

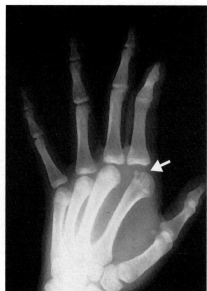

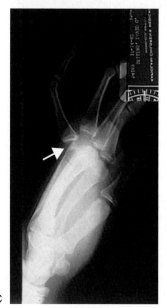

Figure 10-14 X-ray appearance of a dorsal dislocation of the index finger MCP joint. (**A**) The AP view shows only minimal changes at the MCP joint (*arrow*). (**B**) The oblique view shows a widened MCP joint space and some dorsal displacement of the proximal phalanx (*arrow*). (**C**) The lateral view shows a complete dislocation (*arrow*).

interposed structures that either block or trap the proximal phalanx from returning to its anatomic position.

Mechanism of Injury and Pathologic Anatomy

If the thumb collateral ligaments are visualized as structures that suspend the proximal phalanx during flexion and extension, it is easy to speculate that any disruption of the proximal attachments or restraints to hyperextension may result in the proximal phalanx going "over the top" with a sufficient hyperextension force, and becoming locked or trapped on the dorsal surface of the metacarpal. For this to occur, the palmar plate attachment must be disrupted either at its proximal aspect or at its insertion into the base of the proximal phalanx. If the palmar plate is disrupted distally, the accessory collateral ligaments are torn, and this allows the proximal phalanx and the collateral ligaments to swing dorsally to the top of the metacarpal. If the palmar

plate is detached proximally, it and its imbedded sesamoid bones are carried dorsally along with the proximal phalanx.

In addition to the palmar plate, other structures that may be pulled along in this excursion are the adductor pollicis aponeurosis, including the bony insertion on the ulnar base of the proximal phalanx; the abductor expansion; and the two heads of the FPB, which, along with the intact proper collateral ligaments, may form an entrapment noose around the neck of the thumb metacarpal and prevent reduction. The FPL may be entrapped in the joint but usually remains in the sheath.

Diagnosis

■ A radiograph that demonstrates sesamoid bones on the dorsal aspect of the metacarpal and adjacent to the base of the proximal phalanx usually indicates a complex irreducible dislocation of this joint (Figure 10-15).

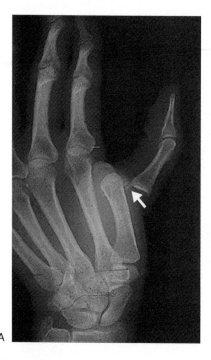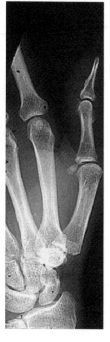

Figure 10-15 Locked dorsal dislocation of the MCP joint of the thumb. (**A**) The sesamoid bones are resting on the dorsal aspect of the neck of the thumb metacarpal (*arrow*). (**B**) An open reduction was required to reduce this locked dislocation.

Treatment

- Closed reduction may be attempted, under appropriate anesthesia, by flexing the wrist and thumb interphalangeal joint and then pushing the hyperextended proximal phalanx distalward.
- Longitudinal traction is avoided because it may "tighten

the noose" represented by the various soft tissues around the neck of the metacarpal and prevent reduction.
- If closed means are not successful, open reduction is indicated through a dorsal or palmar approach.
- Figure 10-16 shows the clinical and x-ray appearance of a dorsal dislocation of the MCP joint of the thumb, and

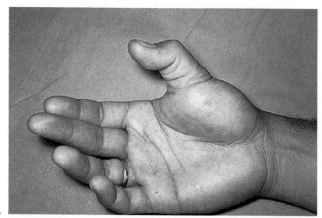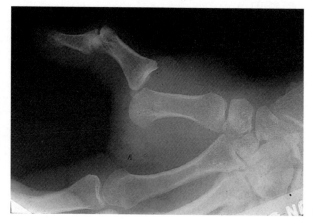

Figure 10-16 Clinical and x-ray appearance of an MCP thumb dorsal dislocation, and technique of reduction. (**A**) Note the hyperextension of the MCP joint. (**B**) The radiograph demonstrates that the proximal phalanx is "perched" on the dorsal aspect of the metacarpal. (**C**) Reduction under suitable anesthesia is achieved by hyperextension of the proximal phalanx and by "pushing" or "sweeping" it off the neck of the metacarpal.

the hyperextension and distal slide technique to reduce the dislocation.

Collateral Ligament Injuries

Ulnar Collateral Ligament Rupture or Avulsion

Mechanism of Injury and Pathologic Anatomy

This injury is due to sudden and forceful radial deviation (abduction) of the proximal phalanx of the thumb, often secondary to a fall on the out stretched hand with the thumb abducted. It may be associated with activities such as skiing or ball sports.

Disruption of the UCL at the distal insertion (with or without a bone fragment) is five times more common than proximal tears or disruptions. Tears in the substance of the UCL occur with less frequency. Associated injuries include tears of the dorsal capsule, partial avulsion of the palmar plate, or a tear in the adductor aponeurosis. In addition to providing lateral stability to the MCP joint, the UCL and RCL play a role in suspending the proximal phalanx. Therefore, disruption of the UCL may result in palmar migration and rotation (supination) of the proximal and distal phalanx on the intact RCL.

Stener Lesion

In 1962, Stener described complete rupture of the UCL with interposition of the adductor aponeurosis between the distally avulsed UCL and its site of insertion. This configuration is easy to understand based on the fact that the UCL is deep to the adductor aponeurosis. Also, with avulsion it is carried proximally, while the leading edge of the adductor aponeurosis is carried distally by the deforming force of injury. When the force abates and the proximal phalanx returns to its normal alignment, the UCL is external rather than deep to the adductor aponeurosis. Even if this configuration did not occur, the natural tension in the ligament and subsequent contracture would place it well proximal to its distal attachment, and beneath the aponeurosis. The Stener lesion is depicted in Figure 10-17.

Diagnosis

- The diagnosis is made by noting the mechanism of injury; identifying tenderness, swelling, or ecchymoses over the ulnar side of the MCP joint; and noting laxity of the UCL with stress testing.
  - Local anesthesia may be used to facilitate the stress test.
- A radiograph is made as part of the stress test to document the degree of opening of the joint. Comparison stress films may be made of the opposite side, as needed.
- It is beyond the scope of this text to discuss the methods of stress testing in detail, except to note that with complete UCL disruption, the MCP joint may be opened with minimal resistance.

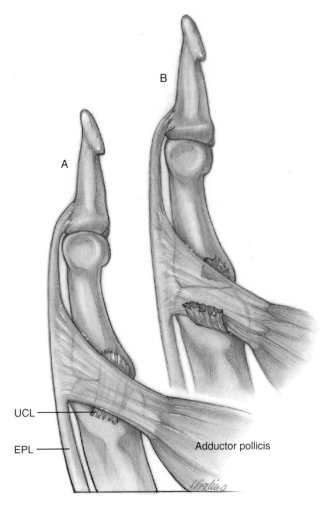

Figure 10-17   The Stener lesion. (**A**) The UCL lies beneath the adductor aponeurosis. (**B**) Rupture of the UCL occurs with sufficient abduction force. When the MCP joint resumes its anatomic position, the proximal portions of the UCL are trapped proximal and superficial to the adductor aponeurosis. The aponeurosis must be surgically reflected, and the UCL rejoined in its anatomic position, to restore stability to the joint.

Treatment

- The basic principle of treatment in complete ruptures of the UCL is to reattach the UCL to its anatomic site of attachment.
- If the anatomic sites of attachment are not duplicated, there may be less range of motion than normal of the MCP joint.

Caveat About Associated Fractures in UCL Injuries

Conventional wisdom has indicated that the position of the so-called avulsion fractures that may be seen with UCL injuries marks the distal aspect of the disrupted UCL. A widely displaced fracture fragment would indicate significant displacement of the UCL, and would suggest the need for surgical intervention. A recent case study reevaluated this concept and found that the location of the fracture fragment did not always indicate the location of the ruptured collateral ligament. The author of this study, quoting reports by Stener in 1963 and 1969, noted that fractures of this type

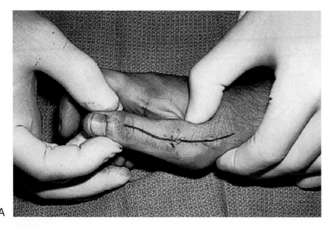
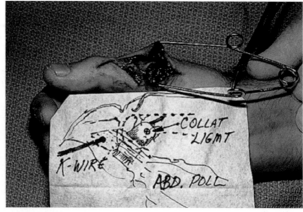

A   B

Figure 10-18   Radial collateral ligament disruption at the MCP joint of the thumb. (**A**) Positive stress test manifested by abnormal deviation of the proximal phalanx. (**B**) The complete avulsion of the RCL was repaired by reattachment of its proximal origin using a small screw. The repair was protected by an oblique transarticular Kirschner wire until healing occurred.

are either *avulsion* fractures due to UCL disruption, or *shear* fractures at the base of the proximal phalanx by the palmar portion of the radial condyle of the metacarpal. If the fracture seen on radiographs is a shear fracture, its position is unrelated to the location of the distal end of the avulsed UCL. A displaced ligament may occur in the presence of an undisplaced fracture.

Radial Collateral Ligament Disruption

Although injuries to the RCL are less common than UCL injuries, they also are associated with significant disability.

Mechanism of Injury and Pathologic Anatomy
The mechanism of injury in disruption of the RCL is forceful adduction or torsion on the flexed MCP joint.

Because the *abductor* aponeurosis is relatively broader compared to the narrower *adductor* aponeurosis, there is no potential for soft tissue interposition (the Stener lesion) with an RCL avulsion. In contrast to the UCL, the RCL is torn with almost equal frequency proximally and distally, and mid-substance disruption is more common in the RCL than in the UCL. The abductor aponeurosis may be disrupted, in addition to the RCL. Disruption of the RCL results in palmar migration and pronation of the proximal phalanx and dorsoradial prominence of the metacarpal head. In my experience, these findings may not be as noticeable immediately after the injury, possibly because initial swelling might mask the deformities, or because these findings may occur progressively and thus may not be prominent in the early phase of this condition.

Diagnosis
- Diagnosis of the acute injury is made based on the history of the injury, findings of ecchymosis or tenderness, and a positive instability test.

- Figure 10-18 demonstrates a positive stress test in an acute RCL avulsion that was repaired by reattachment of the ligament at its proximal attachment.
- In my experience, RCL injuries tend to be diagnosed late rather than early, when compared to UCL injuries.
  - This may be because a complete disruption of the UCL results in immediate and significant disability owing to the functional demands placed on the ulnar side of the thumb, leading to early evaluation.
  - The RCL injury and subsequent dysfunction does not seem to be as disabling, at least in the beginning, but as time passes, it becomes increasingly bothersome and is in fact a significant source of patient complaint and disability.

Treatment
- The basic principle of treatment in complete ruptures is to reattach the RCL to its anatomic site of insertion or repair the tear.
- Late diagnosis may require ligament reconstruction by a tendon graft.

Dorsoradial Capsule Injury

Mechanism of Injury and Pathologic Anatomy
The mechanism of injury includes a direct blow, sports activities, or breaking a fall. Possible predisposing factors are an anatomic variation in the collateral ligaments that allow greater MCP flexion, and an area of relative thinness and weakness in the dorsoradial capsule compared with the ulnar side of the joint.

Diagnosis
- The primary complaint is pain over the dorsum of the thumb and limited use of the thumb. This diagnosis should be considered in patients with persistent pain at the thumb MCP joint.

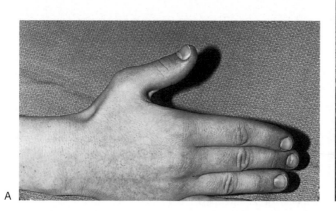

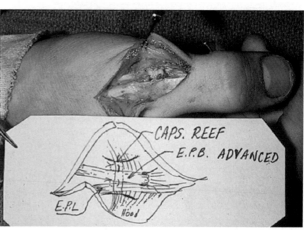

Figure 10-19   Dorsoradial capsular injury at the thumb MCP joint. (**A**) Flexed posture of the thumb MCP joint that represents maximum extension for this patient. (**B**) Repair was achieved by reefing the dorsoradial capsule of the MCP joint, and by advancing the extensor pollicis brevis tendon about 0.5 cm distal to its insertion.

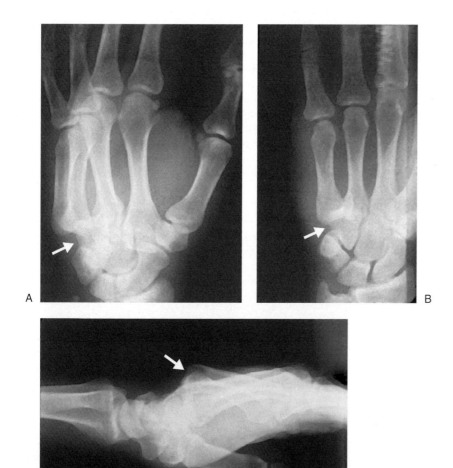

Figure 10-20   X-ray appearance in three views of a dorsal dislocation of the CMC joint of the ring and little fingers (*arrows*). Note that the dislocation is most apparent in the oblique and lateral views.

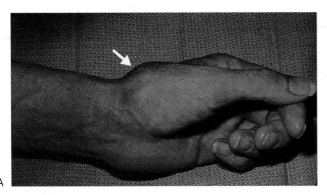
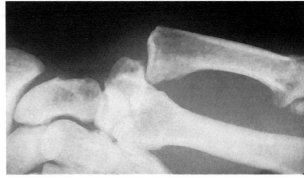

Figure 10-21   Dorsal dislocation of the thumb MCP joint. (**A**) Dorsal prominence at the base of the thumb metacarpal (*arrow*). (**B**) The radiograph reveals complete dislocation without fracture.

■ Patients typically demonstrate tenderness over the dorsoradial aspect of the thumb MCP joint in the absence of laxity of either the RCL or UCL.

■ In some instances, there is minimal palmar subluxation of the proximal phalanx.

■ Some patients experience loss of full active extension of the proximal phalanx.

Treatment

■ Some patients can be treated successfully by immobilization if no palmar subluxation or extensor lag exists.

■ Surgery is indicated for persistent activity-limiting complaints over the dorsoradial capsule, or if findings of palmar subluxation and extensor lag exist.

■ Findings at the time of surgery include thinning or redundancy of the dorsoradial capsule, or an obvious defect in the capsule.

■ Treatment is by reefing (imbrication) or direct closure of the defect in the dorsoradial capsule, and advancement of the insertion of the EPB tendon, if an extensor lag is present. An appropriate period of immobilization to protect the repair should follow.

■ Figure 10-19 shows a patient with this lesion and the surgical intervention that was performed.

CARPOMETACARPAL JOINT DISLOCATIONS

Mechanism of Injury

True dislocations of the carpometacarpal (CMC) joint of the thumb and fingers have been reported, but they are rare. Most are fracture–dislocations, and these injuries have been discussed in the chapter on fractures of the hand. When isolated dislocations of the CMC joint occur, they are usually dorsal and are caused by a longitudinal compression force that produces simultaneous flexion and compression of the metacarpal that drives the metacarpal base from its carpal articulation. Most occur in the little and ring fingers and are even more rare in the thumb.

Diagnosis

■ Figure 10-20 shows the x-ray appearance of a dorsal dislocation of the CMC joint of the ring and little fingers.

■ Figure 10-21 shows the clinical and x-ray appearance of a dislocation of the thumb CMC joint.

SUGGESTED READING

Bean CHG, Tencer AF, Trumble TE. The effect of thumb metacarpophalangeal ulnar collateral ligament attachment site on joint range of motion: an in vitro study. J Hand Surg 1999;24A:283–287.

Becton JL, Christian JD, Goodwin HN, et al. A simplified technique for treating the complex dislocation of the index metacarpal joint. J Bone Joint Surg 1975;57:683–688.

Camp RA, Weatherwax RJ, Miller EB. Chronic post traumatic radial instability of the thumb metacarpophalangeal joint. J Hand Surg 1980;5:221–225.

Doyle JR, Atkinson RE. Rupture of the radial collateral ligament of the metacarpophalangeal joint of the index finger: a report of three cases. J Hand Surg 1989;14B:248–250.

Eaton RG. Joint injuries of the hand. Springfield, Ill: Charles C. Thomas, 1971.

Garroway RY, Hurst LC, Leppard J, et al. Complex dislocation of the proximal interphalangeal joint. Orthop Rev 1984; 8:21–28.

Grant JR. Irreducible rotational anterior dislocation of the proximal interphalangeal joint: a spin dryer injury. J Hand Surg 1993;18B:648–651.

Hughes LA, Freiberg A. Irreducible MCP joint dislocation due to entrapment of the FPL. J Hand Surg 1993;18B:708–709.

Kaplan HJ. The Stener lesion revisited: a case report. J Hand Surg 1998;23A:833–836.

Krause JO, Manske PR, Mirly HL, et al. Isolated injuries to the dorsoradial capsule of the thumb metacarpophalangeal joint. J Hand Surg 1996;21A:428–433.

Lane CS. Detecting fractures of the metacarpal head: the Brewerton view. J Hand Surg 1977;2:131–133.

McLaughlin HL. Complex "locked" dislocation of the metacarpophalangeal joints. J Trauma 1965;5:683–688.

Peimer CA, Sullivan DJ, Wild WR. Palmar dislocation of the proximal interphalangeal joint. J Hand Surg 1984;9:39–48.

Spinner M, Choi BY. Anterior dislocation of the proximal interphalangeal joint, a cause of rupture of the central slip of the extensor mechanism. J Bone Joint Surg 1970;52:1329–1336.

Stener B. Displacement of the ruptured ulnar collateral ligament of the metacarpophalangeal joint of the thumb: a clinical and anatomic study. J Bone Joint Surg 1962;44B:869–879.

Stener B, Stener I. Shearing fractures associated with rupture of the ulnar collateral ligament of the metacarpophalangeal joint of the thumb. Injury 1969;1:12–16.

CARPAL INJURIES

11.1 CARPAL FRACTURES

PERTINENT ANATOMY

The Carpal Bones

The carpus consists of eight carpal bones arranged in a proximal and a distal row, with each row containing four bones. The proximal row includes (from radial to ulnar) the scaphoid, lunate, triquetrum, and pisiform. The pisiform is located palmar to the plane of the remaining three carpal bones of the proximal row, and the pisotriquetral joint is separated from the adjacent articulations. The distal row includes (from radial to ulnar) the trapezium, trapezoid, capitate, and hamate. The carpus is divided into the *radiocarpal* joint and the *midcarpal joints.* The proximal row is convex proximally and concave distally. The proximal row articulates proximally with the distal radius and with the triangular fibrocartilage complex, forming the radiocarpal and ulnocarpal joint. The proximal row articulates distally with the distal carpal row, forming the midcarpal joint (Figure 11.1-1).

The four bones of the distal row articulate distally with the five metacarpal bones and with each other. The bones of the distal carpal row are straighter in alignment across the wrist than the proximal row, especially at their distal articulations with the metacarpal bones.

On the dorsal surface of the carpus, a gentle convex arch is formed by the arrangement of the proximal and distal rows. On the palmar surface, however, a deep concavity is formed, designated as the *carpal groove.* The carpal groove is accentuated by the palmar projection of the pisiform and hook of the hamate ulnarly, and by the projection of the scaphoid tuberosity and trapezial ridge radially. The midcarpal joint and the radiocarpal joint usually do not communicate with each other; if communication does occur, as seen through the flow of dye from an arthrogram, there is a tear or rent in the scapholunate or lunotriquetral ligaments.

Useful External Landmarks and Their Relationships to the Underlying Structures

Figure 11.1-2 is a depiction of the thenar and wrist flexion creases and their relationship to some of the underlying structures.

Lister's Tubercle
The extensor pollicis longus (EPL) tendon courses along the ulnar side of Lister's tubercle on its way from the wrist to the distal phalanx of the thumb. The extensor carpi radial brevis (ECRB) is to the radial side of this tubercle. Lister's tubercle is located 0.5 cm from the radiocarpal joint and is in line with the cleft between the index and middle finger metacarpals. The interval between the proximal pole of the scaphoid and its articulation with the lunate and the scapholunate ligament is just ulnar and distal to Lister's tubercle.

Styloid Process of the Middle Finger Metacarpal
This process, located on the dorsal and radial aspect of the middle finger metacarpal, points to the articular interface between the capitate and trapezoid, and is just proximal to the insertion of the ECRB tendon.

Lunate Fossa
This palpable central depression on the back of the wrist is in line with the middle finger metacarpal, is just distal and ulnar to Lister's tubercle, and marks the location of the carpal lunate.

Radial Styloid
This visible and easily palpated landmark is both palmar and dorsal to the abductor pollicis longus (APL) and extensor pollicis brevis (EPB) tendons that course across its apex.

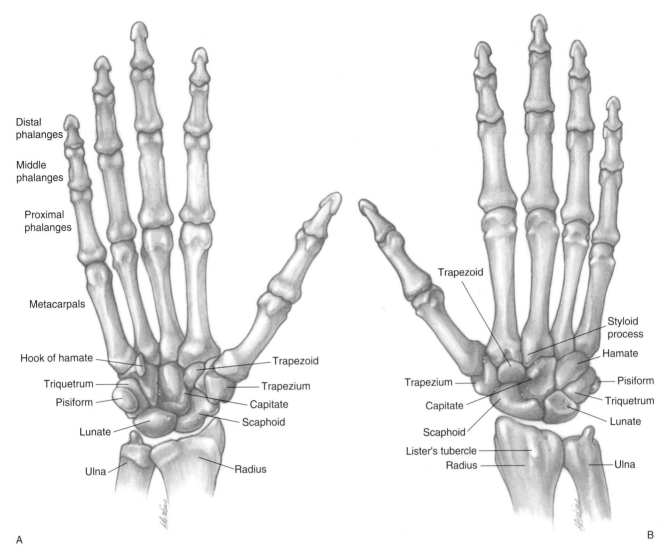

Figure 11.1-1 **A.** Skeletal anatomy of the wrist, palmar aspect. **B.** Skeletal anatomy of the wrist, dorsal aspect.

Distal Head of the Ulna

The slightly expanded distal end of the ulna has a head and styloid process. The head is most visible and palpable when the forearm is in *pronation*; the posteroulnar styloid is most readily palpable in *supination* and is approximately 1 cm proximal to the plane of the radial styloid.

Pisiform Bone

The pisiform bone, located on the ulnar and palmar aspect of the base of the hand, provides a visible and palpable landmark that aids in the identification and location of the flexor carpi ulnaris (FCU) tendon, the underlying ulnar neurovascular bundle, and the hook process of the hamate.

Hook Process of the Hamate

The hook of the hamate, located on the ulnar and palmar aspect of the distal carpus, can be palpated approximately 1 cm radial and distal to the pisiform. Because of its deep location, it may be difficult to palpate in some individuals. The hook of the hamate lies between the ulnar tunnel

(Guyon's canal) and the carpal tunnel. It thus provides a landmark for the ulnar nerve and artery (located just ulnar to the hook), and the ulnar boundary of the carpal tunnel. Point tenderness in this area may indicate a fracture of the hook process, a somewhat common injury in sports that use racquets, clubs, or bats, such as tennis, golf, or baseball.

Scaphoid Tubercle

The scaphoid tubercle is in the distal palmar aspect of the scaphoid. It projects into the palm, and the tubercle is palpable on the radial aspect of the base of the hand, usually just distal to the *distal palmar wrist crease*. It becomes more prominent with the wrist positioned in radial deviation, since the scaphoid assumes a position of more palmar flexion in this position. Conversely, the scaphoid tubercle is less prominent and possibly not palpable when the wrist is in ulnar deviation, since the scaphoid assumes a position of decreased palmar flexion and lies more in the plane of the radius and ulna.

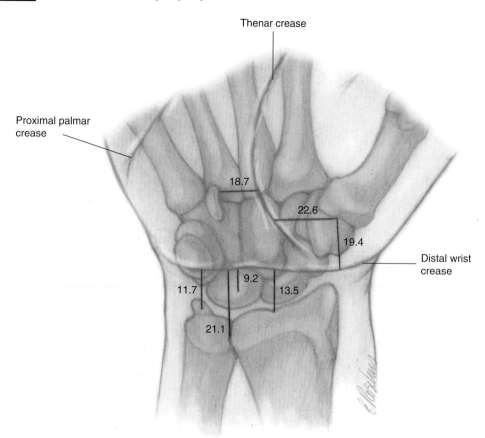

Thenar crease

Proximal palmar crease

18.7

22.6

19.4

Distal wrist crease

11.7

9.2

13.5

21.1

Figure 11.1-2 Flexion crease landmarks. Relationship of the carpal bones and other bony landmarks to the thenar and distal wrist creases. The number indicate the mean distance (in mm) of the structures depicted from the respective creases.

Distal Wrist Flexion Crease

The distal wrist crease is located over the proximal carpal row and passes over the waist of the scaphoid and, 80% of the time, over the pisiform bone. The lunate is proximal to the distal wrist crease with its center an average of 9.2 mm from the crease. The radiocarpal joint is 13.5 mm proximal to the crease and the center point of the distal radioulnar joint (DRUJ) is 21.1 mm proximal to the wrist crease. The base of the ulnar styloid is on average 11.7 mm proximal to the wrist crease.

Anatomic Snuff Box

The anatomic snuffbox is a narrow triangle, with its apex distal, that is bounded dorsoulnarly by the EPL, radially by the APL and EPB tendons, and proximally by the distal margin of the extensor retinaculum. It contains the dorsal branch of the radial artery in the dorsoulnar corner, the tendon of the extensor carpi radialis longus (ECRL) and one or more branches of the superficial branch of the radial nerve. Tenderness in the anatomical snuffbox is associated with fractures of the scaphoid.

Vascular Anatomy of the Carpus

The vascular supply to the carpus is through two main systems, the *dorsal carpal vascular system* and the *palmar carpal vascular system* (Figure 11.1-3). The dorsal and palmar systems consist of a series of dorsal and palmar transverse arches that are connected by anastomoses formed by the radial, ulnar, and anterior interosseous arteries.

Vascular Supply of the Scaphoid

The scaphoid receives its vascular supply mainly from the radial artery (Figure 11.1-4). Vessels enter the scaphoid in limited areas dorsally and palmarly at nonarticular zones of ligamentous attachment. The dorsal vascular supply to the scaphoid accounts for 70% to 80% of the internal vascularity of the bone, *all in the proximal region.* The major dorsal vessels enter the bone through small foramina located at a dorsal ridge in the region of the scaphoid waist.

At the level of the intercarpal joint, the radial artery gives off the intercarpal artery, which immediately divides into two branches. One branch runs transverse to the dorsum of the wrist. The other branch runs vertically and distally over the index metacarpal. Approximately 5 mm proximal to the origin of the intercarpal vessel at the level of the styloid process of the radius, another vessel is given off that runs over the radiocarpal ligament to enter the scaphoid through its waist along the dorsal ridge.

There are consistent major communications between the dorsal scaphoid branch of the radial artery and the dorsal branch of the anterior interosseous artery. No vessels enter the proximal dorsal region of the scaphoid through the dorsal scapholunate ligament, and no vessels enter through the dorsal cartilaginous areas. The dorsal vessels usually divide into two or three branches soon after entering the scaphoid. These branches run palmarly and proximally, dividing into smaller branches to supply the proximal pole as far as the subchondral region.

The palmar vascular supply accounts for 20% to 30% of the internal vascularity, all in the region of the distal pole. At

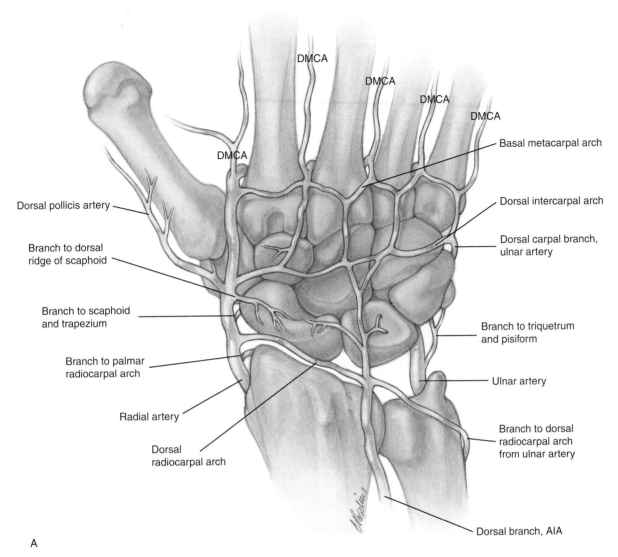

Figure 11.1-3   A, B. Anatomy of the arterial supply to the dorsal and palmar aspect of the wrist.
Figure continues.

the level of the radioscaphoid joint, the radial artery gives off the superficial palmar branch. Just distal to the origin of the superficial palmar branch, several smaller branches course obliquely and distally over the palmar aspect of the scaphoid to enter through the region of the tubercle. These branches, the palmar scaphoid branches, divide into several smaller branches just before penetrating the bone. In 75% of specimens, these arteries arise directly from the radial artery.

Specific Fractures of the Carpus

The majority (80%) of carpal fractures involve the scaphoid, followed by (in descending order of incidence) the triquetrum, trapezium, hamate, lunate, pisiform, capitate, and trapezoid.

SCAPHOID

Mechanism of Injury

The usual history is a fall on the extended wrist. Experimental studies have shown that fractures of the scaphoid can be produced consistently by forces applied to a *hyperextended* (90 degrees or more) and *radially deviated* wrist. Progressively less extension resulted in fractures of the distal radius and forearm.

Diagnosis

■ Initial findings include a history of a fall, complaints of persistent discomfort or pain in the wrist, and tenderness on palpation in the anatomical snuffbox.

■ X-rays are taken in four views: one posterior-anterior (PA), one lateral, and two oblique views.

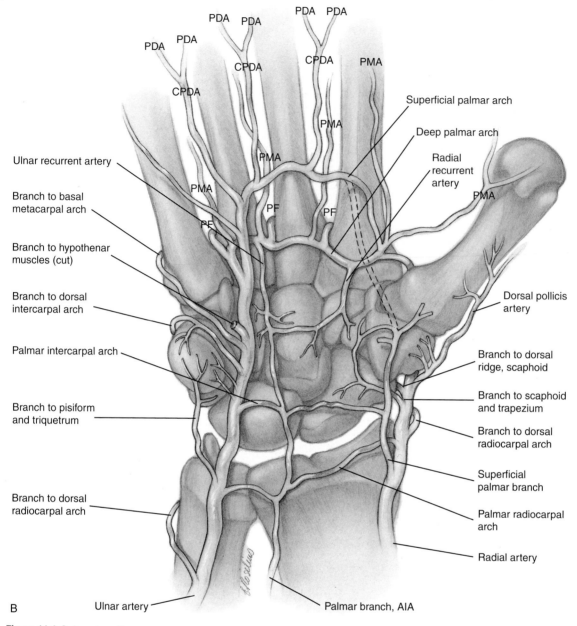

B

Figure 11.1-3 (*continued*)

■ The PA radiograph is best performed with the patient making a fist.

   ■ The fist posture results in slight wrist extension, and promotes ulnar deviation of the wrist that may be useful in opening up the fracture interface.

   ■ This position also places the longitudinal axis of the scaphoid parallel to the plane of the x-ray plate. Figure 11.1-5 demonstrates a fracture of the carpal scaphoid.

■ If radiograph studies do not demonstrate a definite fracture, the wrist is immobilized in a short-arm thumb spica cast, and repeat radiographs made in 2 to 3 weeks.

■ If radiograph studies at 2 to 3 weeks are inconclusive, and positive physical findings are present, a bone scan may be used to further assist in the diagnosis.

■ Some surgeons may use magnetic resonance imaging (MRI) rather than a bone scan, because MRI may detect an occult fracture sooner than a bone scan.

   ■ MRI with gadolinium is useful for evaluating vascularity of the scaphoid.

■ Computerized tomography (CT) is a useful method to define bone anatomy, and may aid in the diagnosis of an angular deformity that may require surgical correction.

Treatment

■ Treatment options may be based on a number of different classification systems that in turn are based on the location of the fracture (distal, middle, or proximal pole), stability, whether the fracture is displaced or nondisplaced,

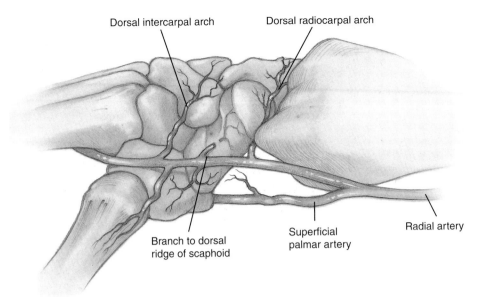

Figure 11.1-4 Anatomy of the arterial supply to the scaphoid and the radial aspect of the wrist.

whether it is angulated or nonangulated, and the plane of the fracture relative to the long axis of the scaphoid.
- The simplest treatment related classification is based on the *location of the fracture*.

Distal-Third Fractures
- Fractures of the tuberosity and distal third may be treated with a short-arm thumb spica cast until union is evident by radiograph or other studies.
- If the fracture is intra-articular and displaced, an open reduction and internal fixation may be considered.

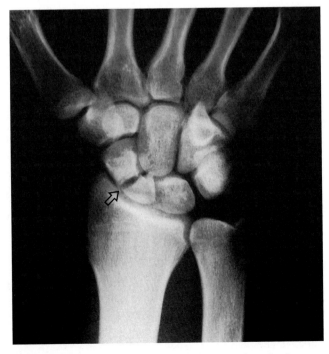

Figure 11.1-5 X-ray view of a fracture of the carpal scaphoid. (Courtesy of H. Relton McCarroll, Jr., MD, San Francisco)

Middle-Third Fractures
- Recent, stable, and undisplaced fractures are managed with a short-arm thumb spica cast.
- Recent undisplaced but *potentially unstable* fractures, including vertical oblique or reduced trans-scaphoid perilunate fracture dislocations, should be managed with a long-arm (above the elbow) thumb spica cast. Some surgeons consider a reduced trans-scaphoid perilunate dislocation to be inherently unstable, and advise internal fixation.
- Displaced or angulated fractures require open reduction and internal fixation by techniques based on the surgeon's experience and choice, including K-wires and or Herbert screws.

Proximal-Third Fractures
- Recent fractures are treated with a Herbert screw followed by a long-arm thumb spica cast.
  - Delayed or nonunion and avascular necrosis is highly likely in spite of the above-recommended treatment, and may require one or more secondary operations including bone grafting, vascularized bone grafting, excision of the proximal pole, or proximal row carpectomy.
- The length of immobilization will vary from injury to injury, and is based on the experience of the surgeon, clinical findings, and suitable diagnostic studies.

Additional Treatment Principles
- Fractures of the scaphoid treated *more than 4 weeks* after injury are less successfully treated by cast immobilization.
- Percutaneous fixation may be a useful technique for fixation of undisplaced fractures.
- Stable and nondisplaced fractures will most likely heal with cast immobilization; unstable and displaced fractures are best treated with some form of internal fixation.
- A gap or fracture offset of 1 mm or greater is considered to be a reliable indicator of *instability,* and is associated with a higher incidence of nonunion and malunion.

- Open reduction and internal fixation are indicated in these fractures.
- Internal fixation of the surgeon's choice is usually indicated in fractures involving the proximal pole due to their propensity for delayed and nonunion.
- The initial determination of stability status may not always be correct.
- Differences of opinion exist regarding the necessity for immobilization of the thumb and elbow in scaphoid fractures, and may vary with the experience and preference of the surgeon.

Palmar Versus Dorsal Surgical Approaches to the Scaphoid

- The major blood supply to the scaphoid enters at the *dorsal and distal* aspect of the bone; based on this fact, *palmar or anterior surgical approaches* to this bone are favored for management of distal pole and waist fractures.
- The blood supply to the distal and middle aspects of the bone is abundant in comparison to the proximal pole whose blood supply is precarious.
  - This poor blood supply is a significant factor in the high rate of nonunion in scaphoid fractures of the proximal pole.
- The palmar approach is recommended for correction of the "humpback" deformity (dorsal angulation and collapse of the scaphoid).
- The *dorsal approach* is preferred for ease of screw placement in proximal pole fractures, and does not compromise the dorsal blood supply if dissection is confined to the proximal pole.
  - It is also the approach of choice for insertion of vascularized bone grafts.

Other Treatment Options

- The treatment of established nonunion (including bone graft techniques), the use of electrical stimulation for delayed or nonunion, and procedures for secondary reconstruction of nonunion or malunion of the scaphoid is beyond the scope of this chapter.

Late Complications of Scaphoid Fracture Nonunion

- If untreated, scaphoid nonunions lead to a predictable pattern of arthrosis in the wrist.
- Scaphoid nonunion may exist with or without avascular necrosis (AVN) of the proximal aspect of the scaphoid; if present, AVN lessens the chances of success in reconstructive procedures.
- Fractures of the waist may collapse, and dorsally angulate to produce the humpback deformity.
- Four progressive stages of *scaphoid nonunion and advanced collapse* (SNAC) have been identified: (1) arthritis of the radial styloid, (2) spread of the arthritis to include the scaphoid fossa of the radius, (3) the addition of capitolunate arthritis, and (4) diffuse carpal arthritis.

Triquetrum

Incidence and Types of Fracture

Triquetral fractures are the most common carpal fractures exclusive of the scaphoid. Two types have been identified: dorsal rim chip fractures (the most common) and fractures of the body.

Mechanism of Injury

Chip Fractures.   Although the exact mechanism of injury is unknown, these injuries may be due to avulsion of the conjoined insertion of the dorsal radiocarpal (dorsal radiotriquetral) and dorsal intercarpal ligaments during hyperflexion and radial deviation of the wrist, or due to impaction from the ulnar styloid or hamate during axial loading and hyperextension of the wrist.

Body Fractures.   These injuries are usually the result of a direct blow to the ulnar aspect of the wrist, which results in a medial tuberosity fracture. Triquetral fractures are often associated with other carpal injuries such as a perilunate dislocation. An anteroposterior crushing injury may result in sagittal fracture. Lunate or perilunate dislocation may cause proximal pole fracture, as the palmar lunotriquetral ligament avulses the proximal pole of the triquetrum. Transverse fractures are usually the result of shear force, and often are associated with scaphoid fractures.

Treatment

- Small nondisplaced or even displaced chip fractures are usually treated symptomatically with a short period of immobilization as needed.
- Larger chip fractures, due to their potential for nonunion or instability if untreated, are immobilized in a cast.
- Open reduction and fixation may be required to restore the insertions of the DRC and DIC ligaments to prevent persistent pain and instability that is sometimes seen in injuries with larger fragments.
- Fractures of the triquetral body or palmar radial fractures are usually minimally displaced, and are treated by cast immobilization—but they may be associated with lunotriquetral or other ligament tears.
- Palmar radial fractures have been associated with volar intercalated segment instability (VISI) collapse, and may warrant fixation and repair or reconstruction of the lunotriquetral ligament complex.

Trapezium

Incidence and Types of Fracture

Fractures of the trapezium are the second-most common nonscaphoid fracture. Five types have been identified, including vertical transarticular (the most common), horizontal, dorsoradial tuberosity, anteromedial ridge, and comminuted. Fractures of the trapezium often occur in combination with thumb metacarpal or distal radius fractures.

Mechanism of Injury

Vertical transarticular fractures are due to a longitudinal axial force transmitted by the thumb metacarpal. Horizontal fractures are due to direct shearing forces, and dorsoradial fractures are the result of vertical shearing as the metacarpal impacts the trapezium into the radial styloid. An object held in the web space (such as the handlebars of a bicycle or motorcycle) may produce a similar injury. Anteromedial ridge fractures result from an anteroposterior force that flattens the transverse carpal arch and causes an avulsion through the transverse carpal ligament of the anteromedial ridge. This fracture may occur in conjunction with a fracture of the hook process of the hamate.

Treatment

- Displaced intra-articular fractures are best treated by open reduction and fixation, but most other fractures are treated by 4 to 6 weeks of cast immobilization.
- The articulation with the adjacent thumb metacarpal is very critical for thumb function, and post-injury arthrosis may be avoided by anatomic reduction of intra-articular fractures.

Hamate

Incidence and Types of Injury

Hamate injuries are most common in stick or racquet sports such as golf, baseball, or tennis. Fracture of the hamate hook presents with pain (and often, point tenderness) distal and radial to the pisiform. Nonunion and the resultant irregularity of the fracture interface may cause attritional rupture of the flexors, and this loss of flexion in the little and ring fingers may be the presenting complaint (Figure 11.1-6).

Two major types of fractures have been identified, and involve the hook process and the body of the hamate. Hook fractures may involve the tip, waist, or base. Fractures of the body may involve the proximal pole, medial tuberosity, or (in the body), be oriented in the sagittal oblique plane or dorsal coronal plane.

Mechanism of Injury

Hook fractures may result from a sudden forceful blow, or from repetitive impacts that may cause a stress fracture. An avulsion fracture may occur by means of traction from the FCU tendon and its extension through the pisohamate ligament. A crush injury in the **AP** plane may result in an avulsion-type fracture mediated through the transverse carpal ligament. Fractures of the body of the hamate may result from direct blows to the ulnar aspect of the hand (medial tuberosity fracture), anteroposterior crush injury (sagittal oblique fracture), or carpometacarpal dislocation of the ring and little fingers that results in a dorsal coronal fracture.

Treatment

- Hook fractures may be treated based on location, degree of displacement, and time from injury.
- Recent nondisplaced fractures, regardless of location, may be treated with immobilization, with the wrist in radial deviation to lessen the possible deforming force of the ulnar finger flexors.
- Displaced avulsion fractures that involve only the superficial tip of the hook may be treated symptomatically.
  - The fragment may be excised if it remains symptomatic after several weeks.
- Fractures of the waist or base of the hook may be excised. Some surgeons advise preservation of the hook by means of ORIF and bone grafting, believing that the hook is important as a mechanical pulley that maintains flexor tendon function.
- Nondisplaced body fractures may be treated by cast immobilization, but displaced fractures, especially those seen with metacarpal subluxation or instability, should be anatomically reduced and fixed.
- The motor branch of the ulnar nerve courses around the base of the hook process, and is at risk during surgery in this region.

Lunate

Incidence, Vascular Supply and Types

Lunate fractures are said to represent about 1% of all carpal fractures, excluding fractures associated with Kienbock's disease.

True lunate fractures are often associated with fractures of the distal radius, scaphoid, capitate, and triquetrum.

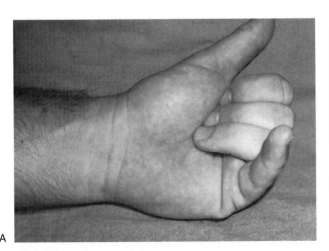
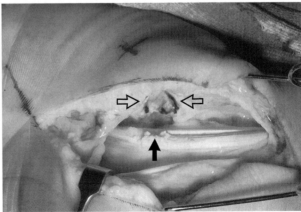

A   B

Figure 11.1-6   Attritional rupture of flexor tendons due to fracture of the hook process of hamate.
A. Loss of flexion in the left little finger. **B.** Fracture of the base of the hook process (*open arrows*) and frayed margin (*solid arrow*) of the flexor tendon.

Twenty percent of lunate bones are vascularized by a single palmar supply, and in the remaining 80%, the vascular supply arises from both palmar and dorsal vessels that anastomose in the body of the lunate.

The five types of fractures that have been identified are based on their location and vascular supply: (1) palmar pole fractures (the most common) affecting the palmar nutrient artery, (2) osteochondral (chip) fractures of the proximal articular surface but not affecting vascularity, (3) dorsal pole fractures possibly affecting the dorsal nutrient artery, (4) sagittal-oblique fractures through the body, and (5) coronal split of the body.

Mechanism of Injury

- Type I palmar pole fractures are due to wrist hyperextension and compression from the capitate and radius, combined with tension on the radiolunate and lunotriquetral ligaments. The palmar pole is avulsed by the lunotriquetral ligaments, and this may produce flexion of the lunate.
- Type II osteochondral fractures may occur following shear-related injuries, as seen in lunate dislocations, subluxations, or in patients with Kienbock's disease.
- Type III dorsal pole fractures result from shear forces in perilunate dislocations (as the capitate displaces dorsally) or from avulsion of the scapholunate ligament in acute rotatory subluxation of the scaphoid.
- Type IV sagittal-oblique fractures between the proximal and distal articular surfaces result from shear forces produced by radiocarpal fracture-dislocation.
- Type V coronal fractures result from wrist hyperextension, which produces tension on the short radiolunate ligament that avulses the palmar pole. This fracture may also be seen following a palmar perilunate dislocation of the capitate.

Treatment

- Most lunate fractures require surgical treatment based on the fracture and its associated ligamentous injury.
- Type I fractures may require correction of a lunate rotatory component if present.
- Type II injuries may require debridement if symptomatic. The specific treatment recommendations are outlined above.
- Type III fractures associated with acute scapholunate dissociation may require operative stabilization of the scapholunate joint.
- Type IV fractures that are displaced require fixation.
- Type V fractures may require surgical intervention, depending on the degree of displacement and the associated carpal instability.
- Kienbock's disease of the lunate should be considered in the absence of significant trauma.

Pisiform

Incidence and Types of Injury

Fractures of the pisiform are uncommon, but four types have been identified: transverse (the most common), parasagittal, comminuted, and pisotriquetral impaction.

Mechanism of Injury

The usual cause of this fracture is a fall or direct impaction on the pisiform, with the wrist extended. Active contraction of the FCU muscle-tendon unit may play a role in separation of the fracture interface. Incongruity of the pisiform may result in pisotriquetral incongruity and degenerative arthritis. As well, a shearing injury may result in intra-articular loose bodies, which may remain symptomatic.

Treatment

- Most fractures may be treated with immobilization, with the expectation that union or fibrous union will occur.
- Wide separation of the fragments may indicate some degree of discontinuity of the FCU, and may be an indication for exploration.
- Some surgeons prefer to excise widely separated or comminuted fractures and restore the integrity of the FCU by suture techniques of their choice.
- Parasagittal and comminuted fractures, as well as pisotriquetral impaction conditions (if symptomatic) may be treated by pisiform excision.

Capitate

Incidence and Types of Injury

Fortunately, capitate fractures are uncommon. They are difficult to treat due to the fact that the proximal pole is entirely intra-articular and without soft-tissue attachment. AVN is likely if the fracture is displaced. Four fracture types have been reported: transverse fracture of the body (the most common), transverse fracture of the proximal pole, and coronal oblique and parasagittal fractures.

Mechanism of Injury

The first two types occur due to compression loading of the hyperextended wrist, which forces the capitate against the dorsal edge of the radius. This mechanism of injury may also produce a concomitant fracture of the scaphoid, and is called the *scaphocapitate fracture syndrome*. The scaphoid fracture may be the only injury evident on the initial radiographs, and the wise examiner will look for clinical evidence of injury to the capitate in addition to the scaphoid injury. Types III and IV usually result from hyperextension and axial loading injuries.

Treatment

- CT is often required to make the diagnosis. MRI is used to evaluate the vascularity of the proximal pole.
- The treatment of capitate fractures requires prompt diagnosis and stabilization. If diagnosed early and it is nondisplaced, cast immobilization may be used.
- If the fracture is displaced or part of *scaphocapitate fracture syndrome*, open reduction and internal fixation is indicated.
  - Vascularity of the proximal pole may be evaluated intraoperatively.
- Restoration of distal carpal row height, anatomic reduction, and careful evaluation for associated injuries are the primary goals of treatment.

TABLE 11.1-1 SUMMARY OF CARPAL FRACTURES EXCLUSIVE OF THE SCAPHOID

Bone (Normal Right PA and Lateral)	Fracture Types	Most Common Treatment	Common Associated Injuries	Treatment Pearls
Lunate 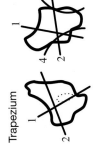	1. Palmar pole 2. Osteochondral (chip) 3. Dorsal pole 4. Sagittal oblique 5. Coronal split	1. Closed treatment and casting for 4–6 weeks if minimally displaced or small fragments. 2. ORIF for intra-articular incongruity or associated instability.	1. Lunotriquetral or radiolunate ligament tears. 2. Kienböck's disease.	1. Beware Kienböck's disease if fracture present independent of significant trauma. 2. Consider MRI for evaluation of vascularity. 3. Injury may suggest carpal instability pattern.

Triquetrum	1. Dorsal rim chip fractures
	2. Body fractures
	  (a) Medial tuberosity
	  (b) Sagittal
	  (c) Transverse proximal pole
	  (d) Transverse body
	  (e) Palmar radial
	  (f) Comminuted
		1. Closed treatment with casting for 4–6 weeks if small chip (Type 1) or minimally displaced.
		2. If large Type 1 or significantly displaced body type may require ORIF.
			1. Dorsal avulsion may represent avulsion from DRC and DIC ligament.
			2. Triquetrum and lunate may secondarily flex if DRCL torn.
			3. Ulnar impaction/TFCC injury may accompany body fracture.
				1. Stabilization of DRC and DIC ligament may be required if large dorsal avulsion.
				2. Arthroscopy may be necessary to evaluate ulnar/TFCC injury after healing of body fracture.

Trapezium	1. Vertical transarticular 2. Horizontal 3. Dorsoradial tuberosity 4. Anteromedial ridge 5. Comminuted	1. Thumb spica casting 4–6 weeks for minimally displaced fractures. 2. Spanning ex-fix if comminuted. 3. ORIF vs. K-wires for displaced intra-articular. 4. Ridge excision for symptomatic Type 4. 5. Trapezium excision or CMC fusion for late arthrosis.	1. 1st MC fractures common. 2. Ridge fractures may secondarily cause CTS. 3. Late 1st CMC arthritis may develop after IA injury. 4. FCR/FPL rupture possible if medial irregularity.	1. Anatomic reduction for intra-articular fractures. 2. May consider primary fusion for combined trapezium and proximal 1st MC intra-articular fractures.
Trapezoid 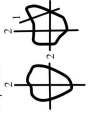	1. Dorsal rim 2. Body	1. Cast immobilization for 4–6 weeks for minimally displaced fractures. 2. May require closed reduction of fracture or 2nd MC and pinning for stabilization. 3. ORIF rarely necessary.	1. Unusual as an isolated injury. 2. Usually associated with 2nd MC dorsal dislocation.	1. Often requires CT or MRI to diagnose. 2. Recurrence of posterior subluxation of 2nd MC must be carefully followed. 3. Fusion of trapezoid–2nd MC may be necessary for late arthrosis and pain.

(continued)

TABLE 11.1-1 (continued)

Bone (Normal Right PA and Lateral)	Fracture Types	Most Common Treatment	Common Associated Injuries	Treatment Pearls
Capitate	1. Transverse (axial) body 2. Transverse proximal pole 3. Coronal oblique 4. Parasagittal	1. Cast immobilization for 4–6 weeks for minimally displaced fractures. 2. Closed reduction and K-wires for extra-articular reducible fractures. 3. ORIF for irreducible displaced, intra-articular, or proximal pole fractures.	1. "Scaphocapitate syndrome"—including scaphoid fracture and lunotriquetral ligament injury. 2. Avascular necrosis (late) of proximal capitate.	1. Proximal capitate is mostly intraarticular, leading to poor vascular supply. 2. Urgent ORIF of displaced or rotated proximal pole fractures. 3. Beware associated (but not apparent) scaphoid fracture, lunotriquetral ligament injury, or other perilunate injury.

Hamate	1. Hook
	  (a) Avulsion (tip)
	  (b) Waist
	  (c) Base
	2. Body
	  (a) Proximal pole
	  (b) Medial tuberosity
	  (c) Sagittal oblique
	  (d) Dorsal coronal fractures
		1. Cast immobilization for 4–6 weeks for minimally displaced fractures.
		2. Hamate hook excision if continued pain after period of immobilization.
		3. Rest, equipment adaptation; and immobilization for stress or repetitive injury fracture.
		4. ORIF of displaced body or intra-articular fractures.
			1. Irritation and eventual rupture of ulnar finger flexors may occur with displaced hook fracture.
			2. May be associated with 4th or 5th MC dislocation.
			3. May occur with avulsion of FCU.
				1. Cast immobilization in slight radial deviation will minimize the deforming force of the ulnar finger flexors.
				2. Hamate hook provides mechanical advantage of ulnar finger flexors.
				3. Hook has watershed blood supply at waist with feeding vessels through tip and base.
				4. Consider hamate hook lateral or carpal tunnel view radiograph for visualization.

Pisiform	1. Transverse (common) 2. Parasagittal 3. Comminuted 4. Pisotriquetral impaction	1. Immobilization for 2–4 weeks for minimally displaced or comminuted fractures. 2. Consider ORIF or excision and tendon reconstruction if FCU disrupted. 3. Excision and tendon reconstruction for arthrosis related to healed (or unhealed) fracture.	1. FCU disruption (partial or complete). 2. Triquetral or hamate impaction injury related to mechanism.	1. Best visualized on lateral radiograph. 2. Fibrous union may be well tolerated if FCU in continuity.

(From Putnam MD, Meyer NJ. Carpal fractures excluding the scaphoid. In: Trumble T, ed. Hand surgery update 3, hand, elbow and shoulder. Rosemont, IL: American Society for Surgery of the Hand, 2003:175–187.)

Late Results of Nonunion of the Capitate

Capitate osteonecrosis may occur due to loss of vascularity. This in turn may lead to distal-row collapse, scaphoid rotatory subluxation, and progressive carpal arthritis with persistent pain and stiffness.

Trapezoid

Incidence and Types

The trapezoid is the least commonly fractured carpal bone. Trapezoid fractures rarely occur alone, and are usually associated with fracture-dislocations involving dislocation of the index metacarpal or the trapezoid itself. Diagnosis may be aided by CT or MRI, since radiographs may not show the fracture. Two types have been identified; they include fractures of the dorsal rim and body.

Mechanism of Injury

This fracture usually results from an axially directed force along the index metacarpal. These fractures are often difficult to identify on plain films, and thus require a high index of suspicion. As noted above, a CT scan or MRI will best characterize this fracture.

Treatment

- Minimally displaced trapezoid fractures are treated with cast immobilization for 4 to 6 weeks, but displaced fractures may require ORIF or closed reduction and immobilization.
- Osteonecrosis may occur in the trapezoid due to its poor blood supply. Trapezoid-index metacarpal arthrodesis may be indicated for late arthrosis.
- Table 11.1-1 depicts the fracture type, treatment, associated injuries, and treatment "PEARLS," and is reproduced with permission of the authors and publisher.

11.2 CARPAL INSTABILITIES AND FRACTURE-DISLOCATIONS OF THE CARPUS

DEFINITION

Carpal instability is defined as loss of carpal ligament integrity due to acute traumatic dislocations or ligamentous laxity. It implies the loss of the ability to maintain normal kinematic and kinetic functions and relationships under static conditions and or functional loads between the radius, carpal bones and metacarpals. In the broader definition of carpal instabilities used in this chapter, they may be associated with certain fracture dislocations of the carpus, and include isolated carpal dislocations and adaptive instabilities secondary to malunions of distal radius fractures.

Carpal instability is further divided into *static* and *dynamic* forms. *Static instability* refers to carpal malalignment that is detectable on standard x-ray views, whereas *dynamic instability* refers to carpal instability that is reproduced or demonstrated on physical examination maneuvers, and may often be demonstrated on *stress* radiographs. Static instabilities are usually associated with complete ligamentous disruption, whereas dynamic instabilities are usually associated with a partial or incomplete ligamentous disruption. Dynamic carpal instability is said to be the most common cause of wrist pain and carpal instability in adolescents and young adults. It is most likely due to attenuation of the palmar radioscaphoid and scapholunate interosseous ligaments.

Dorsal wrist ganglions that most often arise from the region of the SL ligament have been shown to be associated with symptoms and signs of dynamic scapholunate instability.

The Ring Concept

A current theory of carpal kinematics characterizes the carpus as a ring that allows reciprocal motion between the proximal and distal rows during radial and ulnar deviation, and during flexion and extension. The scaphoid is considered to be the stabilizing link between these two rows, and the triquetrum is said to be the pivot point for carpal rotation. Any *interruption* of the ring in the proximal carpal row results in carpal instability.

The Intercalated Segment

This term is used to describe the relationship or position of the proximal carpal row that is *interposed,* or suspended between the radius/ulna and the distal carpal row/hand. Some have called the proximal carpal row a "free body in space." This oversimplification is amplified by noting that the radius

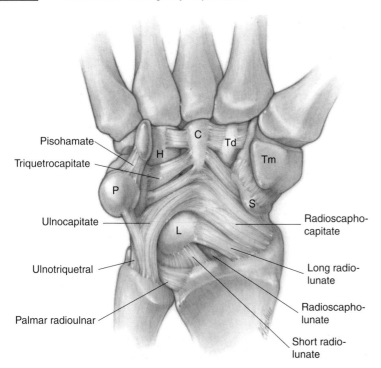

Pisohamate
Triquetrocapitate
Ulnocapitate
Ulnotriquetral
Palmar radioulnar

Radioscapho-capitate
Long radio-lunate
Radioscapho-lunate
Short radio-lunate

Figure 11.2-1   The palmar radiocarpal ligaments (see text for details).

of curvature of the proximal pole of the scaphoid and the lunate are different (the lunate has a greater radius). This finding fits with the interosseous scapholunate ligament anatomy that demonstrates thick and unyielding fibers dorsally compared to the palmar portions of the ligament that are less dense and more elastic. These two facts (among others) account for the different rates or ratios of movement that demonstrate equal rotation of these two bones in wrist extension, but show greater rotation of the scaphoid in wrist flexion. This observation is but a small example of the complexity of the kinematics of the wrist, and the reader is referred to the Suggested Reading list for additional study.

PERTINENT ANATOMY

The reader's understanding of carpal instability and the concepts of carpal kinematics will be enhanced by a review of the current description and terminology of the carpal ligaments.

Palmar Radiocarpal Ligaments

Figure 11.2-1 shows these ligaments, including the radioscaphocapitate, long radiolunate (previously named the radiotriquetral and also the radiolunotriquetral) and short radiolunate, radioscapholunate, pisohamate, triquetrocapitate, ulnocapitate, ulnotriquetral and palmar radioulnar ligaments.

Dorsal Radiocarpal Ligaments

Figure 11.2-2 shows these ligaments, including the dorsal intercarpal, dorsal scaphotriquetral, and dorsoradiocarpal (sometimes called the dorsal radiotriquetral) ligaments.

Palmar Midcarpal and Proximal and Distal-Row Interosseous Ligaments

Figure 11.2-3 shows the capitohamate, triquetrohamate, triquetrocapitate, lunotriquetral, scapholunate, scaphocapitate, scaphotrapezium-trapezoid, trapeziotrapezoid, and trapeziocapitate ligaments. The scapholunate (SL) ligament is divided into three parts: dorsal (the most substantial part), proximal, and palmar. It is the main stabilizer of the scaphoid that prevents it from flexing under load. In contrast to the SL ligament, the lunotriquetral (LT) ligament is more substantial in its palmar aspect.

CLASSIFICATION

A currently accepted classification system is presented as an aid to understanding some of the more common patterns of carpal instability.

Carpal Instability Dissociative (CID)

This compound term is used to describe an injury to one of the major interosseous ligaments involving the same carpal row. It is termed *dissociative* because there is separation or dissociation between at least two carpal bones. Common examples of CID are scapholunate dissociation, lunotriquetral dissociation, unstable scaphoid fracture, and perilunate dislocation. Examples of scapholunate dissociation and lunotriquetral dissociation are given in Figures 11.2-4 and 11.2-5.

The introduction of scapholunate and lunotriquetral dissociation allows us to add two other compound terms that the reader will encounter in descriptions of these injuries.

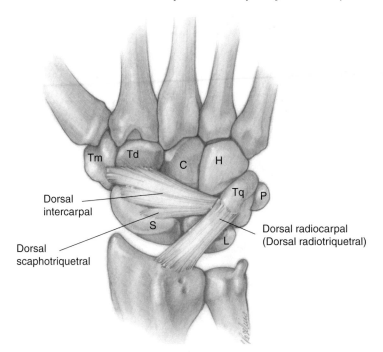

Figure 11.2-2 The dorsal radiocarpal ligaments (see text for details).

Dorsal Intercalated Segment Instability (DISI)

In SL dissociation, a collapse deformity occurs in which the lunate and triquetrum *usually* rotate into an extended posture (they face *dorsally*) that is combined with supination and radial deviation. Figure 11.2-6 demonstrates a chronic scapholunate dissociation showing a DISI deformity.

Volar Intercalated Segment Instability (VISI)

In lunotriquetral dissociation, the lunate rotates into a flexed posture (it faces palmarward, or *volar*).

Late Results of Untreated SL Dissociation

Untreated SL dissociation may often be associated with a condition called *scapholunate advanced collapse* or *SLAC* deformity. If scapholunate dissociation is present for a prolonged period of time, it will result in a scapholunate advanced collapse deformity, with severe arthritis in the radioscaphoid and midcarpal region.

The articular surface of the distal radius that articulates with the scaphoid is elliptical, and dorsal scaphoid dissociation or subluxation results in *incongruity between the scaphoid and the scaphoid fossa* in the radius. This is

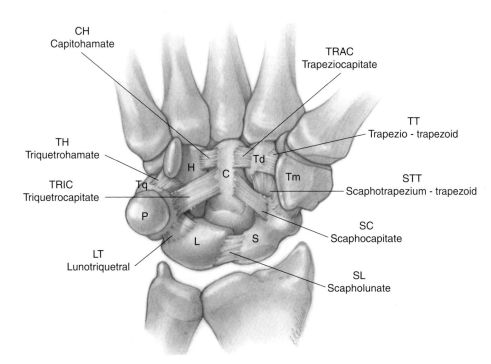

Figure 11.2-3 Palmar midcarpal and proximal- and distal-row interosseous ligaments (see text for details).

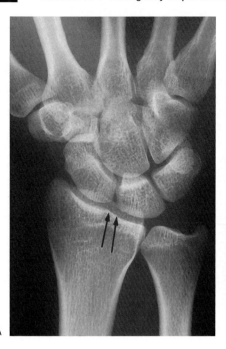

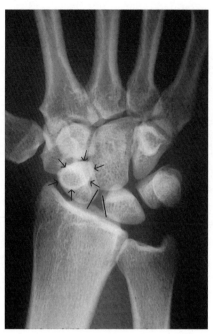

Figure 11.2-4   Comparison of x-ray findings in a normal wrist and in one with a scapholunate dissociation. **A.** The normal appearance of the wrist in the AP view. Note the uniform spacing of the carpal bones, and more specifically, the parallel alignment of the articular interface between the proximal pole of the scaphoid and the lunate (*parallel vertical arrows*). **B.** A scapholunate dissociation showing a widened and nonparallel space between the scaphoid and lunate, a foreshortened scaphoid, and a positive "ring sign" (*arrows in a circle*).

analogous to two superimposed and co-linear tea spoons that normally are co-linear but then one spoon (scaphoid) rotates into noncolinear alignment. The result of this incongruous alignment is arthritis. Figure 11.2-7 demonstrates the mechanism for development of a SLAC arthrosis.

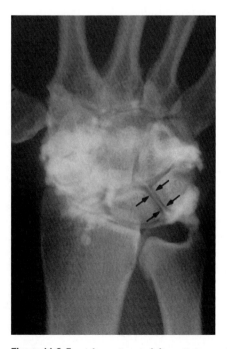

Figure 11.2-5   A lunotriquetral dissociation as shown by an arthrogram. Note the presence of radio-opaque dye in the space between the lunate and triquetrum (*opposing arrows*), indicating disruption of the lunotriquetral ligament.

Carpal Instability Nondissociative (CIND)

It is called *nondissociative* because there is no scapholunate separation or *dissociation* between the proximal pole of the scaphoid and the adjacent lunate or between the lunate and the triquetrum. CIND is often referred to as midcarpal instability. This condition refers to carpal instability that is characterized by a major noninterosseous ligament injury that could be seen in dorsal or palmar carpal subluxation/dislocation and ulnar translation. It is termed *radiocarpal CIND*. Figure 11.2-8 represents an example of CIND in a patient with palmar radiocarpal dislocation.

Midcarpal CIND is characterized by midcarpal instability, such as capitate lunate instability (CLIP wrist), palmar or dorsal midcarpal instability, and medial anteromedial instability (MAMI). Symptoms are often present as a painful wrist clunk that is reproduced by pronation, axial compression, and ulnar deviation. The sequence of events is as follows: with radial deviation, the proximal row palmar flexes; during ulnar deviation, there is loss of the normal synchronous (or smooth) movement of the proximal row, and it "jumps" rather than glides into extension; this precipitous catch-up movement or clunk reproduces the patient's symptoms.

Carpal Instability Complex (CIC)

A useful definition of these injuries is when the instability involves or impairs the relationship of the bones in the same row (CID type) *and* the relationship between rows (CIND type). Dorsal perilunate dislocation, trans-scaphoid perilunate fracture dislocation, trans-scaphoid trans-capitate dislocation, and trans-triquetrum perilunate fracture dislocation are all types of CIC injuries. The first two injuries are the most common.

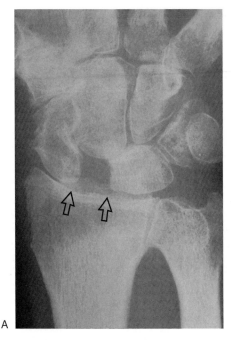
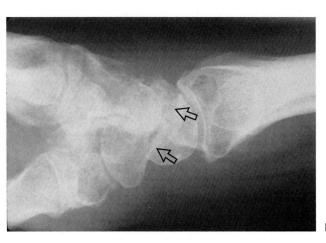

A   B

Figure 11.2-6   DISI deformity as seen in an established scapholunate dissociation. **A.** AP view of the wrist showing a widened scapholunate space (*vertical arrows*). **B.** Note the dorsally rotated lunate (*arrows*) on the lateral view.

Further division of these injuries may be made into *lesser* and *greater arc* injuries (Figure 11.2-9). Lesser arc injuries are defined as purely *ligamentous injuries* without fracture, and greater arc injuries share the same mechanism of injury but are associated with a *fracture* through a carpal bone. A classic example of the latter is the trans-scaphoid perilunate fracture dislocation (Figure 11.2-10). Slower loading forces (injuries) are usually associated with carpal fractures, in contrast to faster loading forces that usually produce a purely ligamentous injury.

Carpal Instability Adaptive (CIA)

The term *extrinsic midcarpal instability* has been used to describe this *secondary* carpal instability that results from dorsal angulation of the distal radius in malunited fractures of the distal radius. This term is used to differentiate or distinguish this instability from those midcarpal instabilities that are intrinsic to the carpus. The deformity in the radius leads to a secondary malalignment of the proximal carpal row, loss of wrist flexion and *radiocarpal* or *midcarpal* instability.

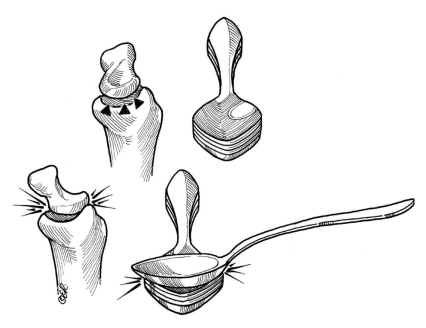

Figure 11.2-7   Artist's depiction of the pathomechanics of the SLAC arthrosis (see text for details).

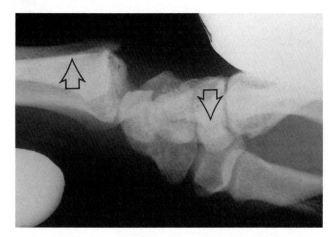

Figure 11.2-8 Lateral x-ray view, showing a radiocarpal palmar subluxation. This was a stress radiograph (*arrows*).

Clinical Findings. These patients present with complaints of pain in the wrist, and there is tenderness over the radiocarpal and midcarpal region, along with an obvious deformity of the wrist. Corrective osteotomy of the radius may help in re-alignment of the carpus.

DIAGNOSIS

Physical Examination

Watson's Scaphoid Shift Maneuver
- This maneuver is a physical examination technique that aids in the diagnosis of scapholunate dissociation. It is performed with the forearm in slight pronation.
- This maneuver is performed by applying pressure over the palmar tubercle of the scaphoid by the examiner's thumb with the wrist in ulnar deviation and slight extension.
- Pressure is maintained on the distal pole of the scaphoid and then the wrist is brought into radial deviation and slight flexion.

- *In wrists with this form of instability (SL), the proximal pole of the scaphoid is displaced dorsally over the lip of the radius.*
- Release of the thumb pressure causes the scaphoid's dorsally displaced proximal pole to return to its *anatomic* position in the scaphoid fossa of the radius, and a palpable (and usually painful) "clunk" or "pop" may be noted (Figure 11.2-11).

Ballottement Test
- The ballottement test or maneuver is used to identify abnormal motion or tenderness at the lunotriquetral junction.
- It is done by firmly fixing the lunate with the examiner's thumb and index finger of one hand while the pisiform and triquetrum are displaced dorsally and volarly with the other hand's thumb and index finger (Figure 11.2-12).
- A positive test is revealed by pain, and indicates lunotriquetral instability.

Other Tests
- Various forms of compression, distraction, and translation may reveal abnormal mobility or pain patterns with these motions, and can be indicative of various types of instability about the wrist as previously described.
- Some patients may be able to reproduce various clunks and abnormal movements about the wrist that may sometimes aid the astute examiner in establishing a diagnosis.

Radiologic Examination

- Imaging techniques include standard x-ray views such as the PA and lateral, PA in radial and ulnar deviation, and lateral views in flexion and extension, as well as AP and lateral views with a fist.
- The Moneim view is taken with the wrist elevated on the ulnar side by a sponge pad.
  - This view facilitates observation of the space between the proximal pole of the scaphoid and the adjacent lunate, and will often reveal a scapholunate separation that may not be seen on the regular PA films.

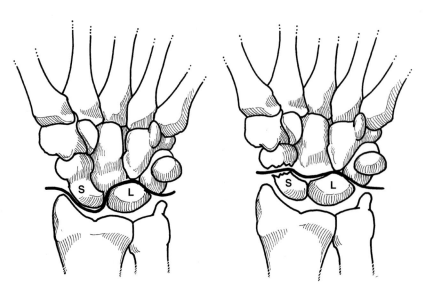

Figure 11.2-9 The lesser and greater carpal arcs (see text for details).

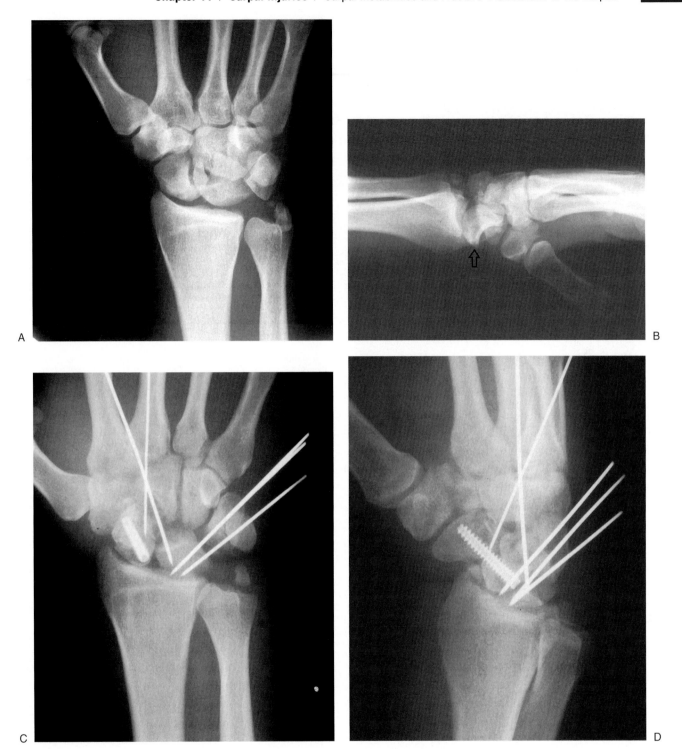

Figure 11.2-10   Trans-scaphoid-perilunate fracture dislocation. **A.** PA view showing the loss of continuity of the carpal arcs described by Gilula (see Figure 11.2-13). **B.** Lateral view of the palmar-flexed lunate (*vertical open arrow*) and dorsal displacement of the remaining carpus around the lunate. **C, D.** Internal fixation techniques used to restore the architectural integrity of the carpus. (Courtesy of H. Relton McCarroll, Jr., MD, San Francisco)

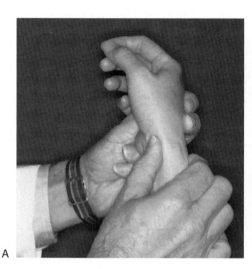
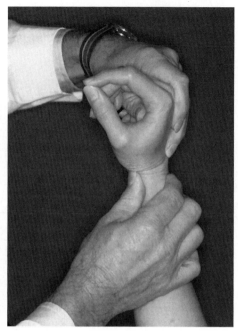

A   B

Figure 11.2-11   The scaphoid shift maneuver for a SL dissociation (see text for details).

- Similarly, PA views with radial and ulnar deviation may show a separation that may not be seen on regular films.
    - Axial loading or compression of the carpus by making a fist often demonstrates a scapholunate separation that might not be present on routine radiographs.

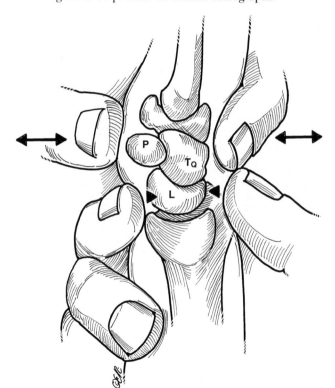

Figure 11.2-12   Ballottement maneuver for LTD (see text for details).

- Additional imaging techniques include arthrography with or without videofluoroscopy, bone scans, tomograms, and a CT or MRI.
    - A tomogram or CT is a useful aid in evaluating associated fractures. At this point in time, an MRI is less helpful.
- An arthrogram is cost effective and, when done as a triple phase injection, may provide useful information about the midcarpal, radiocarpal, and distal radioulnar articulation.
    - Contrast material injected into the midcarpal joint should not extend into the radiocarpal joint unless there is a ligament disruption in the proximal row (see Figure 11.2-5).
- An arthrogram is easy to obtain, and has been most helpful in terms of revealing disruption of the interosseous ligaments.
    - Arthroscopy of the wrist is preferred over an arthrogram by some surgeons, and may be more accurate in determining the extent of ligament injury and the status of the cartilage surface.
- A bone scan is nonspecific, although it may reveal inflammatory changes about the joint.

Defining Normal Carpal Alignment

Carpal Arcs, Carpal Spacing and Lunate Configuration

- Gilula identified three unbroken arcs that mark the articular margins of the proximal and distal carpal row in the PA x-ray view of the wrist. A set-off in any of these arcs or lines indicates an intercarpal derangement at the site where the line is offset (Figure 11.2-13).
- Most articulating bones have a space between them that is usually 2 mm or less, and any overlap greater than 4 mm is suggestive of a carpal joint abnormality.

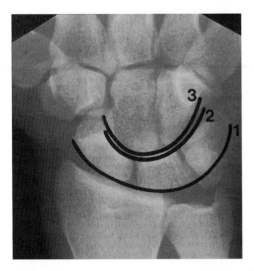

Figure 11.2-13 Gilula lines demarcating the proximal and distal carpal rows.

In PA-neutral x-ray views of the wrist, the lunate normally has a *trapezoidal* shape. If the lunate is *triangular* in shape, it suggests a malrotated lunate (either flexed or extended).

Measurement of Carpal Bone Alignment

- Commonly used measurements made from lateral wrist radiographs are the scapholunate angle, the capitolunate angle, the radiolunate angle, and the lunotriquetral angle.
- These angles are depicted in Figure 11.2-14.

The SL Angle

- The SL angle is measured by a line drawn through the longitudinal axis of the scaphoid from the distal to proximal pole, and by a line drawn through the horizontal axis of the lunate.
- Normal values range from 30 to 60 degrees, with an average of 47 degrees.
- Angles greater than 70 to 80 degrees are a definite indication of SL dissociation.

The Capitolunate (CL) Angle

- Although the longitudinal axes of the radius, lunate, capitate, and third metacarpal are not usually colinear, the CL angle is useful when studying midcarpal (CIND) instabilities.
- A line is drawn that is perpendicular to a line that connects the palmar and dorsal tips of the lunate.

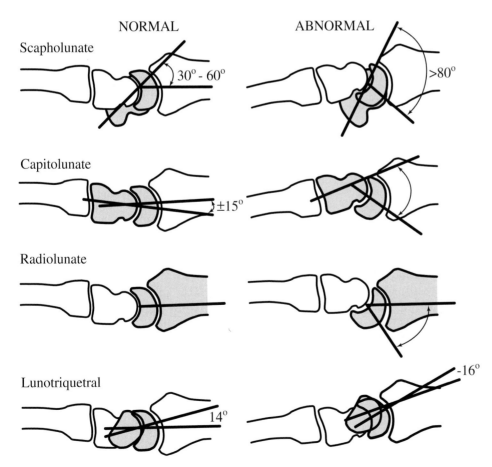

Figure 11.2-14 Useful carpal angles (see text for details).

- The capitate axis is represented by a line drawn from a point in the center of the convexity of the capitate head to a point at the center of its distal articular surface.
- Theoretically, the normal CL axis should be 0 degrees with the wrist in neutral, but what is considered normal ranges to 15 degrees.

The Radiolunate (RL) Angle

- A line is drawn that is perpendicular to a line that connects the palmar and dorsal tips of the lunate.
- The angle formed by this line and the longitudinal axis of the radius is the RL angle.
- An RL angle greater than 15 degrees is abnormal, and such a finding is associated with DISI and VISI deformities.

The Lunotriquetral (LT) Angle

- The lunotriquetral angle represents that angle formed by a line drawn through the horizontal (longitudinal axis) axis of the lunate and a line drawn through the longitudinal axis of the triquetrum.
- The accurate assessment of these axes is difficult to determine.
- The average normal angle is 14 degrees.
- In lunotriquetral dissociation, the angle averages −16 degrees.

Other Useful Diagnostic Findings

- Scapholunate dissociation is one of the most common forms of carpal instability.
- Common findings that may be noted on plain radiographs are foreshortening of the scaphoid, the appearance of a ring in the distal pole of the scaphoid, lack of parallel apposition of the adjacent articular surfaces of the scaphoid and lunate, widening of the space between the proximal pole of the scaphoid and the lunate, and an increased scapholunate angle (Figure 11.2-4).

TREATMENT

- Treatment options may vary according to many factors, which include the location of the instability, the underlying cause, the length of time from injury to treatment, the presence or absence of secondary deformities and arthrosis, and whether the instability is static or dynamic.
- In general, surgical treatment is based on the principles of *carpal realignment* and *restoration of normal carpal kinematics*.
- Attempts to achieve these two principles have included *ligamentous reconstruction* and *capsulodesis* of various

forms, *arthrodesis* of various types, *carpectomy* and *realignment osteotomy* of the radius in CIA types of instability.

- A detailed discussion of these techniques is beyond the scope of this text. New techniques and methods will no doubt evolve as the understanding of this complex joint grows.

SUGGESTED READING

Amadio PC, Taleisnik J. Fractures of the carpal bones. In: Green DP, Hotchkiss RN, Pederson WC, eds. Green's operative hand surgery. 4th Ed. New York: Churchill Livingstone, 1999:809–864.

Blatt G. Capsulodesis in reconstructive hand surgery. Dorsal capsulodesis for the unstable scaphoid and volar capsulodesis following excision of the distal ulna. Hand Clin 1987;3:81–102.

Brahin B, Allieu Y. Compensatory carpal malalignments. Ann Chir Main, 1984;3:357–363.

Burge P. Closed cast treatment of scaphoid fractures. Hand Clinics 2001;17:541–552.

Dovan TT, Gelberman RH, Cooney WP. Carpal Instability. In Trumble TE, ed. Hand surgery update 3, hand, elbow and shoulder. Rosemont, IL: Amer. Soc Surg Hand, 2003:205–216.

Doyle JR, Botte MJ. Surgical anatomy of the hand and upper extremity. Chapter 1, Skeletal anatomy, pp. 1–91; Chapter 4, Vascular anatomy, pp. 237–293; Chapter 9, The wrist, pp. 486–531, Philadelphia: Lippincott Williams & Wilkins, 2002.

Garcia-Elias M. Carpal instabilities and dislocations. In: Green DP, Hotchkiss RN, Pederson WC, eds. Green's operative hand surgery. 4th Ed. New York: Churchill Livingstone, 1999:865–928.

Gilula LA, et al. Roentgenographic diagnosis of the painful wrist. Clin Orthop 1984;187:52–64.

Imbriglia JE, Broudy AS, et al. Proximal row carpectomy: clinical evaluation. J Hand Surg 1990;15:426–430.

Kleinman WB. Dynamics of carpal instability. In: Watson HK, Weinzweig J, eds. The wrist. Philadelphia: Lippincott, Williams and Wilkins, 2001:456–481.

Kleinman WB, Carroll CT. Scapho-trapeziotrapezoid arthrodesis for treatment of chronic static and dynamic scapho-lunate instability: a 10-year perspective on pitfalls and complications. J Hand Surg 1990;15:408–414.

Knoll VD, Trumble TE: Scaphoid fractures and nonunions. In Trumble TE, ed. Hand surgery update 3, hand, elbow and shoulder. Rosemont, IL: Amer. Soc Surg Hand, 2003:161–173.

Park MJ, Cooney WP III, Hahn ME, et al. The effects of dorsally angulated distal radius fractures on carpal kinematics. J Hand Surg 1990;15:721–727.

Putnam MD, Meyer NJ. Carpal fractures excluding the scaphoid. In Trumble T, ed. Hand surgery update 3, hand, elbow and shoulder. Rosemont, IL: Amer. Soc Surg Hand, 2003:175–187.

Taleisnik J, Watson HK. Midcarpal instability caused by malunited fractures of the distal radius. J Hand Surg 1984;9A:350–357.

Tolo ET, Shin AY. Fracture dislocations of the carpus. In Trumble T, ed. Hand surgery update 3, hand, elbow and shoulder. Rosemont, IL: Amer. Soc Surg Hand, 2003:189–204.

Watson HK, Ashmead DT, et al. Examination of the scaphoid. J Hand Surg 1988;13:657–660.

Watson HK, Ballet FL. The SLAC wrist: scapholunate advanced collapse pattern of degenerative arthritis. J Hand Surg 1984;9:358–365.

TENDON INJURIES

12.1 Flexor
Tendon 179

12.2 Extensor
Tendon 190

12.1 FLEXOR TENDON

The results of flexor tendon surgery have improved significantly over the last 40 years, based on an improved understanding of the anatomy and biology of the flexor tendon system, improved sutures and suture techniques, and the development of rehabilitation protocols that facilitated early recovery and improved functional results. Currently accepted general principles of treatment include primary repair of recent clean injuries in the operating room, with repair of both flexor tendons using suture techniques at the repair site that minimally distort the anatomy of the tendons and that are strong enough to allow early protected movement. Additional factors in a successful outcome relate to preservation of the critical portions of the pulley system.

PERTINENT ANATOMY

Figure 12.1-1 depicts the most common anatomical arrangement of the synovial sheaths and flexor tendon pulleys in the thumb and fingers.

Digital Flexor Sheath

The digital flexor tendon sheath is composed of *synovial* (membranous) and *retinacular* (pulley) tissue components. It is a system that allows a tendon to "turn a corner" and maximize the available tendon excursion to produce a significant arc of flexion. Loss of this pulley system results in "bowstringing" of the tendon and loss of flexion.

Membranous Portion

The membranous portion is a synovial tube sealed at both ends. The floor or dorsal aspect of this tunnel is composed of the transverse metacarpal ligament, the palmar plates of the metacarpophalangeal (MCP), proximal interphalangeal (PIP), and distal interphalangeal (DIP) joints, and the palmar surfaces of the proximal and middle phalanges. In the

index, long, and ring fingers, the membranous portion of the sheath begins at the neck of the metacarpals and continues distally to end at the DIP joint. In most instances, the small finger synovial sheath continues proximally to the wrist.

Visceral and parietal synovial layers are present, and a prominent synovial pouch is present proximally that represents the confluence of the visceral and parietal layers. A visceral layer reflection or pouch is also noted between the two flexors at the neck of the metacarpal, but is 4 to 5 mm distal to the more visible proximal and superficial portions of the synovial sheath. The membranous or synovial portions of the sheath are most noticeable in the spaces between the pulleys, where they form plicae and pouches to accommodate flexion and extension of the digits.

Retinacular Portion

The retinacular (pulley) portion is a series of transverse (the palmar aponeurosis pulley), annular, and cruciform fibrous tissue condensations, which begin in the distal palm and end at the DIP joint.

With the exception of the third annular pulley, the pulleys are located between joints; this fact, along with some element of compressibility, allows a large arc of flexion without impingement. The finger pulley system consists of the palmar aponeurosis pulley, five annular, and three cruciform pulleys. The second and fourth annular pulleys are the most important to preserve or reconstruct in flexor tendon surgery. In the thumb, two annular and one oblique pulley are present, and it is the oblique pulley that is most important from a functional perspective.

The reader is referred to the Suggested Reading list at the end of this chapter for references that detail additional anatomic features of the flexor tendon sheath and the biomechanical principles of muscle/tendon excursion, moment arms, radians, work of flexion, lubrication factors, tendon nutrition and healing.

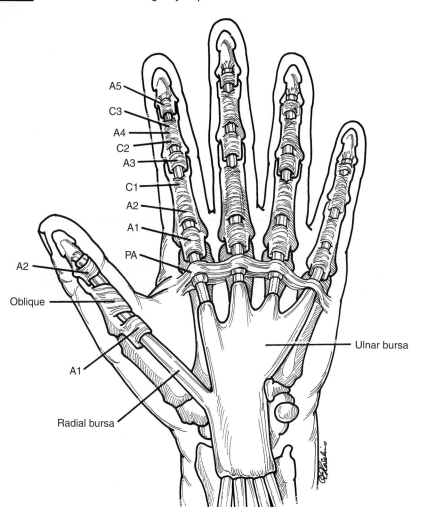

A5
C3
A4
C2
A3
C1
A2
A1
PA
A2
Oblique
A1
Radial bursa

Ulnar bursa

Figure 12.1-1   Composite view of the synovial sheaths and pulleys system of the thumb and fingers (see text for details).

Vascular Supply of the Flexor Tendons

Sources of vascular supply to the flexor tendons are from intrinsic longitudinal vessels that continue from the palm, synovial attachments to the enclosed flexor tendons in the proximal sheath, and specialized forms of mesotendon called the vincula, located inside the sheath (Figure 12.1-2).

Clinical Significance

Removal of the flexor digitorum superficialis (FDS) for a tendon transfer is best performed proximal to or at the proximal edge of Camper's chiasma, since this will preserve the vinculum breve superficialis (VBS) and vinculum longum profundus (VLP). This may have the incidental side benefit of avoiding the potential for hyperextension at the PIP joint, as well as preserving the blood supply of the FDS and flexor digitorum profundus (FDP). See Figure 12.1-3. Core intratendinous sutures are ideally placed in the relatively avascular *palmar* aspect of the profundus tendon, when practical. The comparative role of synovial nutrition and the vascular supply in tendon healing will not be debated here except to put into context the value of avoiding damage to the vascularity of the tendons in the sheath.

ZONES OF FLEXOR TENDON INJURY

Finger Zones

The naming of five zones of injury in the fingers has aided in comparison of results, and to some extent is of prognostic value. The zones are depicted in Figure 12.1-4.

- Zone I is just beyond the insertion of the FDS to the insertion of the FDP. This zone is occupied *only* by the FDP.
- Zone II is from the distal palmar crease to the distal insertion of the FDS, and injuries in this zone more likely than not involve both flexor tendons.
- Zone III begins just distal to the distal edge of the transverse carpal ligament (at the origin of the lumbrical muscles) and ends at the distal palmar crease.
- Zone IV is the region of the carpal tunnel.
- Zone V is at the wrist and distal forearm.

Thumb Zones

The thumb zones of injury are depicted in Figure 12.1-4.

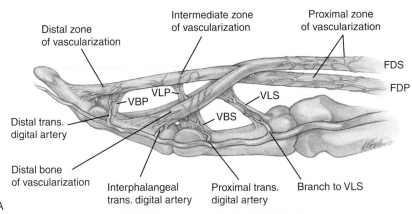

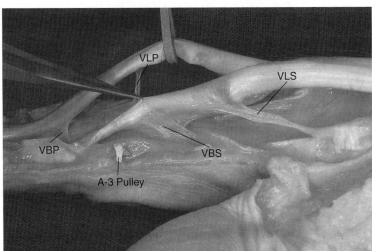

Figure 12.1-2 **A**. Artist's depiction of the blood supply of the finger flexor tendons. **B**. Fresh cadaver dissection of the flexor tendons showing the vincula. VBP, vinculum breve profundus; VLP, vinculum longum profundus; VLS, vinculum longum superficialis; VBS, vinculum breve superficialis.

DIAGNOSIS

Physical Examination

The Finger Cascade

■ Many flexor tendon injuries may be diagnosed by noting the *posture* of the injured hand/digit, and comparing it to that in the opposite hand or adjacent digits.

■ The normal posture of the fingers reveals a progressive flexion posture, or *cascade*, with the little finger being the most flexed, and the index being the least flexed.

■ Figure 12.1-5 demonstrates the loss of the normal finger cascade in this young male with a laceration to the medial side of the left ring finger.

■ Findings at surgery confirmed complete laceration of the FDS and FDP in this zone II injury.

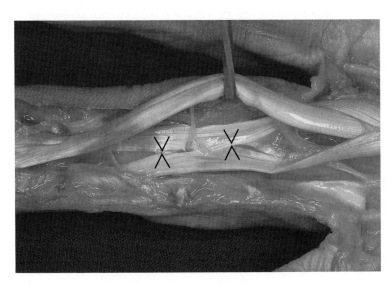

Figure 12.1-3 Fresh cadaver dissection showing Camper's chiasma (*opposing arrows*) in the FDS tendon in the region of the PIP joint (see text for details).

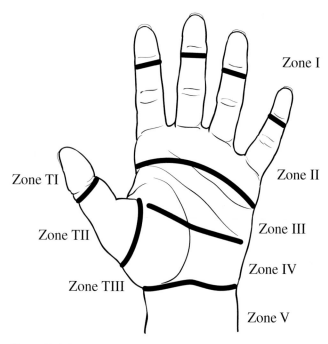

Figure 12.1-4 The zones of flexor tendon injury (see text for details).

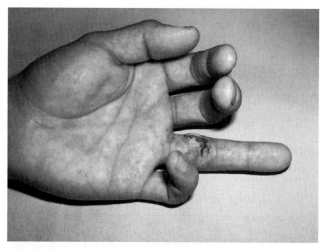

Figure 12.1-5 Note the loss of the normal finger cascade in this young male with a laceration of the proximal phalanx. The preoperative diagnosis of laceration of both flexor tendons was confirmed at surgery.

- Figure 12.1-6 demonstrates a more subtle loss of the normal finger cascade associated with a rupture of the insertion of the FDP (zone I injury) in this teenage flag ball player.
  - There is a comparative lack of flexion in the ring finger (loss of cascade) compared with the adjacent fingers, and a lack of flexion at the DIP joint when making a fist.
  - This is an avulsion of the insertion of the FDP of the ring finger.

Direct Testing of FDS and FDP
- Figure 12.1-7 demonstrates the techniques used to demonstrate the function of the FDS and FDP.

- Trapping the adjacent fingers in *extension* permits only the FDS to flex the PIP joint.
- This maneuver works because the FDS is functionally characterized as four independent muscle bellies with four separate tendons.
- The FDP is easily isolated by blocking motion at the PIP joint.

TREATMENT

- Laceration of the flexor tendons represents a significant and serious injury.
- Surgical repair is best performed by experienced surgeons who have suitable facilities and instruments available for repair.
- Flexor tendon injuries are not considered to be true emergencies, and best results are obtained when such

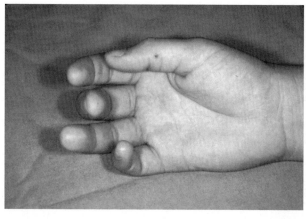

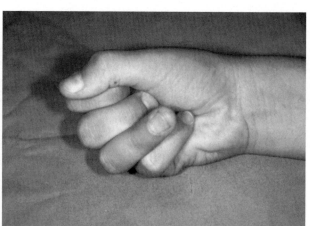

Figure 12.1-6 FDP tendon rupture in a flagball player. **A.** Note the loss of normal finger cascade and the increased extension posture of the right ring finger. **B.** Note the loss of flexion in the DIP joint while making a complete fist.

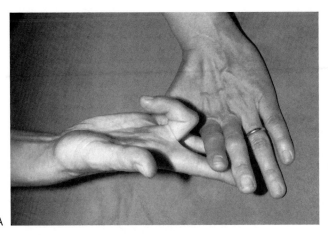 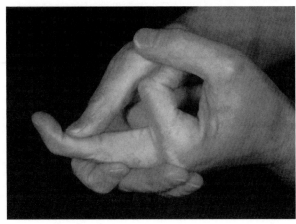

A   B

Figure 12.1-7   Testing for function of the FDS and FDP tendons. **A.** Holding the adjacent fingers in extension permits only the FDS to act on the PIP joint of this middle finger. **B.** Holding the PIP joint in extension permits isolation of the FDP tendon function.

surgeries are performed in a timely fashion but on an elective basis.

■ If both tendons are lacerated, both tendons are repaired.

■ Zone II injuries are the most likely to result in adhesions and loss of function.

■ The post-operative management of these injuries is very important, and should be considered a part of the surgical protocol.

Surgical Exposures

■ Most flexor tendon injuries are due to lacerations of the palmar surface of the digits or palm.

■ These lacerations are more often than not *transverse* in orientation.

■ Figure 12.1-8 demonstrates how these traumatic incisions may be appropriately extended to achieve surgical exposure and at the same time avoid a pernicious scar that might produce a contracture.

■ These elective extensions of the transverse wounds are positioned to utilize the fact that midaxial incisions do not contract and allow the elevation of a thick and well-vascularized flap for exposure.

   ■ The wounds may also be extended by using oblique limbs of extension that also meet the same needs.

Suture Materials

■ Tendon sutures have been fabricated from various materials, including stainless steel, nylon, polypropylene, and polyester.

■ Because of its ease of use, strength, and minimal elasticity, 3-0 and 4-0 braided polyester sutures are commonly used for flexor tendon repairs.

Suture Techniques

■ Many techniques have been developed for reapproximation of the lacerated flexor tendons since Bunnell

developed his well-known tendon-grasping suture more than 50 years ago.

■ Although there may not be an ideal suture technique, there are some underlying principles in all suture techniques: ease of suture placement, secure knots that will not slip or stretch out, a smooth suture junction without gapping or bunching, and sufficient strength to allow early supervised motion programs (see the section on rehabilitation that follows).

■ A suture technique developed by Strickland is depicted in Figure 12.1-9. It begins as a two-strand, core-grasping technique supplemented by a second-core suture and a running and locking epitendinous suture.

■ The strength of a given suture repair is nearly directly proportional to the number of strands of suture material that cross the repair site, and to the size of the suture material.

■ A four-strand repair is stronger that a two-strand repair.

■ The addition of a peripheral epitendinous suture to the core sutures has been found to increase the strength of the repair site in a significant fashion. This helps prevent gap formation that may lead to adhesions and failure to recover useful motion in the digit.

■ The epitendinous suture may also "tidy up," reconform, and "debulk" the repair site to permit easy passage of the repair site through the critical pulleys.

Some Points of Intraoperative Technique

■ *Atraumatic technique* is a useful descriptive term to note that careful meticulous dissection and gentle handling of all tissues is very important in the management of flexor tendon injuries.

■ After extending the wound and opening the sheath *at the anticipated repair site*, it is necessary to retrieve the two tendon ends. The distal end is usually retrieved by flexing the digit.

■ The proximal end retracts due to the physiologic tension of the muscle, and if not retracted too far proximally by

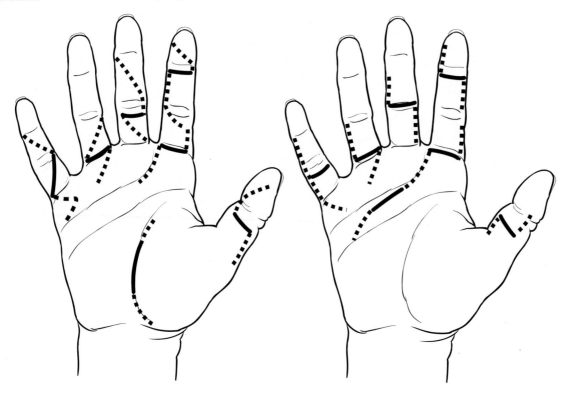

Figure 12.1-8 Useful skin incisions for the extension of traumatic wounds associated with flexor tendon injuries. The solid lines represent the traumatic wound, and the dotted lines represent the safe extensions of these wounds for exposure and repair.

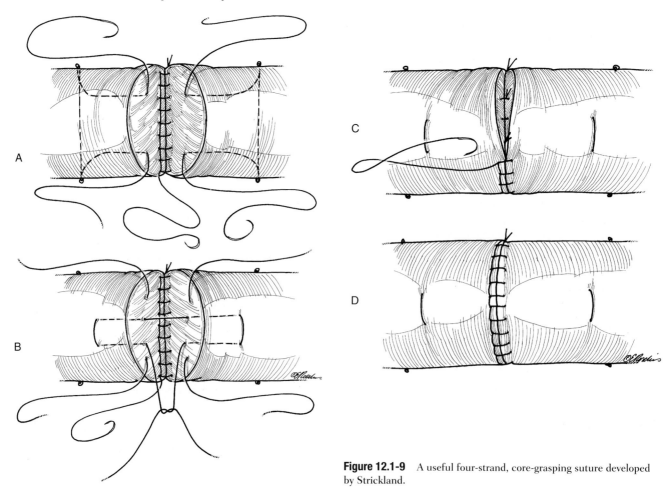

Figure 12.1-9 A useful four-strand, core-grasping suture developed by Strickland.

intact vincula, may be grasped with fine tooth forceps and brought distally.

- *Blind repeated probing up the proximal sheath with a grasping instrument is to be avoided.* If the proximal end cannot be easily grasped or "milked down" by digital massage, then a small and moistened feeding tube catheter is passed proximally (usually into the palm), and the retracted tendon is sutured to the catheter at this level. The catheter is then brought distally into the repair site, carrying with it the proximal tendon stump. When the two stumps are adjacent, a 22-gauge hypodermic needle is passed transversely through the sheath to impale and fix the proximal tendon.
- A repair of the surgeon's choice and experience is performed.
- Indiscriminant excision of the membranous or retinacular portions of the sheath is to be avoided, but portions of the sheath may be incised or excised to promote placement of the sutures.
- Repair of the incised sheath has been advocated by some surgeons, but such repair should not compromise the gliding movement of the repaired tendons in the sheath.

Rehabilitation

Rationale

- Early passive motion is designed to change an unfavorable scar to a favorable one by altering the biologic process of collagen synthesis and degradation.
  - Early passive motion by applying small but frequent forces in opposite directions modifies and elongates restrictive tendon adhesions.
- Studies have shown that early motion stress to repaired flexor tendons results in more rapid recovery of tensile

strength, less adhesions, better tendon excursion, and minimal repair site deformation.

- Load at failure of *mobilized* tendons tested at 3 weeks was twice that of *immobilized* tendons, and the favorable differences continued at all intervals through 12 weeks.
- Studies have revealed that passive MCP joint movement results in little or no motion of the flexor tendons, whereas DIP joint motion results in FDP excursion of 1 to 2 mm/10 degrees of joint flexion.
  - Each 10 degrees of PIP flexion results in FDP and the FDS excursion of about 1.5 mm.

Some Practical Applications of These Principles

- These and other studies and experience have led to the progressive evolution and development of tendon mobilization protocols and techniques that focus on promoting motion at the PIP joint.

Active Extension-Elastic Band Flexion Method

- The first technique is the most widely used at this time. An orthotic device maintains the wrist and MCP joints in slight flexion.
- An elastic band is attached to the fingernail of the involved digit, this elastic band is passed beneath a midpalmar bar and is anchored proximally on a portion of the orthotic device.
- Figure 12.1-10 demonstrates an example of a currently used method.

Controlled Passive Motion Method

- This method involves immobilization of the wrist and digits in a similar orthotic device, but movement is achieved

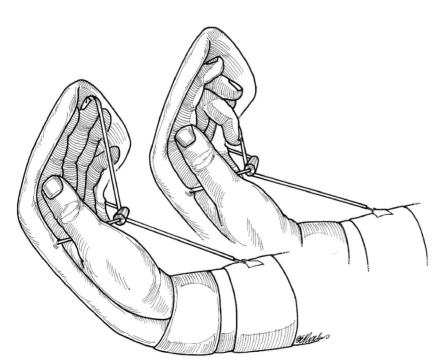

Figure 12.1-10   Active extension-elastic band flexion rehabilitation method for flexor tendon repairs.

by serial passive movement of the DIP, PIP, and MCP joints.

■ Those that use this method state that it is less likely to result in flexion contracture when compared to the elastic band traction method.

Controlled Active Motion Method

■ The introduction and use of 4-6 strand tendon repair methods has made it possible to use this method with a certain level of safety in terms of its major complication of tendon rupture.

■ In any splinting program, it is best to maintain the interdigital joints in extension to minimize the likelihood of flexion contractures.

■ The specific details of these three methods are beyond the scope of this text and will no doubt evolve and change. Also, completely new methods may be developed in response to the need for better final results.

Caveats

■ Utilization of any of these methods requires a team approach with a surgeon and therapist.

■ A cooperative patient is mandatory for success when using any of these methods.

Investigative Methods to Limit Peritendinous Adhesions

■ The methods of early excursion of the tendon repair site just reviewed are a form of *extrinsic mechanical* means to limit adhesions.

■ Investigative methods have included the insertion of polyvinyl alcohol shields (PVA) as an *intrinsic mechanical* shield to limit peritendinous adhesions following flexor tendon repair.

    ▪ The material is semipermeable, allowing passage of synovial fluid nutrients to the tendon repair site—but unfortunately, the method was associated with an increased rupture rate and a diminished strength of site repair.

■ Hyaluronic acid is a glycosaminoglycan normally found in the synovial fluid of the sheath.

    ▪ Studies have suggested that hyaluronic acid (HA) may limit the formation of adhesions following zone II flexor tendon repair, and a recent study found that an HA membrane applied circumferentially around the tendon repair site inhibited the formation of restrictive adhesions.

    ▪ Histologic examination of the tendon repair sites did not demonstrate any interference with intrinsic tendon repair.

■ The application of 5-fluorouracil to the repair site has been reported to result in diminished adhesions, without an increased risk of rupture.

Late Reconstruction

Tenolysis

■ Not all tendon repairs result in useful recovery of function; lysis of adhesions may be required in selected cases.

■ The indications for this procedure are when the patient has reached a plateau in their progress from splinting and therapy.

■ The needs of the patients, as well as their age, occupation, and the digit involved, may aid in the decision-making process.

■ The wise surgeon will recognize that a tenolysis operation may sometimes reveal a disrupted tendon and a severely compromised bed that only a staged tendon reconstruction can solve. Both the surgeon and patient must be prepared for this eventuality.

■ Surgeons vary in their opinion regarding the timing of tenolysis. Most would wait several months after primary repair or tendon grafting before considering this option.

Technique

■ Active participation of the patient is critical to the success of the operation and local anesthesia with intravenous sedation as needed is used.

■ A generous zigzag incision is laid out from the fingertip to the proximal palm, and is used as needed.

    ▪ All adhesions are excised, and the critical portions of the pulley system are preserved.

■ A staged tendon reconstruction should be considered when an adequate pulley system cannot be preserved.

    ▪ During the procedure, the active pull-through of the tendon is noted by having the patient actively flex the digit.

    ▪ The procedure ends when an adequate level of flexion is achieved.

■ Aftercare includes a splint that permits immediate and continued flexion of the digit.

■ In selected patients, an indwelling catheter may be left in place for 4 to 5 days for the instillation of small amounts of local anesthetic during exercise periods.

■ Any concomitant surgical procedures, such as capsulotomy, increase the risk for a poor result.

Two-Stage Tendon Reconstruction

Indications and Contraindications

■ Primary tendon repairs that have failed after repair and tenolysis are associated with joint contracture, have a known loss of critical pulleys, and, in patients in whom conventional tendon grafting is likely to fail, are candidates for two-stage tendon reconstruction.

■ The insertion of a silastic Hunter-tendon prosthesis permits the formation of a scar-free bed and sheath for subsequent insertion of a free tendon graft.

■ Contraindications include those digits with marginal circulation and sensibility, and patients unwilling or unable to engage in a prolonged, often tedious, and difficult rehabilitation process.

First Stage

■ The first stage consists of wide exposure of the flexor sheath and pulley system through a zigzag incision.

■ All useful portions of the pulley system are preserved, the flexor tendons excised, and a 1 cm stump of profundus tendon is left distally.

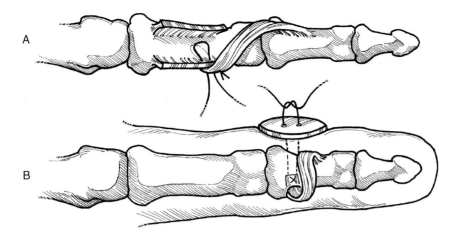

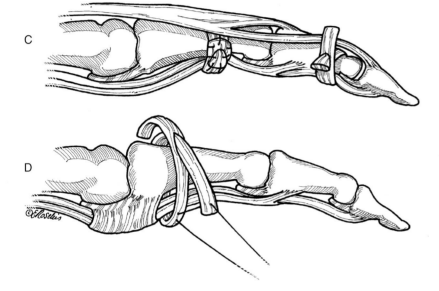

Figure 12.1-11 Methods of digital pulley reconstruction. **A, B.** Hemi-FDS to pulley remnant and to bone. **C, D.** Pulleys formed by single loop or loop and a half around phalanges, using tendon remnants of free tendon grafts. **E.** Pulley formed by using extensor retinaculum. **F, G.** Pulleys formed in palmar plate (Karev pulley) and using free graft tunneled through palmar plate. **H.** Pulley formed by graft interweave through remnants of tendon. *Figure continues.*

- The excised tendon material is kept moist for possible use as material to reconstruct pulleys.
- If available, one or two slips of the superficialis are left attached to use in pulley reconstruction.
- If any joint contractures are present and not corrected by excision of the flexor tendons, then joint release is performed by a palmar plate release and a collateral ligament incision.
- Dissection in the palm is carried to the level of the lumbrical origin.
- A second incision is made at the flexor aspect of the wrist to accept the proximal end of the silastic Hunter-tendon prosthesis.
- A suitably sized prosthesis (3 to 6 mm in width) is inserted from the fingertip to the wrist.
- The end of the Hunter tendon is sutured *beneath* the distal stump of the profundus.
- Pulleys are reconstructed to obtain a minimum of two pulleys (in the A2 and A4 positions) but more than two pulleys are desirable if possible.

- Some methods of pulley reconstruction are illustrated in Figure 12.1-11.
- Prior to closure the tendon is pulled at its proximal end to note that it glides freely and does not bowstring.
  - The tendon should also glide freely when the digit is extended. It should not buckle or bulge.
- Aftercare includes a bulky dressing, followed by a supervised passive exercise program.

Second Stage
- This stage is performed when satisfactory passive motion has been obtained. It usually takes 3 or more months.
- A suitable tendon graft (usually the plantaris, or, if not available, one of the long toe extensors) is attached to the proximal end of the Hunter tendon. The distal end of the Hunter tendon is detached and pulled distally to atraumatically insert the tendon graft into the new flexor sheath.

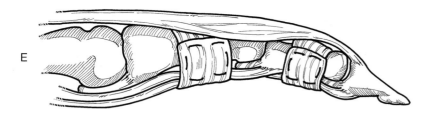

E

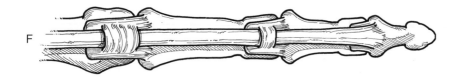

F

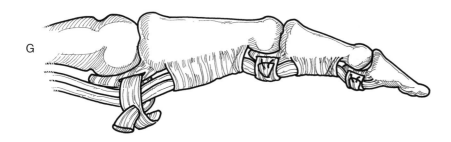

G

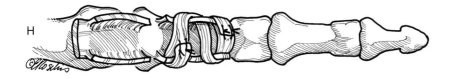

H

Figure 12.1-11 (*continued*)

- The distal anastomosis (first) is made into the stump of the profundus at the DIP joint, and the proximal anastomosis (at the wrist) made by joining the graft to a suitable donor—such as the profundus—to one of the central digits. An interweave technique is used to place the graft in the substance of the donor motor.
- Tension is adjusted prior to insertion of the proximal sutures to match the normal finger cascade.
  - Appropriate tension may be verified by noting *extension* of the operated digit when the wrist is flexed and *flexion* of the digit when the wrist is extended.
- Rehabilitation following the second stage reconstruction is via an active extension-elastic band flexion method, as previously described.
- Figure 12.1-12 demonstrates a two-stage Hunter tendon reconstruction sequence.

SPECIAL SITUATIONS

Partial Tendon Lacerations

- Although adequate tendon strength and function may be maintained after partial tendon lacerations, some partial lacerations may result in entrapment and triggering of the tendon against an adjacent pulley.
- Current recommendations are for repair of lacerations greater than 50% of the tendon, and debridement of the tendon edges in those less than 50%.
- Under no circumstances should the tendon ends be excised or "squared-up" to make the repair technically easier or more "tidy." Any shortening of a flexor tendon may result in the loss of extension of the digit.

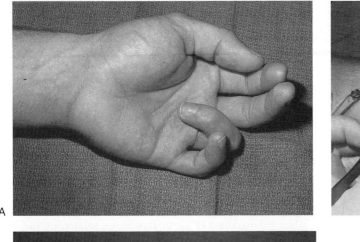
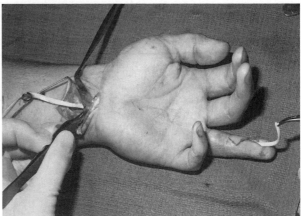
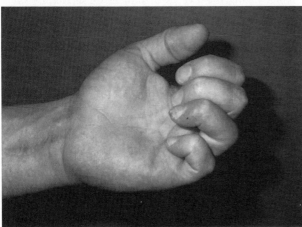
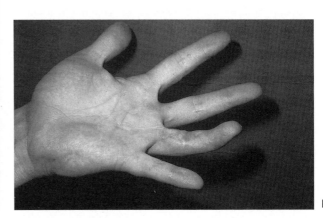

Figure 12.1-12 Two-stage Hunter tendon reconstruction for a fixed-flexion contracture of the ring finger following a failed flexor tendon repair. **A.** Note the fixed flexion contracture of the ring finger; passive extension was not possible. **B.** Insertion of a free tendon graft using the plantaris tendon. The plantaris tendon graft (*left*) is being drawn into the new flexor sheath by the Hunter tendon (*right*), following joint release, pulley reconstruction, and insertion of a Hunter tendon 4 months prior. **C, D.** Note the active flexion and nearly complete extension of the reconstructed finger.

Profundus Tendon Avulsion

- This injury is likely to occur in certain sports such as flag or regular football, in which forceful grasping is used to grab a flag or jersey of an opponent.
- The FDP of the *ring finger* is most often injured, and may be misdiagnosed by coaches and others as a "sprained finger." Radiographs are often negative.
- Figure 12.1-6 shows a classic clinical case that was diagnosed and treated a few days after injury. Function was restored.
- The avulsion may occur with a small or substantial bone fragment. The prognosis is based on the level to which the FDP retracts, the remaining blood supply of the tendon, the length of time between the injury and treatment, and the presence and size of the bone fragment.
- There are three types.
  - *Type I* is characterized by retraction of the profundus tendon into the palm.
    - □ If seen early, it may be threaded back down the flexor sheath and reattached, followed by routine mobilization.
    - □ If not, the treatment choices include leaving it alone (or trimming the tendon stump in the palm if it is symptomatic and interferes with function), performing an arthrodesis of the DIP joint, or performing a tendon graft.
    - □ The latter choice carries with it the risk of compromise to the intact FDS, and may not always be a suitable alternative.
  - *Type II* is characterized by retraction of the tendon to the region of the PIP joint, and a small bone chip may be present in the distal tendon stump.
    - □ These injuries may be reattached as late as 6 weeks after the injury, with satisfactory results.
  - *Type III* injuries present with a large bone fragment that becomes trapped at the distal edge of the A4 pulley, and are comparatively easy to reattach due to the lack of significant retraction, as well as a sizeable bone fragment.
- The key to a successful outcome in this injury is *early diagnosis and treatment*.

12.2 EXTENSOR TENDON

The extensor mechanism in the finger, in comparison to that of the flexors, is thinner, less substantial, and less likely to hold sutures well. At the wrist and forearm, however, the extensors' substance and cross-sectional area are much more like the flexor tendons. Injuries to the extensor tendons are common, owing to their relatively exposed and superficial location. The dorsal aspect of the hand and wrist is covered with a thin layer of supple skin, with minimal subcutaneous tissue. In many areas, such as the distal finger joint, the tendon is very thin and subject to rupture with sufficient force. Injury may be secondary to laceration, deep abrasion, crush, or avulsion, and the majority of extensor tendon injuries are at joint levels. Penetrating wounds that disrupt the tendon are also prone to enter the joint; this is true not only at the interphalangeal joints, but also at the MCP joint. The degree of joint contamination must be evaluated and considered in the treatment plan.

Unlike the flexor tendons, loss of continuity of the extensor mechanism in the hand and fingers is usually not associated with immediate retraction of the tendon ends because of the multiple soft-tissue attachments and interconnections at various levels. Furthermore, the extensor mechanism in the hand is extrasynovial, except at the wrist, where the tendons are covered with a synovial sheath. Paratenon surrounds the extensor tendons over the dorsum of the hand, and tendons covered with paratenon do not separate widely when lacerated. Therefore, divided extensor tendons are usually free to retract only on the dorsum of the wrist. Because of this, many tendon injuries, especially in the fingers, may be treated successfully by splinting alone. In the hand and fingers, any gap in the tendon following laceration or avulsion is usually caused by unopposed flexion of the joints rather than retraction of the tendon.

PERTINENT ANATOMY

Extension of the finger is a complex act and is considered to be more intricate than finger flexion. This mechanism is composed of two separate and neurologically independent systems: the extrinsic extensors innervated by the radial nerve, and the intrinsic systems supplied by the ulnar and median nerves.

The extensor mechanism arises from multiple muscle bellies in the forearm. The extensor pollicis longus (EPL), extensor pollicis brevis (EPB), extensor indicis proprius (EIP), and extensor digiti minimi (EDM) have a comparatively independent origin and action. The proprius tendons at the MCP joint level are usually to the ulnar side of the communis tendons. The little finger proprius tendon (EDM) over the metacarpal and wrist level is usually represented by two distinct tendinous structures (Figure 12.2-1). The extensor digitorum communis (EDC) tendon to the little finger is present less than 50% of the time. When it is absent, it is almost always replaced by a junctura tendinum

from the ring finger to the extensor aponeurosis of the little finger.

Traditional knowledge suggested that independent extension of the index and little fingers was caused *solely* by the proprius tendons to these digits. Loss of independent extension, especially of the index finger, was said to be likely, but in the majority of patients, independent extension of the index is still possible if the EIP is absent due to injury or transfer. Extension lag in the index finger may be avoided when taking the EIP as a transfer by sectioning the EIP proximal to the hood.

The wrist, thumb, and finger extensors gain entrance to the hand beneath the extensor retinaculum through a series of six tunnels—five fibro-osseous and one fibrous (the fifth dorsal compartment, which contains the EDM). The extensor retinaculum is a wide fibrous band that prevents bowstringing of the tendons across the wrist joint. Its average width is 4.9 cm (with a range of 2.9 to 8.4 cm), as measured over the fourth compartment (see Figure 12.2-1). At this level, the extensor tendons are covered with a synovial sheath. The extensor retinaculum consists of two layers: the supratendinous and the infratendinous. The infratendinous layer is limited to an area deep to the three ulnar compartments. The six dorsal compartments are separated by septa that arise from the supratendinous retinaculum and insert onto the radius.

Just proximal to the MCP joint level, the communis tendons are joined together by oblique interconnections called juncturae tendinum. These connecting bands usually run in a distal direction from the ring finger communis to the little and middle fingers, and from the middle to the index finger. The EDM tendon receives a junctura from the ring finger extensor if the little finger EDC is absent. It is because of these interconnections that laceration of the middle finger communis tendon just proximal to this junctura may result in only partial extension loss of the middle finger. The juncturae tendinum have considerable interaction between adjacent fingers, and may also decrease the stress on the web. Sectioning the web virtually abolishes any movement between adjacent fingers, in contrast to transection of the long extensors, which has no effect on the interaction between the fingers. This finding is of significance when evaluating an injured hand, because a lacerated tendon may be overlooked if finger extension is partially maintained through juncturae, intertendinous fascia, or the web structures between the adjacent fingers.

The extensor tendon at the level of the MCP joint is held in place over the dorsum of the joint by the conjoined tendons of the intrinsic muscles and the transverse lamina or sagittal band, which together tether and keep the extensor tendons centralized over the joint (Figure 12.2-2). The sagittal band arises from the palmar plate and the intermetacarpal ligaments at the neck of the metacarpals. Any injury to this extensor hood or expansion may result in subluxation or dislocation of the extensor tendon. The extensor

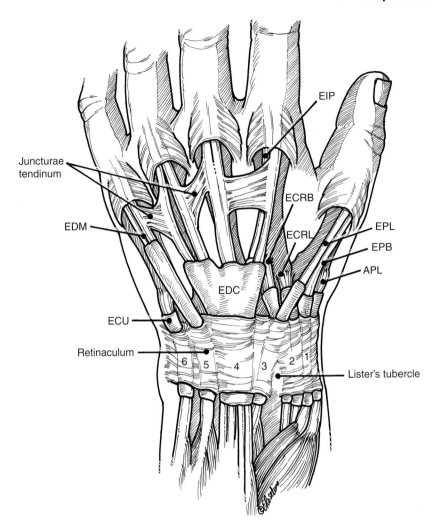

Juncturae tendinum

EDM

ECU

Retinaculum

EDC

EIP

ECRB

ECRL

EPL

EPB

APL

6 5 4 3 2 1

Lister's tubercle

Figure 12.2-1   The extensor mechanism at the wrist, fingers, and thumb. Note the six compartments or canals.

mechanism at the level of the proximal aspect of the finger is composed of a layered, crisscrossed fiber pattern that changes its geometric arrangement as the finger flexes and extends. This arrangement allows the lateral bands to be displaced volarly in flexion and to return to the dorsum of the finger in extension.

The intrinsic tendons from the lumbrical muscles join the extensor mechanism at about the level of the proximal and midportion of the proximal phalanx, and continue distally to the DIP joint of the finger.

At the MCP-joint level, the intrinsic muscles and tendons are palmar to the joint axis of rotation and act as *flexors* of the MCP joint. At the PIP joint, however, they are dorsal to the joint axis, and aid in the *extension* of the PIP joint.

The extensor mechanism at the PIP joint is best described as a trifurcation of the extensor tendon into the central slip, which attaches to the dorsal base of the middle phalanx, and the two lateral bands. The lateral bands pass on either side of the PIP joint and continue distally to insert at the dorsal base of the distal phalanx. The extensor mechanism is maintained in place over the PIP joint by the transverse retinacular ligaments. The extensor tendon achieves simultaneous extension of the two finger joints by a mechanism in which the central slip extends the

middle phalanx, and the lateral bands bypass the PIP joint to extend the distal phalanx. The fibers overlying the PIP joint are differentially loaded as the finger moves. In the flexed position, the most central fibers are tensed, whereas in extension, the lateral fibers are tensed. The most important feature of this mechanism is that the three elements are in balance. Specifically, the lengths of the central slip and two lateral bands must be such that extension of the PIP and DIP joints takes place together, so that when the middle phalanx is brought up into alignment with the proximal phalanx, the distal phalanx reaches alignment at the same time. This mechanism depends on the relative length of the central slip and two lateral bands. This precise and consistent length relationship is what is so difficult to restore when the mechanism has been damaged. Loss of this critical relationship at the PIP joint level, with relative lengthening of the central slip, results in the characteristic boutonniere deformity. A unique arrangement is present at the dorsal aspect of the PIP joint, where the central slip of the extensor tendon invests a fibrocartilage plate prior to its attachment to the dorsal base of the middle phalanx. The average thickness of the central slip at this level is 0.5 mm, but because of the presence of this fibrocartilage plate, the thickness is doubled over the PIP joint. This structure is called the

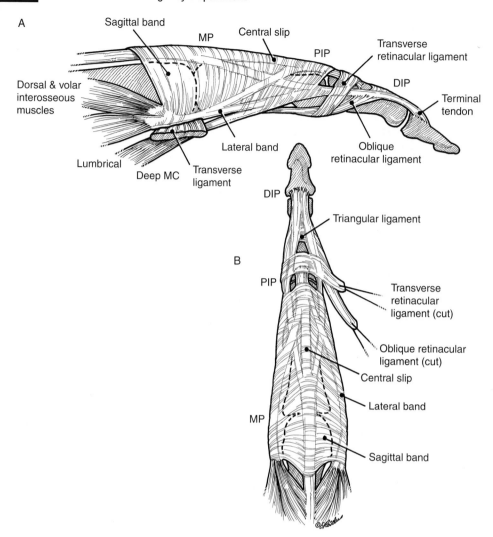

A

Sagittal band

MP

Central slip

PIP

Transverse retinacular ligament

DIP

Dorsal & volar interosseous muscles

Terminal tendon

Lumbrical

Deep MC

Transverse ligament

Lateral band

Oblique retinacular ligament

DIP

Triangular ligament

B

PIP

Transverse retinacular ligament (cut)

Oblique retinacular ligament (cut)

Central slip

Lateral band

MP

Sagittal band

Figure 12.2-2 The extensor mechanism at the MCP, PIP, and DIP joints of the finger.

dorsal plate, and adds to the stability of the extensor tendon and PIP joint. It also increases the moment arm of the extensor tendon at the PIP joint, and prevents attrition of the central slip at the PIP joint. The similarity of the dorsal plate and the patella is striking. In my experience, this dorsal plate adds relative thickness and substance to the extensor mechanism, and aids in the placement of sutures for lacerations in this area.

Zones of Extensor Tendon Injury

The zones of injury are given in Table 12.2-1 and are based on the anatomic characteristics of the extensor mechanism in each zone. This provides a useful basis for establishing a treatment plan and comparing end results following various forms of treatment.

Zone 1 Injuries (DIP Joint; Mallet Finger)

Four types of mallet deformity have been identified, and the classification in Table 12.2-2 is useful in establishing a

treatment plan. Type IV injuries are discussed in the chapter on fractures.

TABLE 12.2-1 THE ZONES OF EXTENSOR TENDON INJURY IN THE FINGERS, THUMB, AND FOREARM

Zone	Finger	Thumb
I	DIP joint	Interphalangeal joint
II	Middle phalanx	Proximal phalanx
III	PIP joint	MCP joint
IV	Proximal phalanx	Metacarpal
V	MCP joint	Carpometacarpal joint/radial styloid
VI	Metacarpal	
VII	Dorsal retinaculum	
VIII	Distal forearm	
IX	Mid and proximal forearm	

DIP, distal interphalangeal; MCP, metacarpophalangeal; PIP, proximal interphalangeal.

TABLE 12.2-2 MALLET FINGER CLASSIFICATION

Type	Description
I	Closed or blunt trauma to the tip of the digit, resulting in sudden forceful flexion of the joint with loss of tendon continuity with or without a small avulsion fracture from the dorsal base of the distal phalanx.
II	Laceration at or proximal to the DIP joint, with loss of tendon continuity.
III	Deep abrasion with loss of skin, subcutaneous cover, and tendon substance.
IV	
A	Transepiphyseal plate fracture in children.
B	Hyperflexion injury with fracture of the articular surface of 20–50%.
C	Hyperextension injury with fracture of the articular surface usually >50% and with early or late volar subluxation of the distal phalanx.

PATHOLOGIC ANATOMY AND DIAGNOSIS

- The most common type of mallet finger is type I, which is caused by loss of continuity—either from tearing the substance of the tendon just proximal to the joint, or from avulsion of the tendon from its insertion, with or without a small piece of bone.
    - The degree of deformity in this injury may vary from a few degrees of extension loss to a 75 to 80 degree flexion posture of the DIP joint (Figure 12.2-3).
- A laceration (type II) over or near the DIP joint that transects the tendon also produces a characteristic mallet deformity.
    - Lacerations directly over the joint more often than not enter the joint; this must be considered in treatment because of the potential for joint contamination.

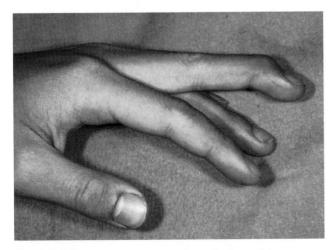

Figure 12.2-3 Clinical appearance of a mallet finger deformity, type I, obtained when a ball struck the tip of the finger.

- Deep abrasion injuries (type III) over the distal joint may result in significant loss of soft-tissue cover, and a loss of a portion or all of the underlying tendon mechanism. The joint is almost always exposed.

TREATMENT

Type I

- Closed type I injuries are treated by continuous splinting of the DIP joint in full extension.
- Only the DIP joint needs to be splinted, but the splinting must be *continuous*. Removal of the splint during the treatment interval and flexing the DIP joint may reverse the healing process.
- When the DIP joint is capable of active extension (usually after 6 to 8 weeks), the splint may be removed, and cautious flexion activity may be started.
- If any recurrence of the deformity occurs, the splint is reapplied for another 2 to 3 weeks.
- Various forms of splinting have been used, and my favorite splints include the commercially available Stack splint, which comes in multiple sizes, and dorsal or palmar splints made from padded aluminum (Figure 12.2-4).
- Reconstitution of the tendon occurs by fibroblastic proliferation, which produces a tendon callus that subsequently contracts and re-forms into a type of tendon that restores continuity.
- The success of this method depends on continuous coaptation of the tendon ends, and avoidance of stretching or tearing of the tendon callus.
- The precarious nature of this healing process is further amplified by noting that the microvascular anatomy of the distal digital extensor tendon often demonstrates an area of minimal or deficient blood supply in this zone.

Type II

- Lacerations over the DIP joint may produce a mallet deformity, and an appropriate suture technique that may be used is given in Figure 12.2-5.
- Splinting is continuous for 6 weeks following surgical repair.

Type III

- The management of this injury is far different from that of a simple closed mallet deformity, and staged surgical reconstruction is required.

Zone II Injuries

DIAGNOSIS

- Injuries in this zone are usually due to lacerations.
- Lacerations over the dorsal aspect of the middle phalanx may result in partial rather than complete laceration of

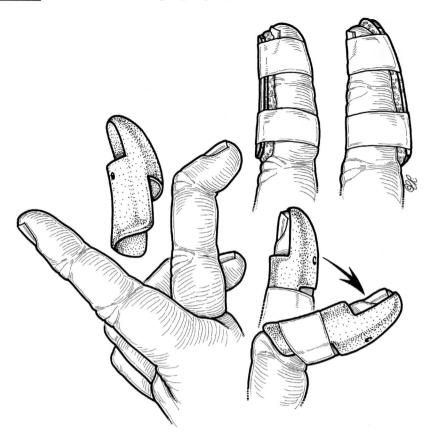

Figure 12.2-4 Useful splints for the treatment of type I closed mallet finger deformity. Note that the PIP joint is left free for motion.

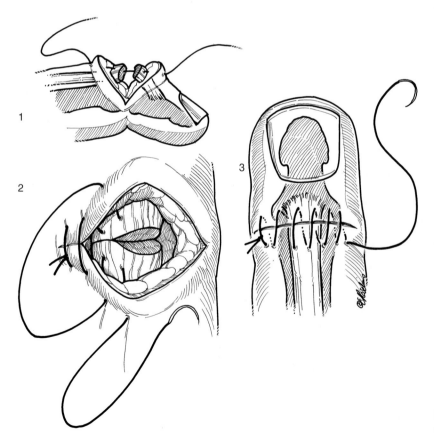

Figure 12.2-5 Suture technique for repairing an extensor tendon laceration over the DIP joint.

the extensor mechanism, due to its increased breadth and curved shape.

■ Incomplete lacerations may not be associated with a mallet deformity.

TREATMENT

■ All wounds in this area should be carefully inspected, and the underlying extensor mechanism evaluated and repaired as indicated.

■ Partial lacerations involving less than 50% of the substance of the extensor may be treated by wound care and skin suture followed by protected range of motion.

■ More extensive or complete lacerations are repaired by a running suture near the cut edge, followed by a cross stitch proximal and distal to the running suture (Figure 12.2-6).

■ Splinting of the DIP joint is performed for 4 to 6 weeks, based on the nature of the laceration and the integrity of the repair.

Zone III Injuries

MECHANISM OF INJURY AND PATHOLOGIC ANATOMY

Injuries to the extensor mechanism in zone III are usually due to closed blunt trauma with acute forceful flexion of the PIP joint, producing avulsion of the central slip from its insertion on the dorsal base of the middle phalanx, with or without fracture and laceration of the extensor tendon at or near its insertion. Volar dislocation of the PIP joint may also result in avulsion of the central slip and subsequent boutonniere deformity. Loss of integrity of the central slip attachment at the dorsal base of the middle phalanx, either from avulsion or laceration, starts a cascade of tendon imbalance that results in a characteristic deformity of flexion at the PIP joint and hyperextension of the DIP joint. This deformity, called the *boutonniere* deformity, illustrates the problem of imbalance in the finger, which is a chain of joints with multiple tendon attachments. This chain collapses into an abnormal posture or deformity when there is an imbalance of the critical forces maintaining equilibrium. This abnormal cascade or sequence begins with flexion of the PIP joint, owing to loss of the central slip and the unopposed force of the flexor digitorum superficialis. Next, with stretching of the expansion (transverse retinacular ligament and triangular ligament) between the central and lateral slips, the lateral bands migrate volarward to a position volar to the axis of joint rotation. Finally, in this position of the lateral bands, the pull of the intrinsic muscles is directed exclusively to the distal joint, which progressively hyperextends. The MCP joint is also hyperextended by action of the long extensor tendon.

DIAGNOSIS

■ Figure 12.2-7 demonstrates the appearance of the boutonniere deformity.

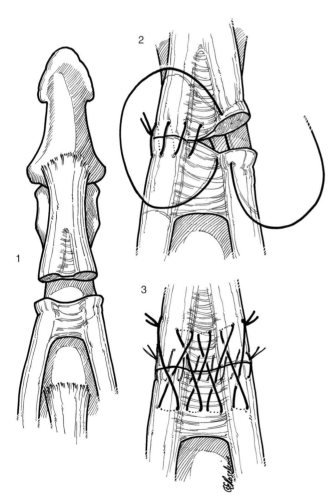

Figure 12.2-6 Extensor tendon suture technique for lacerations over the middle phalanx (zone II).

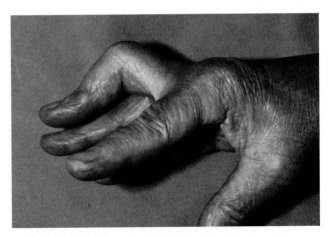

Figure 12.2-7 The clinical appearance of the boutonniere deformity. Note the flexed posture of the PIP joint and the hyperextension of the DIP joint of the middle finger.

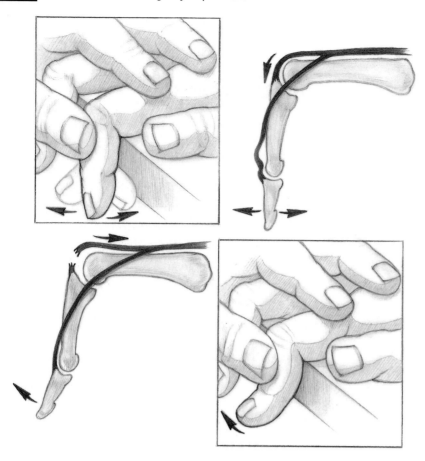

Figure 12.2-8 The Elson test for diagnosis of boutonniere deformity.

- In closed injuries, the characteristic boutonniere deformity may not be present at the time of injury, and usually develops over a 10- to 21-day period following injury.
  - This condition is often missed, even in an open wound.
- A painful, tender, and swollen PIP joint that has been recently injured should arouse suspicion. Active motion is decreased, and the finger is held semiflexed.
- Diagnostic maneuvers include holding the PIP joint in full extension and testing the amount of passive flexion of the distal joint.
- With disruption of the central slip and volar migration of the lateral bands, flexion of the distal joint is markedly decreased.
- Another useful test is the Elson test depicted in Figure 12.2-8.
  - The finger to be examined by the Elson test is flexed comfortably to a right angle at the PIP joint over the edge of a table, and firmly held in place by the examiner. The patient is then asked to extend the PIP joint against resistance.
  - Any pressure felt by the examiner over the middle phalanx can only be exerted by an *intact* central slip.
  - Further proof is that the DIP joint remains flail during the effort because the competent central slip prevents the lateral bands from acting distally. In the presence of a complete rupture of the central slip, any extension effort perceived by the examiner is accompanied by rigidity at the DIP joint with a tendency toward

extension. This is produced by the extensor action of the lateral bands.
  - This test, however, does not demonstrate the presence of a partial rupture of the central slip, and it may be impeded by pain or lack of patient cooperation.
- Consideration may be given to nerve block for pain relief, as indicated.

TREATMENT

Closed Boutonniere

- Correction of this deformity is dependent on restoration of the normal tendon balance, and on the precise length relationship of the central slip and lateral bands.
- In acute cases, before fixed contractures have occurred, this may be achieved by two basic means:
  - Progressively splinting the PIP joint into full extension.
  - Insertion of an oblique transarticular K-wire to maintain the PIP joint in full extension.
- At the same time, active and passive flexion exercises of the distal joint are performed.
- Splinting of the PIP joint, and active flexion of the DIP joint, are believed to draw the lateral bands distally and dorsally, and to reduce the separation of the torn ends of the central slip of the extensor tendon.

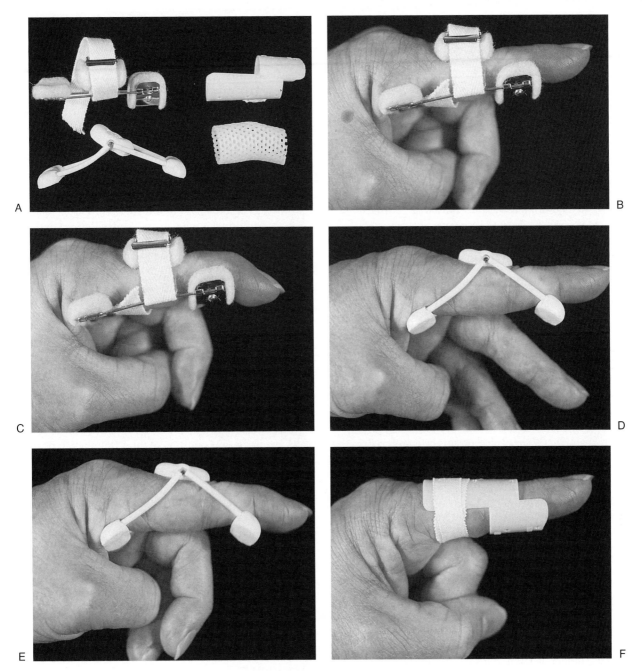

Figure 12.2-9   Various forms of static and dynamic splints used to treat a closed-boutonniere deformity.

■ This allows repair by contracture of the disrupted tendon ends at their anatomic length, and by migration of the lateral bands to their normal anatomic position above the joint axis of rotation at the PIP joint.

■ Positioning and maintaining the PIP joint in extension has been achieved by dynamic and static splinting, K-wire fixation of the joint, and serial plaster casts.

■ When the distal joint can be fully flexed with the PIP joint extended, all components of the extensor mechanism have been restored to their normal relationships and balance. At this point, the splint may be discontinued.

  ■ This may take 6 weeks or more of continuous splinting and DIP joint exercise.

■ Various forms of splints used for treatment of closed boutonniere deformity are depicted in Figure 12.2-9.

■ In closed boutonniere deformity, operative treatment is undertaken in two circumstances:

  ■ The central slip has been avulsed with a bone fragment, and is lying free over the PIP joint. In this case, it should be replaced or excised, and the tendon should be reattached with a pullout suture.

  ■ There is a long-standing boutonnière deformity in a young person.

■ In closed volar dislocations of the PIP joint, there is usually a rupture of the central slip, along with a rupture of a collateral ligament and volar plate and a subsequent boutonniere deformity.

- These potentially disabling soft-tissue injuries must be recognized and repaired by prompt reduction and primary repair of all ruptured structures (central slip, collateral ligament, and volar plate), combined with stabilization of the PIP joint in extension with a K-wire for 3 weeks, followed by gradual mobilization over the next 3 to 4 weeks while the PIP joint is protected.
- Motion of the distal joint is encouraged in the early post-operative period.
- It can be anticipated that this method will produce satisfactory results, although joint stiffness can be a problem because of extensive soft-tissue injury.
- Reconstructions of a chronic, closed boutonniere deformity or of boutonniere lesions caused by burns or rheumatoid disease are beyond the scope of this text.

Laceration of Central Slip at PIP Joint

- Laceration of the extensor mechanism at the PIP joint will result in loss of extension at that joint, which may in turn develop into a secondary boutonniere deformity if not properly treated.
- The average thickness of the central slip just proximal to the PIP joint is 0.5 mm, but this measurement is doubled by the fibrocartilaginous dorsal plate at the point of insertion of the central slip into the dorsal base of the middle phalanx.
- This dorsal plate provides a more substantial substance for suture retention.
- The lateral bands at this level also are approximately twice the thickness of the central slip portion of the extensor tendon, and are likely to retain sutures better than the proximal portion of the central slip.
- A useful repair technique is a modified Kessler suture of 4-0 synthetic suture beginning 1 cm from the lacerated tendon edge.
  - The knot is tied in the substance of the tendon so that two intact strands cross the laceration.
  - This suture begins in the substance of the lateral bands on each side, and ends in the confluence of the lateral bands and the dorsal plate over the PIP joint.
  - Next, a 5-0 synthetic suture is used to perform a cross stitch, as described by Silfverskiold. This is not a circumferential suture, as is used for flexor tendons, because the tendon is flat and thin, but it is placed from margin to margin of the extensor.
  - Both the Kessler and the cross-stitch sutures are placed so that little or no shortening or side-to-side deformity of the extensor mechanism is produced.
- Figure 12.2-10 demonstrates some useful suture techniques for repair of lacerations in the region of the PIP joint.
- Passive motion of the PIP joint in the operating room to 30 degrees, without gapping of the repair site, usually indicates that the repair is satisfactory.
- Some lacerations of the extensor mechanism over the PIP joint are so near the insertion of the central slip that inadequate length is present distally to place or retain the suture material.
  - In these cases, the distal aspect of the suture must be placed through a small transverse tunnel made in the dorsal base of the proximal phalanx with a 0.35 K-wire.
  - A 5-0 cross stitch is placed as space permits to augment the repair (see Figure 12.2-10D, E).
  - Care is taken to ensure that the various components are neither foreshortened nor lengthened, as this may result in contracture or extensor lag, respectively.
  - The PIP joint is splinted in full extension.
- Under ideal circumstances, and when a hand therapist is available, the short arc motion protocol is begun (see Rehabilitation Protocol for Zone III–IV Injuries).
- An alternative treatment option is as follows:
  - A safety-pin splint or a molded, palmar, thermoplast splint, as described for treatment of the closed boutonniere deformity, is applied, and active flexion exercises of the distal joint are started.
  - The splint is maintained on a continuous basis for 5 to 6 weeks with the PIP joint in full extension, and active flexion exercises of the distal joint are performed.
  - When active exercises to the PIP joint are started at 5 to 6 weeks, the patient is advised to support the proximal phalanx in flexion as the PIP joint is extended. This directs the force of the extensor tendon more distally, and the finger is in a more effective position for extension.
  - The PIP joint is splinted in extension between these exercise sessions for another 2 to 4 weeks.
  - At 8 to 10 weeks, active flexion and extension exercises are increased.
  - Dynamic flexion splinting of the PIP joint can be used to augment recovery of flexion if there is no extensor lag at the PIP joint.
  - The recovery of flexion in the DIP joint can be augmented by gentle and intermittent rubber band traction between a dress hook attached to the fingernail distally and a small proximal hook attached to a plaster finger cylinder cast.

Zone IV Injuries (Proximal Phalanx)

MECHANISM OF INJURY AND DIAGNOSIS

- Injuries at this level are usually partial lacerations of the extensor mechanism, because of the broad configuration of the tendon over the curved shape of the underlying phalanx and consequent protection of the lateral bands.
  - Functional loss may be minimal due to this fact.
- These lesions are diagnosed by direct inspection of the wound.

TREATMENT

- Laceration of an isolated lateral band may be repaired with a 5-0 cross stitch, and early protected motion may be started.

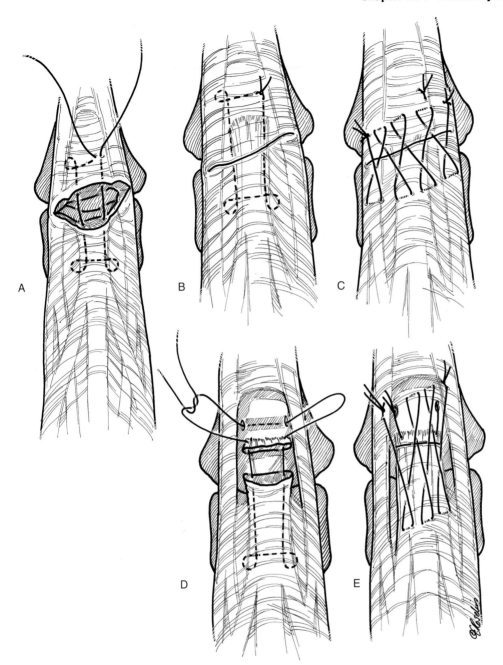

Figure 12.2-10 Suture techniques for repair of lacerations of the central slip at the PIP joint. **A–C.** A Kessler stitch with a crisscross overlay is used if there is sufficient tendon at each end for repair. **D, E.** If sufficient tendon is not available distally, the tails of the Kessler suture are tied through a transverse tunnel made with a 0.035 K-wire through the dorsal base of the middle phalanx. The crisscross stitch is used to complete the repair. The Kessler suture is tied with suitable tension to avoid gapping or undue shortening of the tendon. The distance between the longitudinal components of the suture is adjusted to avoid side-to-side "bunching" or shortening.

- Complete lacerations of the central tendon should be repaired using a modified Kessler suture of 4-0 nonabsorbable material, with a crisscross suture of 5-0 (see Figure 12.2-10A, C).
- Care is taken to avoid relative lengthening or shortening of the central tendon, because this may result in imbalance between the central slip and the lateral bands.
- Because of the relatively large interface between the extensor mechanism and osseous phalanx, and the resultant potential for adhesions, it is ideal to begin short arc motion exercises as described for zone III injuries.

Zone V Open Injuries (MCP Joint)

HUMAN BITE WOUNDS

Mechanism of Injury and Diagnosis

- Tendon injuries at this level are most often associated with open wounds.
- A small, penetrating wound over the MCP joint may be caused by striking someone in the mouth with a clenched fist.

- Although many patients deny this mechanism of injury, a careful history must be taken.
- This is a contaminated wound, and the organisms involved are capable of producing significant wound infection.
  - Gram-positive bacteria (usually staphylococci) alone, or in combination with gram-negative organisms, are most frequently cultured.
- The incidence of complications is directly related to the time span from injury to treatment.

Treatment

- A radiograph is obtained to note the presence or absence of a fracture or foreign body.
- The wound must be extended proximally and distally to permit inspection of the joint, and a culture is taken.
- The wound is debrided, irrigated, and left open.
- Appropriate antibiotics are started immediately (preferably preoperatively).
- Under no circumstances should a human bite wound be closed.
- Most tendon injuries associated with this type of wound are partial, and need not be repaired immediately.
- The hand is splinted, with the wrist in 40 to 45 degrees extension and the MCP joints in 15 to 20 degrees of flexion.
- The soft tissues, including the capsule and extensor hood, are allowed to seek their own position over the joint.
  - Partial or even complete lacerations are seldom—if ever—associated with significant retraction at this level.
- The tendon laceration may be repaired secondarily as needed in 5 to 7 days, or even later depending on the nature of the wound at the time of inspection.
- When the infection is under control, dynamic splinting is started.

LACERATIONS

Treatment

- Lacerations of the extensor tendon or hood at the MCP joint level are repaired using core-type sutures of 4-0 nonabsorbable material.
- Injuries of the extensor tendon at this level are not associated with retraction of the ends, and a modified Kessler with a cross-stitch is used (see Figure 12.2-10A, C).
- Postoperative management includes dynamic splinting using the methods described in the section on Rehabilitation of Extensor Tendon Injuries.

Zone V Closed Injuries (MCP Joint)

CLOSED SAGITTAL BAND INJURIES

Pathologic Anatomy and Diagnosis

- Spontaneous rupture of the radial sagittal band with subsequent ulnarward subluxation or dislocation of the extensor tendon in the nonrheumatoid patient may occur following forceful flexion or extension of the finger.
- The lesion is secondary to a tear of the sagittal band and oblique fibers of the hood, usually on the radial side, although rupture of the ulnar sagittal band and radial dislocation have been reported.
- Ulnar subluxation or dislocation of the extensor tendon, sometimes accompanied by painful snapping of the extensor tendon when making a fist, is the usual finding.
- In some cases, this may be associated with incomplete finger extension and ulnar deviation of the involved digit (Figure 12.2-11).
  - The middle finger is the most commonly involved.
  - This may be the result of an inherent anatomic weakness, because the extensor tendon of the long finger is situated on top of the transverse fibers, and has a comparatively loose attachment at this level.

Treatment

- Patients seen within 2 weeks of the injury may be treated by closed means using a plaster or orthotic device that maintains the MCP joint in a flexion block splint (Figure 12.2-12). The splint maintains the finger in neutral abduction-adduction, allowing full extension but blocking flexion at 10 to 20 degrees.
- The splint is used for 6 weeks.
- Dislocations that are diagnosed long after the injury, or that fail initial splinting, are best treated with surgical release and realignment of the extensor mechanism by one of the methods depicted in Figure 12.2-13.

OPEN SAGITTAL BAND INJURIES

Treatment

- Lacerations of the hood or sagittal bands at this level must be repaired so that the extensor tendon will remain centralized over the dorsum of the joint.
- Failure to repair this type of injury may result in subluxation of the extensor tendon and an associated loss of extension.
- A cross stitch of 4-0 or 5-0 nylon is used to repair these lacerations.
- Gentle flexion and extension exercises are started in 3 to 5 days.
- Abduction and adduction motions are avoided, and these forces are minimized by "buddy strapping" the injured finger to an adjacent finger.

Zone VI Injuries (Metacarpal)

- Zone VI injuries have a better prognosis than more distal lesions (zones II to V) for several reasons:
  - They are unlikely to have associated joint injuries.
  - The decreased tendon surface area in zone VI lessens the potential for adhesion formation.

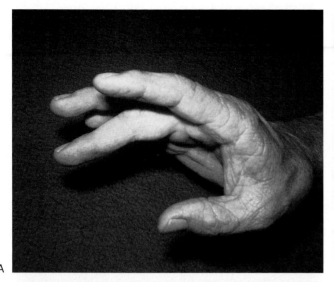

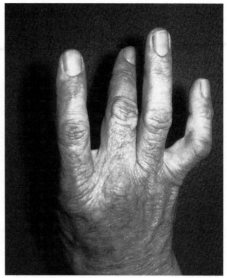

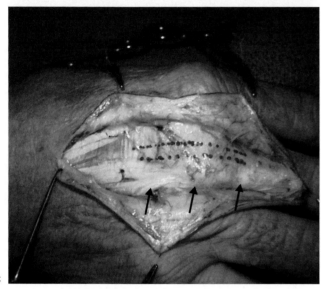

Figure 12.2-11 Traumatic ulnar dislocation of the extensor tendon at the MCP joint. **A.** Note the lack of complete extension of the middle finger. **B.** There is ulnar deviation of the middle finger when the patient attempts to extend the finger. **C.** Operative appearance of the dislocated extensor tendon (*arrows*) and the anatomic or normal position of the extensor (*dotted lines*).

■ The increased subcutaneous tissue lessens the potential for adhesions.
■ There is greater tendon excursion in zone VI.
■ Complex tendon imbalances are less likely to occur.

TREATMENT

■ The extensor tendons in this zone have sufficient substance to accept core-type sutures of the surgeon's choice, and dynamic splinting can be performed with the assurance that disruption of the suture site is unlikely.

■ Postoperative management includes dynamic splinting beginning at 3 to 5 days with the wrist in 40 to 45 degrees of extension and the MCP joints in 0 to 15 degrees flexion. This lasts for 5 weeks. See the section on extensor tendon rehabilitation.

SECRETAN'S DISORDER (PERITENDINOUS FIBROSIS)

This condition is included under extensor tendon injuries in zone VI since it may mimic tendon injuries in this zone.

In 1901, Henri-Francois Secretan described 11 cases of persistent hard edema on the dorsum of the hand, all associated with work-related injuries. All patients were covered by worker's compensation insurance, had sustained trauma insufficient to produce fracture, and had prolonged symptoms and findings. This condition has been called dorsal hard edema of the hand, peritendinous fibrosis of the dorsum of the hand, and factitious lymphedema of the hand. Typically, a worker, usually male, describes a blow to the dorsum of the hand without fracture or laceration and then develops firm, persistent swelling over the back of the hand with subsequent loss of finger flexion and resulting prolonged time out of work.

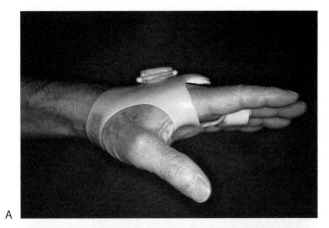

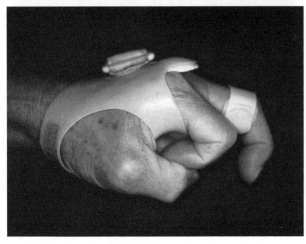

Figure 12.2-12 Orthotic device for treatment of extensor tendon dislocation at the MCP joint. (Courtesy of Inoue and Tamara, from Inoue G, Tamura Y. Dislocation of the extensor tendon over the metacarpophalangeal joints. J Hand Surg 1996;21A:464–469.)

Etiology

A number of factors have been reported in association with this disorder, including proven or suspected self-inflicted trauma, such as repeated blows to the back of the hand or application of tourniquets, compensable work-related injuries, and neurosis, psychosis, or suicidal tendency. Although abnormal tissues have been removed in Secretan's disorder, these tissues are merely the natural response to trauma, and the pathology reports on the tissue specimens and MRI findings are not unexpected. Such findings do not indicate an etiology other than self-inflicted trauma.

Controversy still surrounds this disorder as to etiology and treatment. In my opinion, Secretan's is a disorder with a known etiology and pathogenesis, and it is not a disease, which implies some unique pathologic process that occurs for some as yet undiscovered reason.

Diagnosis

- Diagnosis is based on the history and on physical findings.

- Both T1- and T2-weighted MRI have shown soft-tissue and tendon edema in combination with diffuse peritendinous fibrosis extending to the fascia of the interosseous muscles.
- Operative findings (not advised) have shown fibroadipose tissue with areas of focal myxoid or cystic degeneration similar to ganglion tissue.

Treatment

- Most experts advise nonoperative management of this condition, which has included studious neglect and avoidance of passive manipulation, heat, and massage. They do, however, encourage the patient to exercise by voluntary means.
- The condition may improve by plaster-cast protection.
- This condition must be recognized as a factitious disorder.
  - Patients with factitious disorders are not feigning the disorder; they are causing it.
  - Confrontation in the form of accusation can potentially be harmful to both the patient and the doctor, and should be avoided.
  - The physical problem or lesion may resolve when compensation is terminated. This condition is not a surgical lesion.
  - Best results have been achieved by psychotherapy.
  - Protective casting, although it may result in immediate improvement and can confirm the diagnosis, may not be effective as a definitive treatment, as this disorder is self-inflicted and is characterized by recidivism. However, this technique may somehow demonstrate, in a conscious or unconscious way, the self-inflicted nature of the problem.
  - Active physical therapy may be useful in many cases when combined with psychotherapy.

Zone VII Injuries (Wrist)

ANATOMY

Injuries of the extensor mechanism at the wrist level are associated with damage to the retinaculum. The retinaculum prevents bowstringing of the extensor tendons, and lacerations of the extensors at this level are thought to be associated with subsequent adhesions to the overlying retinaculum. For this reason, many authors in the past advised that portions of the extensor retinaculum located over the site of tendon repair be excised to prevent adhesions. However, some surgeons have noted no statistical differences in their results when comparing zones VI, VII, and VIII. They repaired each retinacular rent primarily, and used traditional postoperative immobilization. The excellent results with early dynamic splinting suggest that excision of portions of the retinaculum over the tendon repair site may not be as important as previously believed. However, *limited excision* of portions of the retinaculum does no harm, and may facilitate tendon exposure and gliding, especially in repairs

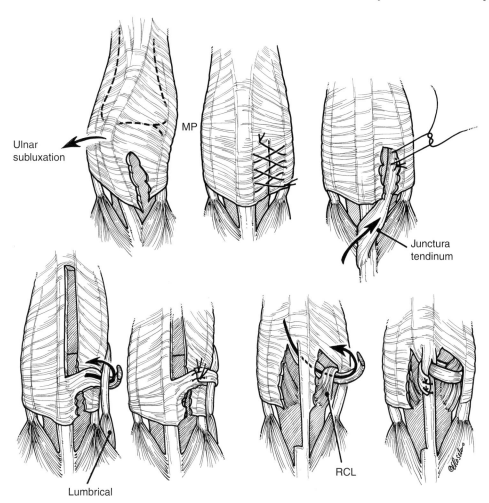

Figure 12.2-13 Techniques for secondary reconstruction of extensor tendon dislocation at the MCP joint.

in which there might be some impingement between the suture site and the adjacent retinaculum.

TREATMENT

- If the surgeon is concerned about maintaining the anatomic integrity of the retinaculum, the traumatic openings in the retinaculum may be extended distally and proximally at each end of the retinacular laceration to facilitate tendon repair and then reapproximated.
- The tendon is repaired using a standard core-type suture of appropriate nonabsorbable material.
- The adequacy of the retinacular restraint is verified by passive flexion and extension of the fingers and wrist.
- Multiple tendon injuries at this level may be dealt with by appropriate excision of the retinaculum as needed.
- Portions of the retinaculum should be preserved either proximal or distal to the suture line to prevent bowstringing; this is usually technically feasible.
- Although it has been recommended that complete excision of the extensor retinaculum be performed in lacerations at multiple levels, it is my opinion that complete excision of the retinaculum is seldom, if ever, necessary,

even in this type of injury. Some portion of the retinaculum can usually be preserved, and adhesions that limit function are unlikely, especially if early dynamic splinting is used.
- Tendons lacerated at this level retract, and traumatic wounds must be extended proximally and distally to find the tendon ends.
- In many instances, the surgeon must deal with multiple tendon lacerations, and the sorting out and matching of these tendon ends for later suture may be quite tedious and time consuming.
- A method of intraoperative tendon labeling has been described, and avoids the repetitive identification of tendon ends and thus saves operative time.
  - The method involves the placement of a 4-0 nonabsorbable suture into each cut end using a grasping suture technique such as the two-suture, modified Kessler.
  - The free ends of the suture material are then clamped in a hemostat and a Steri-Strip is placed through the thumb or finger hole, or around one of the proximal shanks of the hemostat. It is then folded on itself.
  - A sterile marking pen is used to write the name of the tendon on the Steri-Strip.

■ After all tendons have been labeled, they are easily matched and repaired using the same suture that initially tagged the tendon ends.

EXTENSOR TENDON RUPTURE

Mechanism of Injury

In addition to injury by laceration, the extensor tendons may rupture following a closed fracture or may dislocate following injury to the retinaculum. The EPL and EDC tendons may rupture following a Colles' fracture, and the extensor carpi ulnaris (ECU) tendon may dislocate ulnarward with forceful supination, palmar flexion, and ulnar deviation. The radially situated extensor tendons (EIP and EDC to index and EPL to the thumb) may be entrapped, and may rupture in Smith's and Galeazzi's fractures. In Galeazzi's fracture, the ECU may be trapped between the dorsally displaced ulnar head and avulsed ulnar styloid, or the extensor digiti minimi (EDM) tendon may be caught beneath the radial border of the dorsally dislocated ulnar head.

Treatment

■ Impending rupture of the EPL has been treated by subcutaneous transposition from its canal.
■ Treatment of acute ruptures of the EPL tendon is by transfer of the EIP tendon (or intercalary graft) and the ruptured communis tendons by intercalary graft, or by suturing the distal tendon stump to the adjacent extensor tendons.
■ Dislocation of the ECU tendon is treated by repairing the fibro-osseous sheath with a free tendon graft or a portion of the extensor retinaculum.

Zone VIII Injuries (Distal Forearm)

MECHANISM OF INJURY

Injuries at the musculotendinous junction may be caused by laceration or traumatic rupture. Although extensor tendon rupture at the musculotendinous junction is rare, such injuries may be due to sudden, forceful traction forces caused by gloves caught in revolving machines.

TREATMENT

■ In lacerations, the distal aspect of the junction (the tendon) accepts and holds sutures satisfactorily, but the muscle component is less likely to retain the suture.
■ Although it is theoretically possible to place the sutures in the muscle through the fibrous tissue origins of the tendon in the muscle belly, it is not always possible to obtain a suitable repair.

■ If such repairs are tenuous, the surgeon may elect to restore function by tendon transfer or by side-to-side suture, as recommended for management of musculotendinous ruptures.

Zone IX Injuries (Proximal Forearm)

MECHANISM OF INJURY AND PATHOLOGIC ANATOMY

The wrist and common finger extensors, as well as the little-finger proprius, arise from the region of the lateral epicondyle at the elbow. The thumb extensors and abductors, along with the proprius tendon of the index finger, arise from the forearm below the elbow. Injuries at this level are usually caused by penetrating wounds with knives or pieces of broken glass. The size of the skin wound may give little indication of the magnitude of the injury. Single or multiple functional units may be injured. The demonstrated loss of function may be the result of muscle transection, nerve injury, or both. Such loss of function in a penetrating injury in the proximal forearm may defy accurate preoperative diagnosis. The radial nerve at the level of the distal arm gives off branches to the brachialis, brachioradialis, and the extensor carpi radialis longus (ECRL). A major division of this nerve then occurs into the sensory branch and the posterior interosseous nerve (PIN). The superficial (sensory) branch continues distally under cover of the brachioradialis into the forearm, wrist, and hand areas. The posterior interosseous nerve gives branches to the extensor carpi radialis brevis (ECRB) and supinator, which it penetrates and supplies, and then innervates the remainder of the extensor muscle group.

TREATMENT

■ Experimental data on repaired muscle lacerations in laboratory animals (rabbits) imply that useful but incomplete function can be restored with adequate repair of skeletal muscle.
■ A muscle segment totally isolated from its motor point may not contribute to the contractile function of the innervated muscle.
■ In a series of patients with forearm flexor muscle lacerations, it was noted that tendon grafting was an effective method of repair to overcome extensive defects.
■ The indication for this technique is laceration of two or more muscle bellies with at least 50% of the muscle substance lacerated.
■ A penetrating wound with functional loss in the proximal third of the forearm must be carefully explored to determine the exact etiology of the loss.
■ Under tourniquet control and appropriate anesthesia, the wound margins are debrided and then extended proximally and distally and the extent of damage noted.
■ If it can be determined that the wounds extend only into the muscle belly, a careful repair of the muscle

belly is performed with multiple figure-of-eight sutures of polyglactin (Vicryl, Ethicon).

- For muscle grafting, the palmaris longus and long toe extensor tendons are used and passed through the superficial epimysium, muscle belly, and deep epimysium proximally and distally and sutured to themselves with a Pulvertaft side-weave technique.
  - One to three grafts are used, as required.
- The limb is immobilized for 3 weeks, with the elbow at 90 degrees.
- Protected motion is started at 3 weeks, and progressive motion is started at 6 weeks.

NERVE INVOLVEMENT

Diagnosis

- Many times it is impossible to determine nerve damage at the time of surgery in the immediate postinjury period.
- After 7 to 10 days, however, a denervated muscle will spontaneously contract for several minutes under the influence of succinylcholine used during induction of general anesthesia.
- Additional information may be gained by electrodiagnostic studies at 3 to 4 weeks postinjury.

Treatment

- The decision to undertake secondary nerve repair or reconstruction versus tendon transfer depends on the judgment and experience of the surgeon.
- If there is evidence of nerve involvement, the appropriate branches are identified and traced out to their insertions.
- Penetrating wounds often injure the nerve at or near its entrance into the muscle belly.
  - Retraction of the distal nerve stump into the muscle belly may occur, and may defy location and subsequent repair.
- If the lesion is confined to the muscle belly, definitive repair is carried out using sutures or tendon grafts and sutures, as previously described.
- The muscle is usually quite hemorrhagic, and muscle planes are difficult to identify.
  - Identification is aided by evacuation of the hematoma, irrigation, and gentle sponging of the cut muscle ends.
  - Identifying intramuscular fibrous septa and fascia for the placement of sutures aids in preventing the sutures from pulling out of the muscle.
- Coaptation of the cut ends of those muscles that arise at or distal to the elbow is aided by wrist extension.
- If suitable repair cannot be obtained by these methods, tendon transfers may be required.

Postoperative Management

- Postoperatively, the extremity is supported in a plaster splint or cast that maintains the wrist in 45 degrees of extension and the MCP joints in 15 to 20 degrees flexion.
- The elbow joint is immobilized in 90 degrees of flexion if the muscles involved arise at or above the lateral epicondyle.
- Immobilization is continued for 4 weeks postinjury, and then protected range of motion is permitted—but a night splint is used to maintain the wrist in extension for another 2 weeks.

Rehabilitation of Extensor Tendon Injuries

HISTORY AND GENERAL PRINCIPLES

Repaired extensor tendon injuries have traditionally been immobilized in extension for 3 to 4 weeks. However, in some instances, this has resulted in adhesions between the extensor tendon and the surrounding tissues. This has been especially true when the tendon injury was associated with a crush injury, surrounding soft-tissue loss, infection, underlying fracture, or joint-capsule or flexor-tendon injury. Significant and extensive research (both basic and clinical) has focused on the best methods of postoperative management of flexor tendon injuries, and controlled and early passive motion of the tendon suture site provided by dynamic splinting has proved to be a useful method to promote a well-healed, smooth, nonadherent, gliding flexor tendon surface, with improved tensile strength. This body of evidence regarding the rehabilitation of flexor tendon injuries with dynamic splinting is applicable to extensor tendon injuries, and many clinical studies have supported this concept.

At this time, there are many accepted protocols for dynamic splinting and early active motion in extensor tendon injuries, even in the most problematic zone III injuries. At this time, only zone I and II injuries and zone III closed boutonniere injuries are treated by static splinting. The protocols that follow have proven to be useful in my practice. However, the reader should note that improvements and changes might be made to these protocols in the future as more experience is gained.

These principles of dynamic splinting may be especially applicable when multiple extensor tendons are injured beneath the extensor retinaculum and when there are associated injuries. The extensor tendons at the wrist level are surrounded by a synovial sheath and constrained by fibro-osseous and fibrous tunnels. Indiscriminate sacrifice of the extensor retinaculum results in altered biomechanics and poor function. The use of controlled passive motion has been clearly shown to improve results in flexor tendon injuries, and these principles are now applied to extensor tendon injuries:

- Extensor tendon injuries can be placed in an outrigger splint that maintains passive extension using elastic traction, but that allows limited active flexion (Figure 12.2-14).
- Excursion of the repaired extensor tendon is achieved by active flexion.

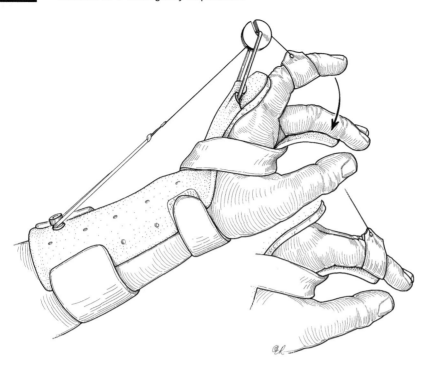

Figure 12.2-14   Dynamic splint for early motion of extensor tendon injuries in zones V to VI.

- Splinting is started 3 to 5 days after surgery and is maintained for 5 weeks.
- Active flexion is performed 10 times an hour.

REHABILITATION PROTOCOLS

Zone III and IV Injuries

Extensor tendon injuries in zones III and IV have historically demonstrated higher percentages of extensor lag and loss of flexion. This led to the development of a rehabilitation protocol based on protected movement of the injured finger. The efficacy of the short arc motion for zone III extensor injuries was based on the fact that 30 degrees of flexion at the PIP joint results in a calculated tendon excursion of 3.75 mm.

- In this protocol, developed by Evans, a thermoplastic palmar static splint is used to immobilize the PIP and DIP joints in full extension, except during exercise.
  - The splint is taped directly over the PIP and DIP joints.
  - Two thermoplastic exercise splints are used:
    - Type I, for PIP joint motion, is a palmar splint with 30 degrees of PIP flexion and 20 to 25 degrees for the DIP joint.
    - Type II, for DIP flexion, is a palmar static splint that maintains the PIP joint in full extension and keeps the DIP joint free.
- The exercise regimen is as follows:
  - First 2 weeks:
    - The static splint is removed on the hour for 20 repetitions of PIP and DIP joint exercise, with the wrist at 30 degrees of flexion and the MCP joint at or near 0 degrees of extension.

  - The patient holds the type I splint in place beneath the proximal phalanx, maintains the MCP joint in full extension, and, beginning from full extension, actively flexes the PIP and DIP joints to the restraints of the splint.
  - Each exercise is performed slowly and sustained briefly in full extension for 20 repetitions.
  - The type II splint is then held in place to maintain the PIP joint in full extension, and the DIP joint is fully flexed and extended.
  - If lateral band repair was required, the flexion is limited to 30 to 35 degrees.
  - The patient is instructed in what Evans terms "minimal active muscle tendon tension," which represents a force of about 300 g.
- Third week:
  - The type I splint is altered to allow 40 degrees flexion at the PIP joint if no extensor lag has developed.
- Fourth week:
  - The type I splint is altered to allow 50 degrees of flexion if no extensor lag is present.
  - This is increased to 70 to 80 degrees by the end of the 4th week if the PIP joint is actively extending to 0 degrees.
  - If an extensor lag develops, flexion increments should be less, and active extension exercises and extension splinting should be emphasized.

Zone V to VII Injuries

Caveat: This protocol, along with other dynamic protocols for extensor tendon injuries, is most suitably used in patients who are reliable and well-motivated, and is based on the availability of an experienced and capable hand therapist.

Studies have found that 5 mm of passive tendon glide is safe as well as effective in limiting adhesions after extensor tendon injury. This amount of gliding is achieved by active MCP-joint flexion ranging from 27.5 degrees to 40.9 degrees (index, 28.3 degrees; long, 27.5 degrees; ring, 40.9 degrees; little, 38.3 degrees).

■ The method of postoperative management for extensor tendon injuries in finger zones V to VII begins with dynamic splinting 3 to 5 days after surgery.
■ The wrist is positioned in an appropriate amount of extension to relieve tension at the repair site. This is usually 40 to 45 degrees.
■ The MCP and IP joints are supported at 0 degrees in elastic traction slings attached to an outrigger device (see Figure 12.2-14).
■ A palmar block limits MCP flexion to the arc of motion previously noted to result in 5 mm of extensor tendon excursion.
■ The patient is instructed to actively flex the MCP joints, but to allow the elastic traction on the outrigger device to passively return the digital joints to 0 degrees. This exercise is done 10 times per hour.
■ Dynamic splinting is discontinued between the 3rd and 4th weeks; active motion is then started using gentle active and active assistive exercises that emphasized extension at the MCP joint with the wrist supported in extension.
■ Between 4 and 5 weeks postsurgery, individual finger extension and the claw position are emphasized to direct controlled stress to the adhesions.
■ At 5 to 6 weeks, finger flexion is emphasized.
■ At 7 weeks, resistance, functional electric stimulation, and dynamic flexion splinting are used as needed to encourage full finger flexion.
■ During the phase of dynamic splinting, resting the digital joints at 0 degrees prevents extensor lag. Controlled MCP motion prevents extension contractures, maintains the integrity of the collateral ligaments, and lessens the effects of adhesions at the repair site.
■ With the wrist and MCP joints fully extended, passive movement of the IP joints may be performed without affecting tendon excursion in zones V, VI, and VII, thus avoiding stiffness in these joints.

Wrist Extensor Tendon Injuries in Zone VII

■ Postoperative management of lacerations of the ECRL, ECRB, and ECU includes immobilization of the wrist at 40 to 45 degrees extension for 4 to 5 weeks with the fingers free.
■ Progressive active and gentle passive range of motion is started after 4 to 5 weeks, and a night splint that keeps the wrist in 40 to 45 degrees of extension is used for an additional 2 weeks.

Zone VIII Injuries

■ Postoperative management includes static immobilization of the wrist in 40 to 45 degrees of extension and the MCP joints in 15 to 20 degrees of flexion for 4 weeks, followed by a static night splint that maintains the wrist in extension for an additional 2 weeks.
■ Flexion of the MCP joints may be started at 2 weeks against elastic traction resistance.

SUGGESTED READING

Angeles JG, Heminger H, Mass D. Comparative biomechanical performance of 4-strand core suture repairs for zone II flexor tendon lacerations. J Hand Surg 2002;27:508–517.

Botte MJ, Cohen MS, von Schroeder HP. Method of tendon labeling in forearm injuries. J Hand Surg 1991;16A:763–764.

Botte MJ, Gelberman RH, Smith DG, Silver MA, Gellman H. Repair of severe muscle belly lacerations using a tendon graft. J Hand Surg 1987;l2A:406–412.

Diao E. Experimental studies of tendon injuries. In: Trumble TE, ed. Hand surgery update 3, hand, elbow and shoulder. Rosemont, Il: Amer. Soc Surg Hand, 2003:233–251.

Doyle JR. Boutonniere deformity. In: Strickland JW, ed. Master techniques in orthopedic surgery: the hand. 2nd Ed. Philadelphia: Lippincott Williams & Wilkins, 2005.

Doyle JR. Extensor tendons-acute injuries. In: Green DP, Hotchkiss RN, Pederson WC, eds. Green's operative hand surgery. 4th Ed. New York: Churchill Livingstone, 1999:1950–1987.

Doyle JR. Palmar and digital flexor tendon pulleys. Clin Orthop Rel Res, 2001;383:84–96.

Doyle JR, Botte MJ. Palmar hand. In: Surgical anatomy of the hand and upper extremity. Philadelphia: Lippincott Williams & Wilkins, 2002:532–641.

Doyle JR, Semenza J, Gilling B. The effect of succinylcholine on denervated skeletal muscle. J Hand Surg 1981;6:40–42.

Evans RB. An update on extensor tendon management. In: Hunter JM, Schneider LH, Mackin EJ, et al., eds. Rehabilitation of the hand, 4th Ed. St. Louis: CV Mosby, 1996:655–706.

Evans RB. Early active short arc motion for the repaired central slip. J Hand Surg 1994;19A:991–997.

Evans RB, Thompson DE. An analysis of factors that support early active short arc motion of the repaired central slip. J Hand Ther 1992;5:187–210.

Inoue G, Tamura Y. Dislocation of the extensor tendon over the metacarpophalangeal joints. J Hand Surg 1996;21A:464–469.

Leddy JP, Packer JW. Avulsion of the profundus tendon insertion in athletes. J Hand Surg 1977;2:66–69.

Newport ML. Extensor tendon injuries in the hand. J Acad Orthop Surg 1997;5:59–66.

Peterson WW, Manske PR, Bollinger BA, et al. Effect of pulley excision on flexor tendon biomechanics. J Orthop Res 1986;4:96–101.

Rayan GM, Murray D. Classification and treatment of closed sagittal band injuries. J Hand Surg 1994;19A:590–594.

Schneider LH. Flexor tendons-late reconstruction. In: Green DP, Hotchkiss RN, Pederson WC, eds. Green's operative hand surgery. 4th Ed. New York: Churchill Livingstone, 1999:1898–1949.

Secretan H. Oedeme sur et hyperplasie traumatique du metacarpe dorsal. Rev Med Suisse Romande 1901;21:409.

Seiler JG. Flexor tendon repair. In: Trumble TE, ed. Hand surgery update 3, hand, elbow and shoulder. Rosemont, Il: Amer. Soc Surg Hand, 2003:253–259.

Silfverskiold KL, Andersson CH. Two new methods of tendon repair: an in vitro evaluation of tensile strength and gap formation. J Hand Surg 1993;18A:58–65.

Strickland JW. Flexor tendons-acute injuries. In: Green DP, Hotchkiss RN, Pederson WC, eds. Green's operative hand surgery. 4th Ed. New York: Churchill Livingstone, 1999:1851–1897.

Widstrom CJ, Johnson G, Doyle JR, et al. A mechanical study of six digital pulley reconstruction techniques: part I. Mechanical effectiveness. J Hand Surg1989;14A:821–825.

NERVE INJURIES

Our peripheral nervous system is our mediator to, and interpreter of, our external environment. This system, along with the optic nervous system, makes it possible for us to not only survive, but to flourish in our environment.

This chapter will discuss the evaluation and treatment of acute nerve injuries as seen in the hand, wrist, and forearm, and will emphasize the diagnosis of acute nerve injuries and the management of commonly encountered injuries of the three major upper extremity nerves and their branches.

This chapter will also describe the classic hand deformities, and findings seen following nerve injuries, repair techniques, and some of the tendon transfers used to treat irreparable nerve injuries.

The discussion of nerve injuries begins with the pertinent anatomy and physiology of nerve injury and repair.

PERTINENT ANATOMY

Gross Anatomy of the Nerves of the Upper Extremity

The anatomic configuration and relationships of the median, ulnar, and radial nerves in the upper extremity are depicted in Figure 13-1. These figures represent the most usual or common arrangement of the nerves, and do not depict anatomic variations. The distribution of the cutaneous nerves in the upper extremity given in Figure 13-2 and Figure 13-3 indicates the most common distribution of the cutaneous branches of the three major nerves in the hand.

Peripheral Nerves

Neural Components

The peripheral nerves contain motor, sensory, and autonomic fibers. The motor fibers originate from the motor neurons in the anterior horn of the spinal cord. The sensory fibers originate from the sensory neurons in the dorsal root ganglia. The autonomic fibers are either preganglionic, arising from the neurons in the brainstem/spinal cord, or postganglionic, arising from the neurons in paravertebral ganglia.

Spatial Organization

There is a significant degree of topographical localization in the peripheral nerve trunk that correlates to distal function. Motor neurons serving a single muscle are found grouped together within the anterior horn of the spinal cord.

Macroscopic and Microscopic Anatomy

Figure 13-4 illustrates the macroscopic anatomy of a typical peripheral nerve as seen in the upper extremity. The following descriptive terms are useful anatomic points of understanding about nerve injury and repair.

The Three Concentric Layers

Epineurium. Epineurium is a loose, collagenous connective tissue that represents the outermost layer of the nerve as well as an internal investing layer that surrounds fascicles and groups of fascicles. The epineurium is an elongation of the dural sleeve of the spinal nerve roots, and is divided into external and internal layers. The external epineurium surrounds the peripheral nerve, and anchors blood vessels entering from the surrounding tissue. The internal epineurium is present between fascicles, and cushions them from external force. It also contains blood vessels. The percentage of nerve cross-sectional area represented by the epineurium may vary, and greater amounts may be found in the nerves in the region of joints and in more exposed locations. This layer may thicken or enlarge in response to trauma, and may represent a large portion of the scar seen after nerve injury. The epineurium is surrounded by a loose collection of areolar tissue that under normal circumstances (absence of extrinsic scar tissue) accounts for the longitudinal excursion of the nerve and the avoidance of traction injuries.

Perineurium. The perineurium surrounds individual fascicles, and is composed of up to 10 concentric lamellae of flattened cells, with prominent basement membranes that are linked tightly together. Longitudinally and obliquely oriented collagen fibers are present between these lamellae. The perineurium functions as an extension of the blood-brain barrier, controlling the intraneural ionic environment by limiting diffusion, blocking the spread of infection to the endoneurium, and maintaining a slightly positive intrafascicular pressure. The perineurium surrounds each fascicle

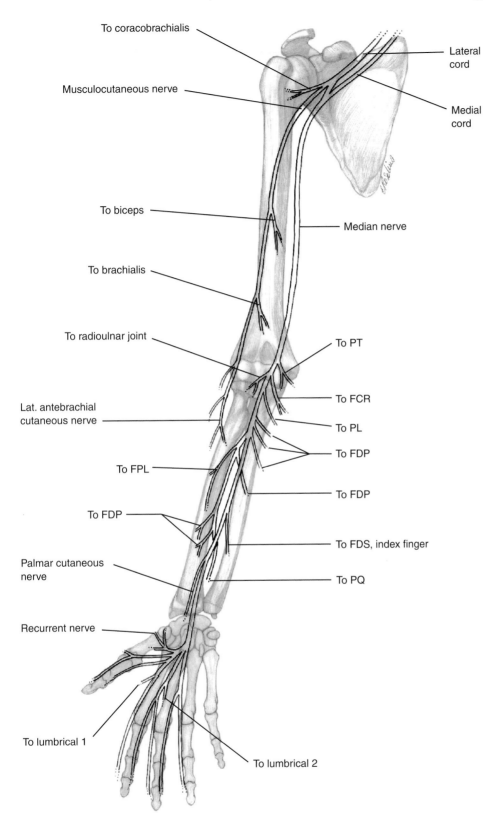

To coracobrachialis

Musculocutaneous nerve

Lateral cord

Medial cord

To biceps

Median nerve

To brachialis

To radioulnar joint

To PT

To FCR

Lat. antebrachial cutaneous nerve

To PL

To FDP

To FPL

To FDP

To FDP

To FDS, index finger

Palmar cutaneous nerve

To PQ

Recurrent nerve

To lumbrical 1

To lumbrical 2

Figure 13-1 The configuration and anatomic relationships of the three major nerves of the upper extremity, and their branches showing distribution and muscles innervated. *Figure continues.*

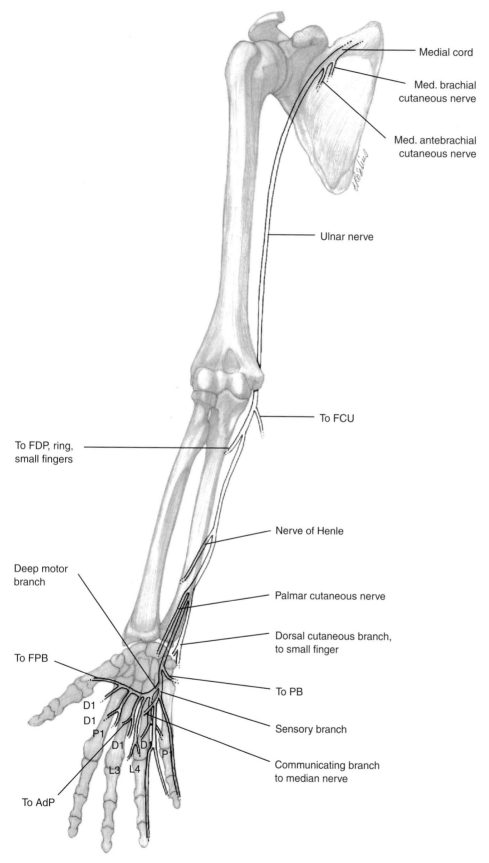

Medial cord

Med. brachial
cutaneous nerve

Med. antebrachial
cutaneous nerve

Ulnar nerve

To FCU

To FDP, ring,
small fingers

Nerve of Henle

Deep motor
branch

Palmar cutaneous nerve

Dorsal cutaneous branch,
to small finger

To FPB

To PB

D1

D1

Sensory branch

P1

D1   D   P

L3   L4

Communicating branch
to median nerve

To AdP

Figure 13-1 (*continued*)

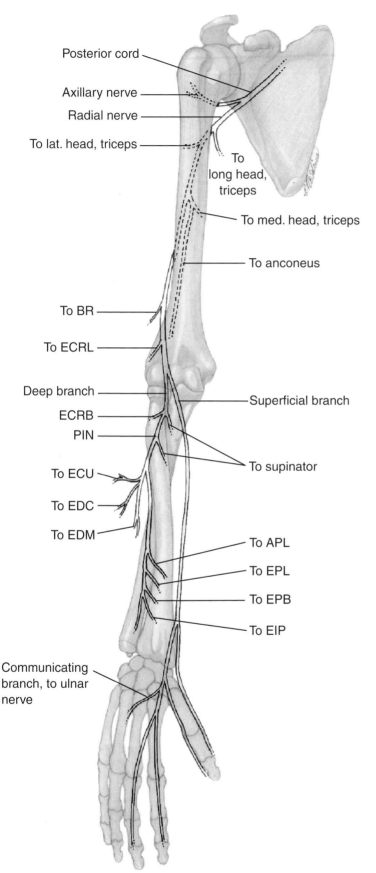

Posterior cord

Axillary nerve

Radial nerve

To lat. head, triceps

To long head, triceps

To med. head, triceps

To anconeus

To BR

To ECRL

Deep branch

ECRB

PIN

To ECU

To EDC

To EDM

Superficial branch

To supinator

To APL

To EPL

To EPB

To EIP

Communicating branch, to ulnar nerve

Figure 13-1 *(continued)*

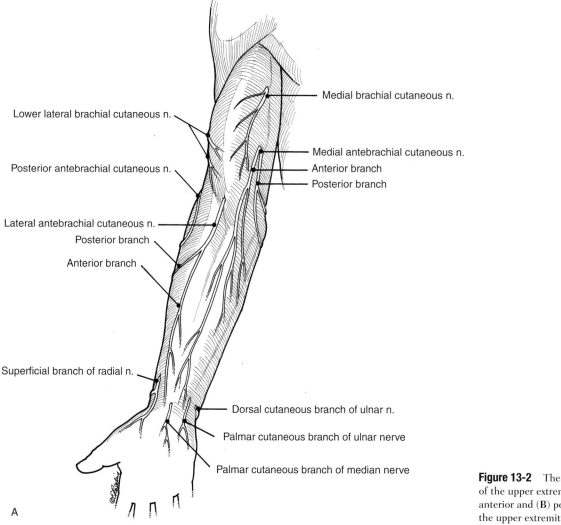

Lower lateral brachial cutaneous n.

Posterior antebrachial cutaneous n.

Lateral antebrachial cutaneous n.
Posterior branch
Anterior branch

Superficial branch of radial n.

Medial brachial cutaneous n.

Medial antebrachial cutaneous n.
Anterior branch
Posterior branch

Dorsal cutaneous branch of ulnar n.

Palmar cutaneous branch of ulnar nerve

Palmar cutaneous branch of median nerve

A

Figure 13-2   The cutaneous nerves of the upper extremity of the (**A**) anterior and (**B**) posterior aspects of the upper extremity. *Figure continues.*

and provides a diffusion barrier. This layer maintains a positive pressure gradient that is manifested by the bulging fascicles of a freshly cut nerve.

Endoneurium.   The endoneurium is the collagenous tissue that acts as "packing" among axons within the perineurium. The endoneurium participates in formation of the Schwann cell tube that contains the myelinated axon and its associated Schwann cells. Schwann cells form membranous expansions around axons, and form the myelin sheath that, in oversimplified terms, represents the "insulation" around the axon and promotes efficient conduction and velocity of action potentials. Large myelinated axons have two layers of collagen (endoneurium); the outer is longitudinally oriented and the inner is arranged randomly and is associated with reticulin. Small myelinated axons have only the outer, longitudinal layer. The Schwann cell basement membrane forms the inner lining of this tubular structure. Endoneurial collagen resists longitudinal stress, and the Schwann cell participates in a complex homeostatic relationship with the axon.

The Fascicle
The fascicle is the smallest unit of nerve tissue than can be manipulated surgically; it contains axons enclosed by endoneurium and is in turn wrapped in perineurium (Figure 13-4). The number of fascicles in a given nerve may vary in number and size. Interconnections may occur between fascicles. Fascicular group mapping has permitted more accurate reapproximation of nerves, and identification of these fascicular groups as to size and axial orientation may allow the surgeon to more appropriately reconnect or join severed nerves either primarily or with nerve grafts.

Vascular Supply
Peripheral nerves are very vascular, and segmental nutrient vessels join a plexus of predominantly longitudinal vessels in the epineurium. These, in turn, supply a second plexus that lies among the lamellae of the perineurium. Perineurial vessels may travel for long distances before entering the endoneurium. This longitudinal plexus of blood vessels allows a nerve to be mobilized for a significant distance without ischemic compromise.

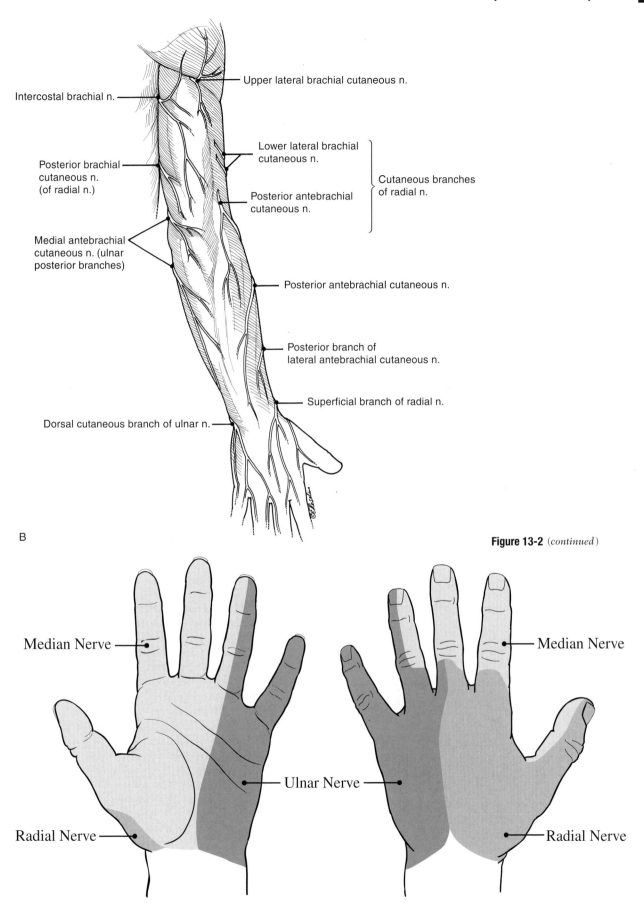

Upper lateral brachial cutaneous n.

Intercostal brachial n.

Posterior brachial cutaneous n. (of radial n.)

Medial antebrachial cutaneous n. (ulnar posterior branches)

Lower lateral brachial cutaneous n.

Posterior antebrachial cutaneous n.

Cutaneous branches of radial n.

Posterior antebrachial cutaneous n.

Posterior branch of lateral antebrachial cutaneous n.

Superficial branch of radial n.

Dorsal cutaneous branch of ulnar n.

B

Figure 13-2 (*continued*)

Median Nerve

Median Nerve

Ulnar Nerve

Radial Nerve

Radial Nerve

Figure 13-3   The terminal (cutaneous) distribution of the median, ulnar, and radial nerves in the palm and back of the hand.

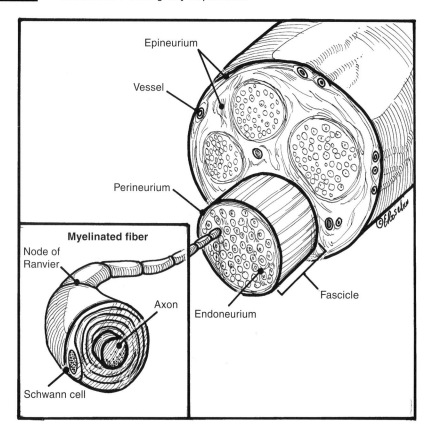

Figure 13-4 Typical cross-sectional anatomy of a peripheral nerve showing the nerve axons surrounded by the investing layers of endoneurium, perineurium, and epineurium. Note the grossly visible vascular network in the perineurium (see text for details).

The Neuron

The neuron is the basic functional and morphological unit of the peripheral nerve. Each neuron consists of a cell body with cytoplasmic extensions, called dendrites, and an axon (Figure 13-5).

The cell body contains a single nucleus with one or more nucleoli, ribosomes, endoplasmic reticulum, and the

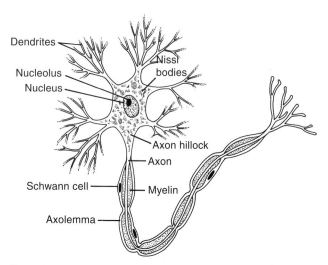

Figure 13-5 The basic functional unit of the peripheral nerve is the neuron, which consists of a cell body, an axon, and dendrites. The axon and dendrites are protoplasmic extensions of the cell body. Some axons are unmyelinated and some are myelinated.

Golgi apparatus. It synthesizes structural components of the neuron.

The axon is a special cylindrical extension arising from the neuron at a confluence of cytoplasm called the axonal hillock. The axon contains axoplasm, microtubules, and neurofilaments surrounded by the axolemma, which serves as the surface membrane. The axon functions as a means of bidirectional axonal transport and nerve conduction.

In general, Schwann cells surround all axons—but only the larger axons have a myelin sheath. In larger myelinated axons, Schwann cells are present along the entire length, and are said to be the glial cells of the peripheral nervous system. The myelinated axon has characteristic indentations at uniform intervals; these are called the *nodes of Ranvier* and are myelin-free zones that facilitate ionic exchange and propagation of electric conduction. The diameter of the axon is one factor that may determine the presence or absence of myelin. The size of the axon may determine the thickness of the myelin layer. Motor fibers have thicker myelin sheaths than sensory fibers.

In an unmyelinated nerve, each Schwann cell surrounds several small axons, and in a myelinated nerve, Schwann cells surround a single axon. The myelin sheath is a complex proteophospholipid that promotes conduction efficiency and the velocity of action potentials. Myelinated axons have four distinctive regions: *the node of Ranvier, paranode, juxtaparanode,* and *internode.* Each of these zones is characterized by a specific set of axonal proteins. Voltage-gated sodium channels are clustered at the nodes, whereas potassium channels are concentrated at juxtaparanodal regions.

Sensory Receptors

There are three common types of mechanoreceptors, and their roles in sensory perception are noted as follows.

Merkel Cell

The Merkel cell is a disc-shaped cell that is clustered around the sweat duct. This complex consists of several receptors served by the branches of a single axon.

This receptor is *slowly adapting,* and is very sensitive to the perpendicular indentation of the skin. The Merkel cell has a well-circumscribed receptive field of 2 to 4 mm, and responds to a small area of skin pressure, such as *static 2-point discrimination.*

Meissner Corpuscle

The Meissner corpuscles are located in the superficial dermis, and are most highly developed in the finger pulp or pads. They are egg-shaped lamellar structures situated closely below the dermis at the sides of the intermediate ridge, and are anchored by thin strands of connective tissue.

These receptors are innervated by several terminal axons, and are *rapidly adapting.* They provide information about rapidly fluctuating mechanical forces acting on the palmar surfaces of the hands and feet.

They fire briefly at the start of stimulus and at times at the end, and respond to flutter vibration at 30 cps. The Meissner corpuscle is well equipped for analysis of motion, such as *moving 2-point discrimination.*

Pacinian Corpuscle

The Pacinian corpuscle lies in the subcutaneous tissue of the palmar and plantar surfaces, and is visible to the naked eye; it reaches up to 2 mm in length.

A single axon innervates the corpuscle and is surrounded by 40 to 60 concentric lamellae.

The Pacinian corpuscle is *rapidly adapting,* and is especially sensitive to vibration with a receptive field that is up to several centimeters in diameter.

PHYSIOLOGY OF NERVE INJURY AND REPAIR

Classification of Injury

Sir Herbert Seddon and Sir Sydney Sunderland both devised a classification system of nerve injury based on degree of disruption of the internal structures of the peripheral nerve. These systems are simple and widely used today because of their correlation to the degree of nerve injury and thus provide a useful basis for comparison of results with various treatments and lend themselves, to some degree, as prognostic factors following nerve injuries. Sunderland noted that nerve injuries may be represented by more than one degree of injury, and that a nerve injury may not always fall into a single category. Table 13-1 compares these two classification systems.

Degeneration and Regeneration

Events in the Neuron and Proximal Axon Following Nerve Injury

The following sequence represents a cursory summary of the events that may occur in the neuron and proximal axon after axotomy.

1. Signals from the periphery turn on the genes in the neuron for successful reinnervation. The neuron receives specific signals from the axonal injury site, which in turn prime the cell to initiate the process of degeneration and subsequent regeneration.
2. The *first phase* is characterized by the arrival of action potentials generated at the injury site. This burst of action potentials opens gated calcium channels, causing an influx of calcium ions that activate calcium-sensitive protein kinases. These kinases regulate various transcription factors.
3. In the *second phase,* protein kinases and other intrinsic constituents activated at the injury site are transported retrograde, promoting synthesis of proteins required for

TABLE 13-1 COMPARISON OF SUNDERLAND AND SEDDON CLASSIFICATION OF NERVE INJURIES

Author	Descriptive Term	Nature of Injury/Neuropathology
Sunderland Seddon	First Degree Injury Neurapraxia	Demyelinating injury with a temporary conduction block
Seddon Sunderland	Second Degree Injury Axonotmesis	Distal degeneration of the injured axon but with almost always complete regeneration due to intact endoneurium
Sunderland Seddon	Third Degree Injury Neurotmesis	Sunderlands third degree injury is less severe than the neurotmesis category of Seddon since the perineurial layer is intact. Regeneration occurs but is incomplete due to endoneurial scarring and loss of end-organ specificity within the fascicle
Sunderland	Fourth Degree Injury	Axon, endoneurium, perineurium are disrupted with extensive scarring that blocks axonal regeneration and often results in a neuroma-in-continuity.
Sunderland	Fifth Degree Injury	Severed nerve trunk without possibility of spontaneous regeneration.

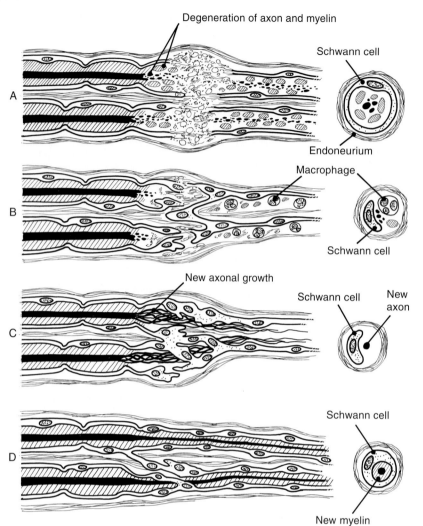

Degeneration of axon and myelin

Schwann cell

Endoneurium

Macrophage

Schwann cell

New axonal growth

Schwann cell   New axon

Schwann cell

New myelin

Figure 13-6 Wallerian degeneration and regeneration. **A.** Breakdown of axoplasm and cytoskeletons into granular, ovoid particles. **B.** Macrophages appear, and in 2 to 3 days they phagocytize and clear away these particles. **C.** Schwann cells proliferate by mitosis, and form a line known as Bunger's band. **D.** Schwann cells wrap around and myelinate newly regenerating axons. (After Chiu DTW, Choi M, Dellon AL. Nerve Physiology and Repair. In: Trumble TE, ed. Hand surgery update 3: hand, elbow & shoulder. Rosemont, IL: American Society for Surgery of the Hand, 2003:287–297).

regeneration. Growth-specific proteins are synthesized, and are transported distally.

4. The *third phase* is mediated by neurotrophic factors, growth-promoting surface molecules, and cytokines released by the extrinsic cells, such as the macrophages and Schwann cells at the injury site. These are then taken up by the injured axon and transported back to the neuron.

5. The *last phase* marks the end of regeneration. Growth factors produced by the target organ arrive.

Axon Sprouting

Within hours of an injury, so-called *collateral sprouts* begin to develop from the most distal node of Ranvier proximal to the site of injury. The sprout formation site may be close to the injury site (in a sharp transection) or farther away (in an avulsion/crush-type injury). *Terminal sprouts* arise from the tip of the surviving axon.

Events in the Distal Axon Following Nerve Injury

Wallerian Degeneration. Wallerian degeneration is a breakdown and cleanup process that occurs in the distal

axon in response to nerve injury (Figure 13-6). It is summarized as:

1. Axoplasm and cytoskeletons break down.
2. Macrophages appear in the injured area and begin to phagocytize the breakdown material.
3. Schwann cells proliferate by mitosis, forming a line known as Bunger's band.
4. Schwann cells envelope and form myelin around new regenerating axons.

Step one is initiated by the influx of calcium ions immediately following an injury. Circulating macrophages and those within the nerve are attracted to the injured area in large numbers. After 2 or 3 days, they start to phagocytize these particles and clear them away.

Schwann cells start to proliferate by mitosis, forming a line known as Bunger's band. This degenerative process takes at least 1 to 2 weeks, and electrodiagnostic tests performed during this period may not pick up any abnormality.

The known key players for Wallerian degeneration are macrophages, Schwann cells, various neurotrophic factors, the injured neuron, and end organs. They influence each other in an intricate interplay, which is currently only partially understood.

If an axon does not regenerate in a timely fashion, the distal endoneurial tube may collapse, rendering regeneration of the axon difficult, if not impossible.

This may be the main reason that muscles fail to be reinnervated following a delayed surgical nerve repair, rather than due to degeneration of muscle fibers and motor end plates, as previously thought.

Regeneration. During regeneration, Schwann cells and neurons are interdependent. This relationship is mediated by both neurotrophic factors and neurite outgrowth promoting factors.

Neurotrophic factors facilitate bidirectional communication between neurons and Schwann cells. Neurite outgrowth promoting factors facilitate attachment of growing axons to other axons and/or Schwann cells, and thus guide nerve regeneration.

Neurotrophic factors are peptides, three major groups of which have been identified: neurotrophins, neurokines, and the transforming growth factor (TGF).

The details of axoplasmic transport, nerve conduction, and neuromuscular transmission are beyond the scope of this text. For more details of these complex processes, refer to the Suggested Readings—particularly the chapter on Nerve Physiology and Repair in *Hand Surgery Update*.

DIAGNOSIS

■ Peripheral nerves are most always *mixed* nerves (they contain both motor and sensory nerve fibers), but the injury may not always involve both components of the nerve.

■ Nerve injuries may be *partial,* and may spare some vital nerve pathways while injuring others.

■ The appraisal of peripheral nerve injuries involves the examination of both *sensory* and *motor* components of the nerve that is being evaluated.

■ Sensory evaluation is based on examination of a nerve's *autonomous zone* of innervation (the anatomic site least likely to have any overlap with another nerve).

■ Motor evaluation is focused on the functional motor unit that is the last or most terminal muscle to be innervated by the nerve under evaluation, or sometimes by the ease of examination of a muscle known to be innervated by that nerve.

■ In an acute situation in the emergency room, the sensory evaluation of an injured nerve is best determined by *light touch* rather than by a pin or needle (especially in children). Two-point discrimination is a valuable tool for evaluation of sensation, but it may be difficult to achieve in an acute injury in the emergency room.

■ Both sensory and motor evaluations are made before any form of local anesthesia is given.

■ In most, if not all instances, the diagnosis of a peripheral nerve injury may be made without inappropriate exploration of the wound in an emergency room setting. The diagnosis is made based on knowledge of the anatomy involved and on a focused examination that utilizes that knowledge.

■ When in doubt as to the extent or nature of injuries to the nerve from lacerations, explore the wound under appropriate anesthesia in an operating room.

The Hoffman-Tinel Sign

■ This is a clinical sign that's useful for determining the level of nerve injury or recovery based on the presence of injured or regenerating axons.

■ The test is performed by digital percussion of the nerve distal to the site of nerve injury, with proximal advancement of the percussion until the site of injury is reached or the zone of regeneration is identified.

■ The percussion, performed gently with the examiner's fingertip, progresses along the course of the nerve until the endpoint is identified by paresthesia localized either to the zone of injury in cases of complete nerve interruption, or distally into the zone of cutaneous innervation.

■ Some clinicians prefer to percuss from proximal to distal to the site of the lesion downward until the paresthesia disappears.

■ The paresthesia, or "pins and needles" sensation, is caused by the regenerating axons that are sensitive to percussion, in part because of the loss of the myelin sheath as part of *Wallerian* degeneration.

■ A positive response over a long segment of nerve may be due to unequal growth rates of various sensory fibers.

■ The sign may be absent in the first 4 to 6 weeks after nerve suture, and the onset and progress of the sign may be inversely proportional to the severity of the injury.

■ Steady distal progression of the endpoint is a favorable sign in nerve regeneration, but it must be recognized that the sign is *qualitative,* not *quantitative.*

CONVENTIONAL TERMS USED IN PERIPHERAL NERVE INJURIES

■ A nerve laceration is said to be *high* or *low* (proximal or distal).

■ More than one nerve may be injured in a *combined* injury. An example is a median and ulnar nerve laceration at the wrist.

■ Combined injuries are often associated with injuries to the vascular supply, which may complicate treatment and recovery. Furthermore, in some unusual instances, the injured nerves may be at different anatomic levels.

SPECIFIC NERVE INJURIES

■ Figures 13-1 and 13-3 show the classic patterns of motor innervation and sensory distribution of the specific nerves.

■ The three major nerves may be injured at any level, but our discussion is confined to nerve injuries in the forearm, wrist, or hand.

- The loss of motor function and sensation will depend on the level of injury.
- Lesions may be represented by contusion, crush, or partial or complete lacerations.
- Our discussion will assume that the injuries are complete, and that motor and sensory components are completely lacerated.

Median Nerve

High Lesions
Sensory Deficits

- Sensory deficit in the flexor aspect of the thumb, index finger, middle finger, and radial half of the ring finger.
- The *autonomous zone* of deficit evaluation is the flexor aspect of the terminal phalanx of the index finger (Figure 13-7).

Motor Deficits

- Loss of pronation of the forearm, flexion at the interphalangeal (IP) joint of the thumb, distal interphalangeal (DIP) joints of the index and middle fingers,

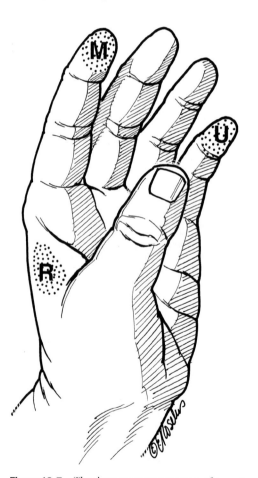

Figure 13-7 The three autonomous zones of sensation in the hand. These are the areas least likely to have any sensory nerve overlap, and thus may be considered reliable areas to test for sensation of the respective nerves involved. M, median, flexor aspect of the terminal phalanx of the index finger; R, radial, web space between the thumb and index finger; U, ulnar, flexor aspect of the terminal phalanx of the little finger.

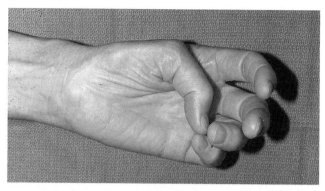

Figure 13-8 Several week old median nerve laceration showing loss of opposition of thumb, and atrophy of the thenar muscles.

proximal interphalangeal (PIP) joints of the four fingers, and abduction-opposition of the thumb.

Dynamic Posture

- Ulnar deviation of wrist with wrist flexion.
- There is also an inability to perform pulp-to-pulp contact between the thumb and the adjacent digits (opposition).
- The thumb stays adducted in the palm during attempted opposition (Figure 13-8).

Low Lesions
Sensory Deficit

- Sensory deficit in the flexor aspect of the thumb, and index finger, middle finger, and ulnar half of the ring finger.
- The autonomous zone of deficit is the flexor aspect of terminal phalanx of the index finger (see Figure 13-7).

Motor Deficit

- Loss of abduction-opposition of thumb.
- Isolated injury of the motor branch of the median nerve will result in loss of thumb abduction-opposition without sensory deficit (Figure 13-8).

Ulnar Nerve

High Lesions
Sensory Deficit

- Loss of sensation in the flexor/dorsal aspect of the little finger, ulnar half of the ring finger, and flexor/dorsal aspect of ulnar half of the hand.
- The autonomous zone of deficit is the flexor aspect of the terminal phalanx of the little finger (Figure 13-7).

Motor Deficit

- Loss of flexion of the flexor digitorum profundus (FDP) of the ring and little fingers; loss of function in all intrinsic muscles except for the lumbricals of the index and middle fingers; and loss of flexion in the flexor carpi ulnaris (FCU).
- Profound wasting of the intrinsic muscles is noted (Figure 13-9).

Dynamic Posture

- Wrist flexion is associated with slight radial deviation.
- Attempts to extend the ring and little fingers result in hyperextension at the metacarpophalangeal (MCP) joints,

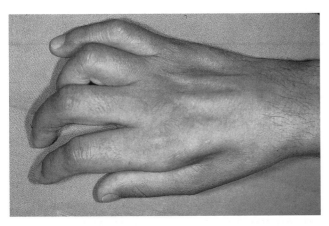

Figure 13-9   High ulnar nerve laceration showing profound atrophy of the intrinsic muscles of the hand.

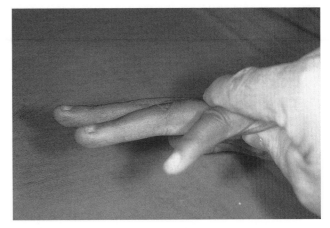

Figure 13-11   Pressure or downward force over the proximal phalanges of the clawed ring and little fingers (low ulnar nerve palsy) reproduces the action of the intrinsic muscles and corrects most of the claw deformity. This finding is called Bouvier's maneuver.

and in flexion at the PIP joints. This is called *Duchenne's sign* (Figure 13-10).

■ Pressure or force over the proximal phalanges of these digits by the examiner promotes extension of the PIP joints; this is called *Bouvier's sign or maneuver* (Figure 13-11).

■ A weak and unstable pinch, with hyperextension of the thumb MCP joint (*Jeanne's sign*) and with hyperflexion of IP joint (*Froment's sign*), are also classic signs of ulnar nerve palsy (Figure 13-12).

■ There is an inability to cross the middle finger over the index finger or to cross the index over the middle finger. This indicates a loss of function in the second and first dorsal interosseous muscles, respectively.

■ The claw deformity may not be as prominent in high ulnar lesions compared to low lesions since both the flexor digitorum superficialis (FDS) and the FDP extrinsic finger flexors are intact in low lesions, and since they account for a stronger flexion deformity in the ring and little fingers.

Low Lesions
Sensory Deficit

■ Loss of sensation in the flexor/dorsal aspect of the little finger, ulnar half of the ring finger, and flexor/dorsal aspect of the ulnar half of the hand.

■ The autonomous zone of deficit is the flexor aspect of the terminal phalanx of the little finger.

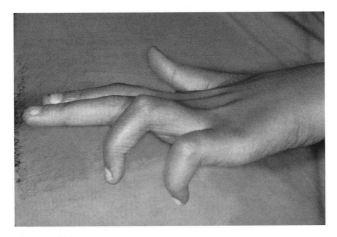

Figure 13-10   Note the claw deformity of the ring and little fingers in this patient with a low ulnar nerve lesion. This deformity is characterized by hyperextension of the ring and little finger MCP joints and flexion of the PIP joints, and is called *Duchenne's sign*. The deformity is due to loss of the ulnar-nerve-innervated lumbricals and the dorsal and palmar interosseous muscles that normally flex the MCP joints and extend the PIP joints, and thus "balance" the effects of the extrinsic flexors of the fingers.

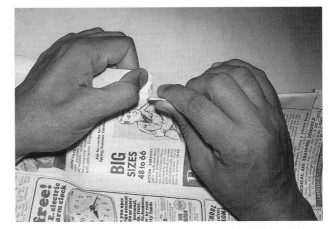

Figure 13-12   Froment's and Jeanne's signs as seen in ulnar nerve palsy in the left hand. Note the compensatory hyperflexion of the IP joint (Froment's sign) and hyperextension of the MCP joint of the thumb (Jeanne's sign) during pinch. This posture is due to loss of the stabilizing force of the adductor muscle on the MCP joint of the thumb and compensatory hyperflexion of the thumb IP joint. Note also the atrophy of the first dorsal interosseous muscle in the thumb-index web space.

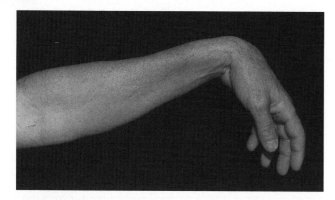

Figure 13-13 This patient demonstrates a high radial nerve palsy. Note the loss of extension of the wrist, thumb, and fingers secondary to a laceration of the radial nerve above the elbow.

Motor Deficit

■ Motor deficits are the same as in high ulnar nerve lesions, except that the FDP function to ring and little fingers is intact, and may accentuate the claw deformity.

Dynamic Posture

■ The dynamic posture is the same as in high ulnar nerve lesions.

Radial Nerve

High Lesions
Sensory Deficit

■ There is loss of sensation over the dorsal radial aspect of the hand and thumb.
■ The autonomous zone is in the web space between the thumb and index finger.

Motor Deficit

■ There is loss of extension of the wrist, fingers, and thumb mediated by the EDC, EDM, EIP, ECRB, ECRL, ECU, EPL, EPB and APL.

Dynamic Posture

■ A high radial nerve lesion results in the loss of wrist, finger, and thumb extension, and is commonly called a "wrist drop" (Figure 13-13).
■ This represents a total and high radial nerve lesion before its division into the motor and sensory components.
■ This division may occur in a region that is 2.5 cm above or 3.0 cm below a line drawn in the coronal plane between the medial and lateral epicondyle of the humerus (Hueter's line).

Low Radial Nerve Palsy
Sensory Deficit

■ The high and low lesion convention has worked well for the median and ulnar nerves, but works less well for the radial nerve because the motor and sensory components are widely separated in the proximal forearm.
■ The *sensory component* of the radial nerve may be injured in a "high or low" anatomic position. This results in the same clinical manifestations that are noted for the high lesion.

Motor Deficit

■ The motor deficit will vary according to the level of injury and the sequence or order of innervation of the respective muscles.
■ The sequence of innervation order is quite *variable*, but Figure 13-1 shows a common one.
  ■ A common sequence is the innervation of the ECRL, supinator, and ECRB, in that order.
  ■ The EDC is most always innervated before the EIP, APL, and EPL.
  ■ The EDM is usually innervated before the EIP, and the APL before the EPL.

PRINCIPLES OF NERVE REPAIR

Primary, Delayed Primary, and Secondary Repair

■ Primary repair is defined as repair within hours of injury.
■ Delayed primary repair is repair performed 5 to 7 days after injury.
■ A repair performed more than 1 week after injury is called a secondary repair.
■ Primary nerve repair has emerged as the treatment of choice when conditions permit (Box 13-1). If these conditions cannot be met, it is better to delay repair.
■ Secondary repair under favorable conditions is usually associated with improved outcomes compared to nerve repair done under less than ideal circumstances.
■ In cases where timely repair cannot be performed, the nerve ends should be sutured together to prevent retraction. This will facilitate a future definitive repair.

Techniques of Nerve Suture

Epineurial Suture

■ Magnification improves the results of nerve suture and the operating microscope is a useful tool to facilitate nerve suture.

BOX 13-1 CONDITIONS THAT FAVOR PRIMARY REPAIR

■ Sharp transections without any element of crush injury
■ Absence of significant tension at the repair site when the ends are joined
■ Minimal wound contamination; a suitable bed of viable muscle, fat, or tenosynovium
■ Absence of other injuries that preclude timely restoration of circulation, skeletal stability, or soft tissue cover
■ A suitable operating room and equipment, including magnification
■ A patient in suitable metabolic and emotional condition to undergo surgery
  ■ An intoxicated patient or a patient who has just attempted suicide is not an ideal candidate for primary repair.

- Placement of the proximal and distal nerve stumps on suitable background material in a bloodless field aids in visualization.
- Correct rotational orientation is obtained by matching the fascicular bundles with respect to size and position, and matching the orientation of the vascular landmarks.
- The cut ends are trimmed perpendicular to their long axis to remove any damaged tissues and to form a uniform surface for contact between the ends.
- A smooth and uniform transection prior to repair may be achieved by devices that hold or stabilize the nerve during the transection.
- A single suture is placed to join the epineurial edges furthest from the surgeon.
- A second suture is then placed at 180 degrees from the first to form equal halves.
- Done properly, this will result in matching opposing surfaces, without bulging, retraction, or twisting of the individual fascicles.
- An 8-0 or 9-0 suture is used for these two critical stitches in a major peripheral nerve, and the tails are left long to permit rotation of the nerve.
- The inability to bring the nerves ends together with 8-0 sutures indicates excessive tension, and further mobilization or grafting should be considered.
- Additional interrupted sutures of 10-0 are used to bisect the 180-degree arc formed by the first two sutures.
- Additional sutures are added in a similar fashion to complete the repair but a "watertight" repair is neither necessary nor desired.

Group Fascicular Suture

- Group fascicular suture requires greater magnification and is technically more challenging than epineurial suture.
- This suture technique is less tolerant of repair under tension due to the less substantial nature of the *internal epineurium* and *perineurium*.
- The proximal and distal stump surfaces are inspected to identify fascicular groups. Fascicular groups tend to separate from other fascicular groups, and with gentle traction and dissection with curved microscissors, fascicular groups may be identified.
- Matching fascicular groups are trimmed at right angles to their longitudinal axis and separated for a distance of 3 to 4 mm in the proximal and distal stumps.
- A retention suture placed in the posterior epineurium is useful to control tension and permit rotation of the nerve to aid in placement of sutures in the various fascicular groups.
- The fascicular groups are joined from back to front by sutures placed in the internal epineurium or perineurium. Only the minimum number of sutures necessary to produce uniform coaptation of the fascicular group is placed.

Individual Fascicular Suture

- The separation of individual fascicles is technically challenging and is less commonly used for nerve suture.
- Large fascicles may accept two 10-0 sutures, but a single suture may be appropriate for smaller fascicles.

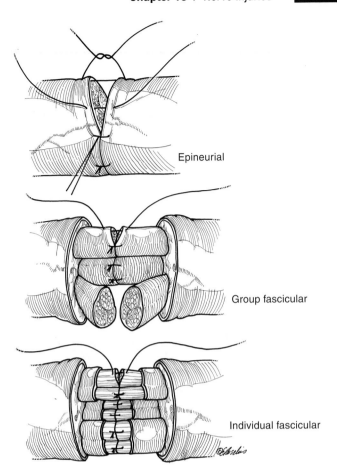

Figure 13-14   The three techniques of peripheral nerve repair.

- This technique may be most useful in partial nerve lacerations where only a portion of a group fascicle has been lacerated.
- Figure 13-14 demonstrates the three techniques of peripheral nerve repair.

Fascicle-Matching Techniques

- Accurate matching of sensory and motor components of a severed nerve is an important factor in the outcome of nerve repair.
- Techniques that aid in matching include using intraneural mapping, intraoperative nerve stimulation, and histochemical identification of the motor and sensory components.
- The later two techniques have time constraints and technical aspects in their performance that limits their use. They may be most useful in secondary nerve reconstruction.

The details of these techniques are beyond the scope of this chapter.

Nerve Grafting

- There are many instances in nerve repair where loss of nerve substance does not permit a *tension free* rejoining of the injured nerve.

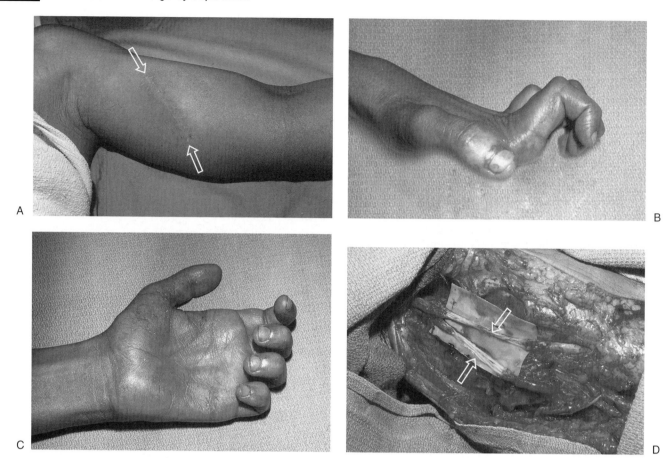

Figure 13-15 **A.** This 22-year-old man sustained a deep laceration to the inner aspect of his left arm. **B, C.** This resulted in sensory deficits in the median and ulnar distribution and a median and ulnar claw hand (a combined high median and ulnar palsy). **D.** He was treated with fascicular bundle nerve grafts (sural nerves) to the median and ulnar nerves, with recovery of wrist and finger flexion and protective sensation in the hand.

- This is most often seen in secondary nerve repair where excision of the scarred and damaged nerve ends results in a significant gap that mitigates against a tension-free union.
- Earlier efforts at nerve graft included interposition of trunk grafts that matched the size of the injured nerve; cable grafts composed of smaller nerves, bundled together, to fill the gap; and a pedicle nerve graft in which one major nerve was sacrificed and used to replace what was considered to be a more important nerve.
- The current technique to restore continuity in a nerve with a significant gap is called group fascicular nerve grafting.
- The technique consists of removing all interposed scar tissue between the two ends of the involved nerve, and interposing autogenous nerve grafts (usually the sural nerve or nerves) to matching fascicles in the proximal and distal stumps.
- Matching of fascicles is most easily achieved in gaps of 4 to 6 cm, although larger gaps may be filled and suitable results obtained (Figure 13-15).
- The lateral antebrachial cutaneous nerve in the forearm may be used to fill gaps in digital nerves.

A discussion of the role of free vascularized nerve grafts, nerve conduits, and neurotropism is beyond the scope of this chapter.

Prognosis and Timing of Nerve Repairs

- In general terms, the results following nerve repair are best within the first 3 months after injury—but reinnervation may be expected within 1 year following injury.
- No reinnervation can be expected after 3 years.

Tendon Transfers in Nerve Injury

- In some instances, nerve repair is not possible—but useful upper extremity function may be restored by tendon transfers.
- In some instances following nerve repair, a useful level of *sensory recovery* (protective sensation or better) may be anticipated *without motor recovery*. It is in these cases that tendon transfer may be most useful.
- Tendon transfers work best in supple joints without fixed contracture and when suitable soft tissue beds are available for passage of the tendons.

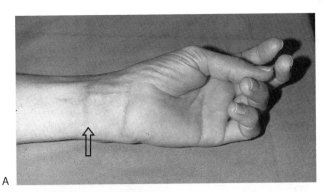

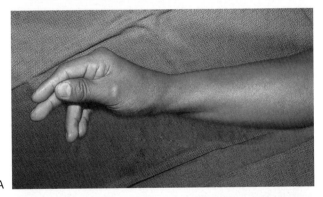

A

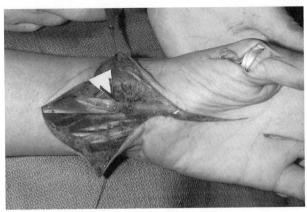

B

Figure 13-16   **A.** Wrist scar, loss of opposition, and thenar eminence atrophy can be seen in this 65-year-old male with complete sensory loss in the median nerve distribution. **B.** Epineurial repair of the median nerve was performed along with a FDS opponensplasty.

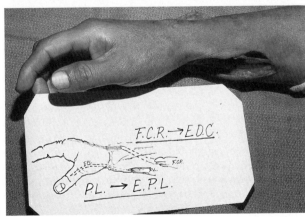

B

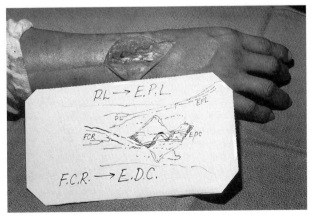

C

Figure 13-17   Intermediate level radial nerve palsy. **A.** Preoperative appearance of an injury to the posterior interosseous branch of the radial nerve (PIN) with loss of thumb and finger extension. **B, C.** Function was restored by transfer of the PL to the rerouted EPL and transfer of the FCR to the EDC tendons.

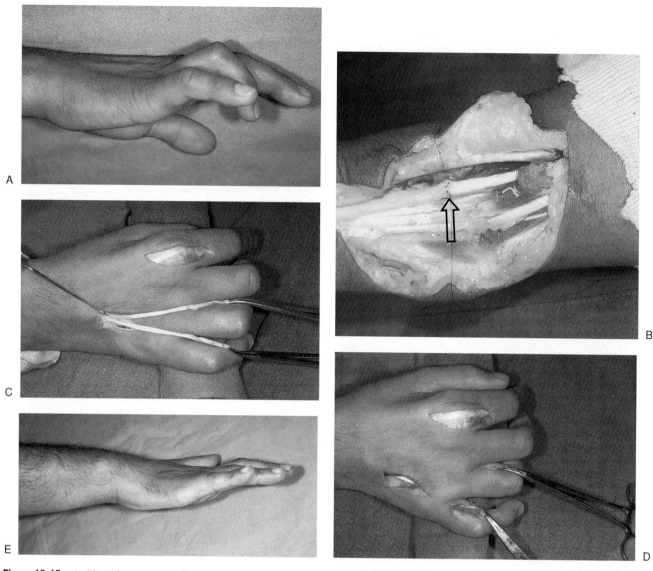

Figure 13-18   **A.** Clinical appearance of an ulnar claw hand. **B.** Secondary epineurial repair of the ulnar nerve was performed. **C, D.** The EIP tendon was split into two tails, passed through the interosseous spaces beneath the axis of rotation of the MCP joints, and sutured to the radial lateral bands of the ring and little fingers. **E.** This transfer replaced the function of the interosseous muscles, rebalanced the extrinsic flexors and extensors, and corrected the claw deformity.

■ The simple treatment algorithm is: (1) what function is lost, and (2) what expendable muscle/tendon units are available for transfer.

■ Selection of an appropriate muscle tendon unit is based on its cross-sectional area (strength) and excursion (fiber length), in order to mimic as much as possible the muscle tendon/unit being replaced.

■ Mechanical factors include orientation of the transfer for a straight-line pull, one transfer to perform one function, appropriate tension, placing the transfer in the proper relationship to the joint axis, and when needed, a strong and suitably placed pulley or fulcrum.

Examples

These transfers are only examples of the many tendon transfers used to restore function in the upper extremity. Refer to the Suggested Reading list for a more comprehensive discussion of the topic.

Low Median Nerve Palsy.   Figure 13-16 demonstrates the preoperative appearance of a 65-year-old male with a one-year-old laceration of the flexor aspect of the left wrist. There was loss of sensation in the median nerve distribution and loss of opposition of the thumb. Treatment included excision of the median nerve neuroma, epineurial repair, and opponensplasty using the FDS of the ring finger to the abductor position of the thumb. Opposition was restored along with protective sensation in the median nerve distribution.

Intermediate Level Radial Nerve Palsy.   Figure 13-17 demonstrates the preoperative appearance of an injury to the posterior interosseous branch of the radial nerve (PIN), with loss of thumb and finger extension. The level of injury was distal to the innervation of the wrist extensors, so wrist extension was maintained. Restoration of thumb and finger extension was achieved by transfer of the PL to the rerouted EPL and transfer of the FCR to the EDC tendons.

Low Ulnar Nerve Palsy. Figure 13-18 demonstrates a typical claw deformity of the ulnar nerve. It resulted from a laceration of the ulnar nerve at the distal forearm. Treatment was by secondary ulnar nerve repair (epineurial) and transfer of a two-tailed tendon graft using the EIP sutured to the radial side of the lateral bands in the ring- and little-finger proximal phalanges.

SUGGESTED READING

Brushart TM. Nerve repair and grafting. In: Green DP, Hotchkiss RN, Pederson WC, eds. Green's operative hand surgery. 4th Ed. New York: Churchill Livingstone, 1999:1381–1403.

Buck-Gramcko D, Lubahn JD. The Hoffmann-Tinel sign. J Hand Surg 1993;18B:800–805.

Chiu DTW, Choi M, Dellon AL. Nerve physiology and repair. In: Trumble TE, ed. Hand surgery update-3, hand, elbow and shoulder. Rosemont, IL: American Society for Surgery of the Hand, 2003:287–297.

Doyle JR, Botte MJ. Surgical anatomy of the hand and upper extremity. Philadelphia: Lippincott Williams & Wilkins, 2002.

Jabaley ME. Internal anatomy of the peripheral nerve. In: Hunter JM, Schneider LH, Mackin EJ, eds. Tendon and nerve surgery in the hand. St. Louis: Mosby-Year Book, 1996:19–25.

Millesi H, Meissl G, Berger A. Further experience with intrafascicular grafting of the median, ulnar, and radial nerves. J Bone Joint Surg 1976;58A:209–218.

Omer G. Combined nerve palsies. In: Green DP, Hotchkiss RN, Pederson WC, eds. Green's operative hand surgery. 4th Ed. New York: Churchill Livingstone, 1999:1542–1555.

Seddon HJ. Surgical disorders of the peripheral nerves. Baltimore: Williams and Wilkins, 1972.

Sheppard JE. Tendon transfers. In: Trumble TE, ed. Hand surgery update-3, hand, elbow and shoulder. Rosemont, IL: American Society for Surgery of the Hand, 2003:353–370.

Smith KL. Anatomy of the peripheral nerve. In: Hunter JM, Schneider LH, Mackin EJ, eds. Tendon and nerve surgery in the hand. St. Louis: Mosby-Year Books, 1996:11–18.

Sunderland S. Nerve and nerve injuries. 2nd Ed. New York: Churchill Livingstone, 1978.

Williams PL. Grays anatomy, 38th Ed. New York: Churchill Livingstone, 1995, Chapter 8, The nervous system.

14 AMPUTATIONS

GENERAL PRINCIPLES

The management of thumb or finger amputation is a complex topic with many variable methods of treatment. Digital amputations may involve the terminal aspect of the digit or a substantial portion of the ray, and general principles of management will be presented in this chapter. This chapter will also include a section on replantation.

The goals of treatment include restoration of adequate sensibility without hypersensitivity, good function and appearance, and a short period of recovery.

The treatment of each case is based on the patient's age, occupation, functional needs, the digit injured, and the surgeon's experience with various techniques.

Treatment methods range from healing by secondary intention with dressing changes, to primary closure (without tension) with local tissue, to split-thickness or full-thickness skin grafts, to various forms of local or distant flaps.

PERTINENT ANATOMY

Terminal Phalanx

Most amputations in the hand involve the terminal phalanx, and this chapter will focus on that level of amputation. The anatomy of the terminal phalanx represents a complex functional unit that consists of bone and soft tissue in the form of thick skin that covers a fat pad with fibrous tissue elements that separate the fat into compartments. This complex structure includes nerves and specialized end organs that provide sensibility to the digital tip in the form of pressure, pain, temperature, and identification of form and texture.

It is the hand, through the digital tips, that obtains information from the environment, which it passes to the brain and ultimately executes a given function in conjunction with the remaining components of the upper extremity. The hand is under central control, mediated by specialized end organs and nerve endings in and beneath the skin, as well as by joint receptors. Although the hand also may be under visual control, this modality is a less effective control method compared to the modalities of sensibility and proprioception:

compare the effective use of the hand by a blind person to the relatively poor hand function in a sighted person who has lost sensibility due to Hansen's disease. Thus, it should be readily apparent that the tips of our digits are critically important to hand function. *The contour of the terminal phalanx with its nail is multiplanar and its shape and specialized end organs can never be restored surgically in spite of our best efforts at reconstruction.*

Nail Unit

The nail unit consists of the nail plate, the nail fold, the nail bed (sterile and germinal matrix), a vascular supply, and nerves. The nail unit assists in digital pad sensibility by providing support and counter pressure for the digital pad. Grasping and pinching are aided by the nail unit, which provides dorsal and peripheral anchoring, and provides stability to the palmar pad. The functional spectrum may include everything from scratching an itch to picking up and manipulating small objects. The anatomy and terminology of the nail unit is depicted in Figure 14-1.

Nail Plate

The hard, often shiny, fingernail or thumbnail is called the nail plate. The nail plate is homologous to the stratum corneum of the epidermis, and consists of compacted, anucleate, keratin-filled squames with dorsal, intermediate, and palmar layers. It is slightly convex in the longitudinal axis and more convex in the transverse axis. The lunula is a white opacity immediately distal to the central aspect of the proximal nail fold, and is said to be due to comparatively poor vascularization of the germinal matrix.

Nail Fold

Proximally, the nail plate extends under the semilunar nail fold, which is lined with dorsal and palmar epidermis. The stratum corneum layer of the dorsal layer of epidermis extends distally over the nail plate to form the cuticle or eponychium.

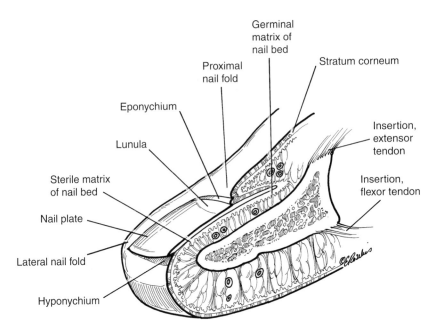

Figure 14-1 The anatomy and terminology of the nail unit and terminal phalanx.

Nail Bed

The nail plate rests on the nail bed (sterile and germinal matrix), which is defined as all the soft tissue immediately beneath the nail plate that participates in nail generation and migration. The nail bed is a specialized form of epithelium, with a proximal zone of germinal matrix and a distal zone of sterile matrix. The germinal matrix is proximal, and the distal margin of the lunula is approximately at the junction between the germinal and sterile matrix. A sagittal section of the distal phalanx reveals a wedge-shaped collection of germinal cells within the proximal portion of the nail bed. Dorsal and palmar components of the matrix are noted. The palmar matrix cells are continuous distally with the nail bed. The nail bed is grooved and ridged longitudinally, which matches a similar pattern on the undersurface of the nail plate, and which may help stabilize the nail for functional demands. Beneath the epithelium of the nail bed is a dermis layer that is anchored to the underlying periosteum of the distal phalanx by fibrous tissue. Keratinized cells are extruded from the dorsal and palmar germinal matrix cells to produce the nail plate, with the major production coming from the palmar cells. The area of epidermis under the distal edge of the nail plate is called the hyponychium. The stratum corneum layer is undulant and constantly being shed. The hyponychium provides an important barrier against entry of bacteria.

Clinical Significance

A smooth nail bed is essential for the regrowth of a normal nail plate. In nail-bed injuries, primary healing cannot occur if the bed is not accurately reapproximated. If the scar is in the dorsal matrix, a dull streak may appear in the nail plate; if the scar is in the intermediate portion of the germinal matrix, a split or absent nail may occur; if the scar is in the palmar nail or sterile matrix, a split or nonadherence of the nail beyond the scar may occur.

Blood Supply and Drainage

The arterial blood supply to the nail bed comes from two dorsal branches from the common palmar digital artery; the proximal vessel is a dorsal branch to the nail fold, and the second courses along the lateral nail plate margin and sends branches to the nail bed (Figure 14-2). These vessels anastomose dorsally with their counterparts to form arcades.

Branches from these vessels and the arcades form sinuses surrounded by muscle fibers, and help to regulate the blood pressure and blood supply to the extremities. These networks have been identified as papillary, reticular, and subdermal, and correspond to the general architecture of the vessels of the skin. The dermis of the nail bed is well vascularized, and includes large arteriovenous shunts (glomera). There is reduced vascular density in the region of the germinal matrix, in contrast to an increased vascular density in the sterile matrix. The comparatively less-vascularized germinal matrix demonstrates a well-developed subdermal network located near a zone of loose connective tissue that is poorly vascularized near the proximal part of the distal phalanx. This zone may be a sliding apparatus between the nail and the distal attachment of the extensor tendon. A coalescence of veins in the skin, proximal to the nail fold, that course proximally in a random fashion over the dorsum of the digit, provides venous drainage. These veins are of sufficient size for microvascular anastomosis.

Nerve Supply

Branches from the paired digital nerves innervate the nail unit. The most common pattern (70%) is represented by a branch that passes beneath the nail plate and into the nail bed at approximately the level of the lunula and a second branch that passes distally to end at the hyponychial area. There are numerous sensory nerve endings, including Merkel discs and Meissner corpuscles.

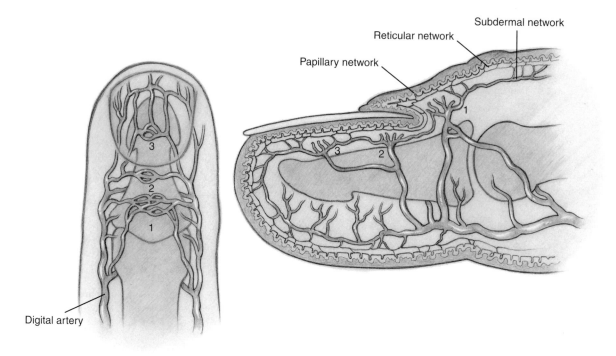

Figure 14-2 Arterial supply of the distal phalanx. 1, Network of nail wall; 2, arcade of germinal matrix; 3, arcade of sterile matrix. See text for details.

Nail Plate Growth

Growth rate is determined by the turnover rate of the germinal matrix, which varies with age, digit (the long finger nail grows faster than the small fingernail), environmental temperature, season, time of day, and nutritional status. Rate of growth in the long finger is approximately 0.1 mm/day. As the matrix cells enlarge, they grow distally due to the confinement of the nail fold, and they are flattened by the pressure of newly forming cells beneath them. This pressure and confinement result in a nail plate that is flat and grows distally. The dorsal layer of the germinal matrix produces nail cells that are relatively shiny, and if these cells are removed or damaged, the nail surface will appear dull.

Relationship of the Germinal Matrix to the Extensor Tendon Insertion

Based on microscopic dissection, the distance from the terminal aspect of insertion of the extensor tendon and the proximal edge of the germinal matrix was found to average 1.2 mm, with a range of 0.9 to 1.8 mm.

The clinical significance of this fact is that when the extensor tendon insertion is visualized during operative procedures on the dorsum of the distal phalanx, care should be taken to avoid damage to the germinal matrix. Conversely, when the germinal matrix is being removed for total ablation of a nail, dissection does not need to be carried proximal to the most distal fibers of the extensor tendon.

TREATMENT

Digital Tip Amputations With or Without Bone Involvement

- These injuries may occur in a variety of planes in relationship to the long axis of the digit. The osseous phalanx may or may not be exposed.
- The following discussion and case presentations illustrate various techniques that may be used based on the nature of the injury.
- The reader should understand that there is no ideal treatment for fingertip amputations, and that differences of opinion exist among the surgeons who treat these injuries.
- Many of the following procedures are technically challenging, and most, if not all, may have cosmetic and functional issues related to the procedure.
- The choice of a given technique may relate to the surgeon's experience and preference.
- *The procedure should be matched to each patient and his or her cosmetic and functional needs.*

Nonsurgical Treatment

- Fingertip avulsions in children may be treated by sterile dressing changes as the primary form of treatment.
- Most, if not all, soft tissue avulsions of the digit tips in children will rapidly regrow the lost skin. This may be the only treatment required.

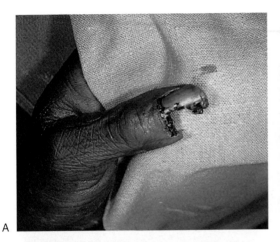
A

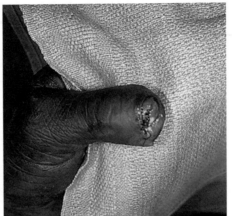
B

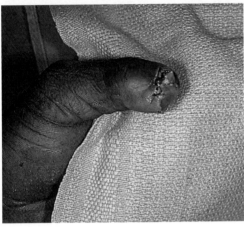
C

Figure 14-3 A. Significant loss of the terminal pulp of the thumb as a result of a power saw injury to the non-dominant left thumb. **B, C.** Treatment was via primary closure, by "folding over" the remaining local tissues. This provided for excellent tissue coverage with good sensibility and circulation. Rapid healing occurred in this unemployed elderly male.

■ In some instances the avulsed part may be reapplied as a biologic dressing with the understanding that it may or may not survive.

■ Significant bone protrusion, if evident, may need to be trimmed back.

■ Secondary reconstruction may be used as necessary.

Surgical Treatment
Primary Closure by Local Tissue

■ Suitable local tissues, if present, may provide very satisfactory tissue for primary coverage of amputation defects.

■ The advantage of this method includes rapid healing with minimal and acceptable shortening, and coverage of the defect with substantial and sensate skin.

■ This technique is illustrated in Figure 14-3 and Figure 14-4.

Primary Closure With Shortening of the Bone. The shortening of the osseous phalanx to obtain satisfactory soft tissue coverage is illustrated in Figure 14-5.

■ After shortening the bone and smoothing its edges with a rasp to round its contour, dorsal and palmar flaps are fashioned and then closed in the coronal plane.

■ The key to closure by this method is to *shorten the bone sufficiently to achieve closure of the skin and soft tissues without tension.*

■ Prior to closure, the digital nerves are identified and gently retracted distally and cut with a scalpel so that they retract proximally into the soft tissues.

Closure by Skin Graft

■ Split-thickness skin graft may be used to promote rapid healing of fingertip amputations.

■ The use of a split-thickness skin graft removed from the forearm with a sterile razor blade and sutured into place over the defect is shown in Figure 14-6. Rapid healing occurred.

  ■ It might be argued that sterile dressings (without a skin graft) might have achieved the same end result, but it may have taken a little longer.

Caveat: Figure 14-7 illustrates the result of a skin graft removed from the forearm of an African American and sutured to a skin loss defect at the tip of his index finger. This resulted in a poor color match, and should be avoided. Figure 14-7B shows a suitable location for removal of a full-thickness skin graft with a suitable color match. The longitudinal axis of the graft is parallel and in the proximal palmar crease. The resultant defect may be closed after limited

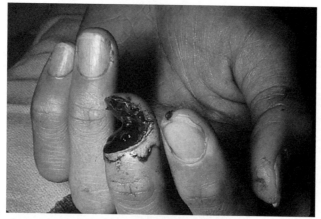
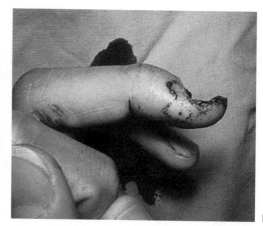
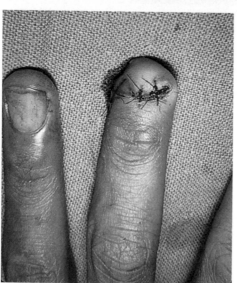

Figure 14-4 **A, B.** A high-speed router blade removed the distal and dorsal aspect of this self-employed carpenter's left middle finger. **C.** Rapid healing with good tissue coverage was achieved by "folding over" the remaining portions of the terminal phalanx.

excision of the palmar fascia in the base of the wound and minimal undermining of the edges. Another suitable source of skin graft is from the "instep" region of the plantar surface of the foot.

Figure 14-8 shows a young African American female with skin loss at the tip of her left thumb, which was treated by application of a full-thickness skin graft from the "instep" on the plantar surface of her foot. The skin graft and donor site healed with minimal scarring, and a good color match was achieved.

Closure by Local Flaps. Local flaps include the VY-plasty, the Kutler, and the Moberg advancement flaps.

VY-Plasty
- This flap is used for closing transversely oriented amputations, and is an alternative to the "fishmouth" closure. Figure 14-9 shows a patient with a three-finger amputation who was treated with a VY-plasty in the ring and index fingers and with a fishmouth closure in the middle finger.
- A V-shaped flap is developed as shown in Figure 14-9B,

and is mobilized and advanced distally to form a Y-shaped configuration.
- Mobilization of the V is carefully performed to avoid loss of its blood supply.
- Bone shortening is used as required.
- Figure 14-9C demonstrates the end result of the VY-plasty in the index and ring fingers, and the end result of the "fishmouth" closure in the middle finger.
- The VY technique is depicted in Figure 14-10.

The Kutler Bilateral VY Advancement Flaps
- This bilateral flap is also a VY advancement flap that is formed on both sides of the digit.
- The flaps are advanced to meet in the midline of the amputation.
- Figure 14-11 illustrates the technique, and Figure 14-12 shows a clinical example.

The Volar Advancement Flap
- This flap is also known as the Moberg flap.
- It is a palmar neurovascular advancement flap that has the potential for excellent sensibility for, and substantial coverage of, an amputated digit.

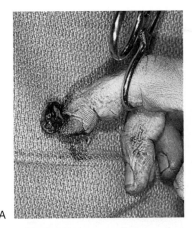
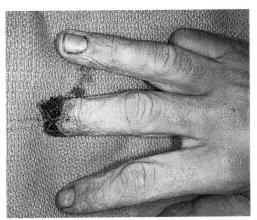
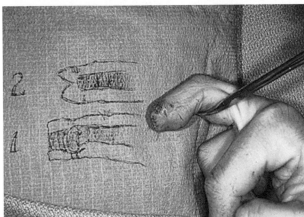
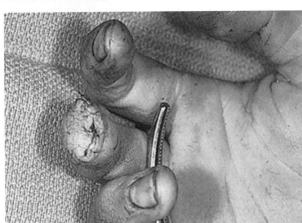

Figure 14-5   **A, B.** Preoperative and injury views of a crush injury to the terminal phalanx of the right middle finger. **C, D.** Revision was accomplished by shortening the osseous phalanx and closing the wound using the "fishmouth" technique, which consists of the formation of dorsal and palmar flaps that are sutured together in the midline.

- It is ideally used in the thumb, and may not be successful in the fingers for a variety of reasons, including flexion contracture and occasional loss of vascularity in the flap.
- Figure 14-13 shows the excellent coverage that can be obtained with this advancement flap.
- The details of the technique are depicted in Figure 14-14.

Closure by Distant Pedicle Flaps

Thenar Flap
- This distant pedicle flap is useful for covering the distal aspect of the index and middle fingers, and, like other distant pedicle flaps, is intended to maintain the length of the digit.
- This flap is best used in those patients who do not have any proclivity for joint stiffness. Some have indicated that it is best used in younger patients who do not have as significant a potential for stiffness as older patients.

Figure 14-15 shows a clinical sequence of a male Pacific Islander with amputations of the tips of the middle and ring fingers. Significant loss of pulp was noted in the middle fin-

ger. A thenar flap was used to restore the pad on the middle finger, and a full-thickness skin graft from the hypothenar eminence was used to cover the amputation at the tip of the ring finger. This graft site was selected as a ready source of full-thickness skin that provided durable coverage for the palmar side of the finger. It also provided an excellent color match for this dark-skinned patient. The end result is noted in Figure 14-15D. A good color match is noted in both digits, the flap and full-thickness donor sites are barely noticeable, and good hand function was recovered. Figure 14-16 is an artist's depiction of the technique.

Cross-Finger Flap
- The cross-finger flap is another technique to cover the tip of an amputated finger; as with other flaps, it is designed to maintain finger length and cover the defect with durable and sensate skin.
- It is very useful for restoring the loss of the pulp on the flexor aspect of the finger.
- Figure 14-17 depicts the sequence of a cross-finger flap used to restore an avulsion of the pulp lost on the flexor surface of the terminal phalanx on the left little finger.

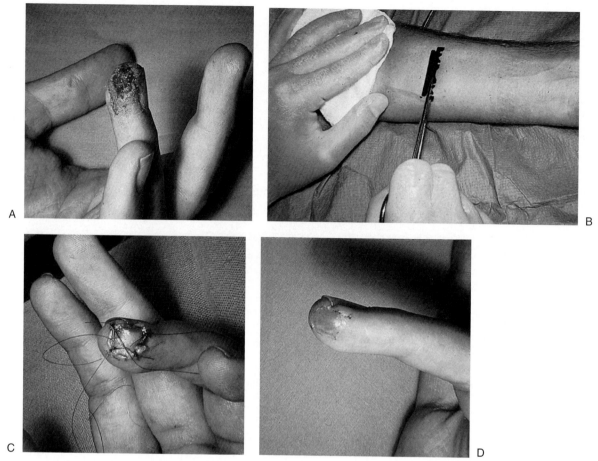

Figure 14-6 **A.** The clinical appearance of a skin defect on the ulnar side of the terminal phalanx of the left ring finger. **B.** A sterile razor blade is used to remove a split-thickness skin graft from the forearm. **C.** The skin graft is sutured into place, and the tails of the suture are left long enough to tie over a cotton stent (not shown) in order to keep the graft firmly applied to its bed. **D.** A complete take of the graft was noted at 10 days.

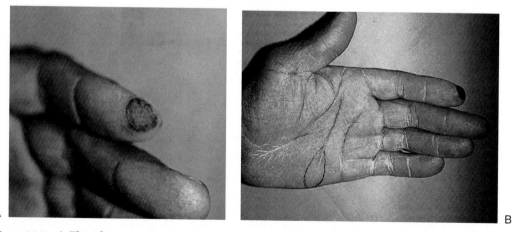

Figure 14-7 **A.** This African American male had a split-thickness skin graft removed from his forearm and applied to a defect at the tip of his left index finger. Note the poor color match. **B.** Area of a more suitable donor site.

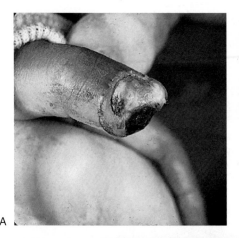

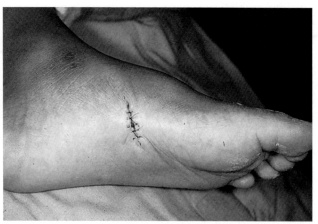

A   B

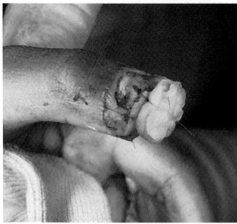

C

Figure 14-8   **A**. This young African American female had a skin defect on the tip of her left thumb. **B**. A full-thickness skin graft was removed from the "instep" region of the plantar surface of her foot and closed primarily. **C**. The graft was sutured in place over the defect beneath a stent, with excellent healing and color match.

- The pedicle flap is raised from the dorsum of the adjacent ring finger down to the paratenon of the extensor mechanism, and it includes the skin and subcutaneous tissue.
- The flap is hinged on the ulnar side of the ring finger, and then sutured to the defect on the little finger.
- The defect on the ring finger is covered with a moderately thick, split-thickness skin graft.
- The flap is divided in 12 to 14 days, and the free margin further inset into the defect.
- Figure 14-18 is an artist's depiction of the cross finger pedicle flap.

Nail Bed Injuries

Subungual Hematoma
- Subungual hematoma may occur following crushing-type injuries due to the abundant blood supply of the nail bed. It may cause severe pain in the digit. It is discussed here because of its association with fingertip injuries.
- Drainage of the hematoma with the incandescent end of a paper clip is a painless way to relieve this condition.
- A radiograph to rule out an associated fracture is useful.
- Some have argued that draining a subungual hematoma in the presence of a fracture may result in an "open fracture," but if a fracture is present by radiograph, sterile dressings may be used until the drainage site closes.

Lacerations and Avulsions
- Nail-bed injuries may occur in conjunction with digit amputations.
- They may occur as simple or complex lacerations and avulsions.
- The nail plate may be present in whole or part, and should not be discarded. Instead, it should be used as a stent following the repair of the nail bed.
- Secondary or delayed reconstruction of these injuries is unpredictable, and the best results are achieved by treatment at the time of the initial injury.

Lacerations
- Some surgeons advocate removal of an attached or partially intact nail plate to facilitate the repair of the underlying nail bed.
- In most cases, however, it may be left in place, where it will act as a biologic stent to recontour and promote the healing of the underlying laceration. Often, the nail is partially avulsed and elevated from its bed. In those cases, the nail may be removed and saved for later reapplication as a biologic stent.
- Simple lacerations of the nail bed are repaired under digital anesthesia and a suitable tourniquet.
- Loupe magnification is useful, and the laceration is sutured with 6-0 or 7-0 chromic or plain gut.
- Following repair, the nail plate is replaced over the repaired nail bed and under the proximal nail fold.

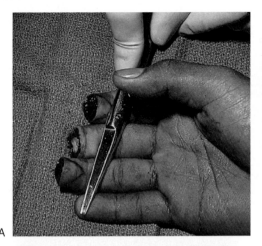

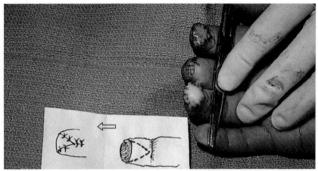

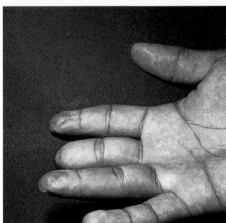

Figure 14-9 **A**. Triple amputation in a patient's right hand. **B**. A VY-plasty has been performed on the index and ring fingers, and a "fish-mouth" closure has been performed on the middle finger. **C**. Note the final result in the three fingers.

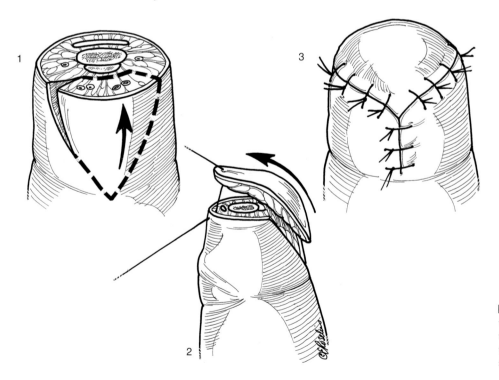

Figure 14-10 Artist's depiction of the VY-plasty technique. The technique is most useful in transverse amputations. Bone shortening is performed as required.

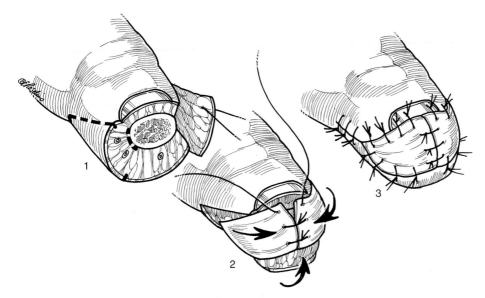

Figure 14-11 Artist's depiction of the Kutler bilateral VY-plasty technique for fingertip amputations.

- This will act as a biologic stent, and will help to contour the nail bed.
- Replacement of the nail plate will prevent scar formation between the proximal nail fold and the bed.
- If the nail is not available, a thin piece of sterile silicone sheet may be cut to duplicate its shape and may be inserted as a replacement.
- The replaced nail will be pushed out as the new nail grows.
- Local wound care and dressings are used to protect the nail bed until the new nail plate covers the matrix.

Avulsions
- Small avulsion defects may be repaired by undermining and advancing the surrounding nail bed to close the defect.
- If a portion of the nail bed remains attached to the undersurface of the nail, it may be reapplied to fill the defect as a free graft.

- If insufficient tissue is available, the great toe can be used with minimal morbidity. The toenail is removed, and a split graft is removed from the nail bed.
- A split graft satisfies the needs of the injured nail bed, and allows healing of the great toe nail bed without side effects.
- The graft is sutured into the defect with fine absorbable sutures as previously described.

Late Reconstruction
- Nail deformities may occur in spite of appropriate treatment, and may be related more to the nature of the original injury than the treatment.
- Common deformities seen are *hook nails*, *split nails* and *non-adherent nails*.

Hook Nail
- Loss of bony support to the distal aspect of the nail bed and plate often results in "hooking," in which the distal aspect of the nail grows towards the palm.

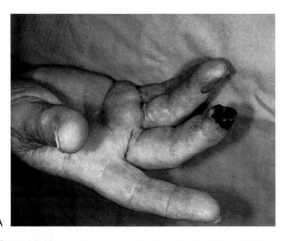
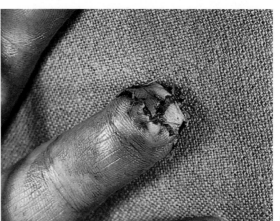

A   B

Figure 14-12 A clinical example of the Kutler bilateral VY-plasty.

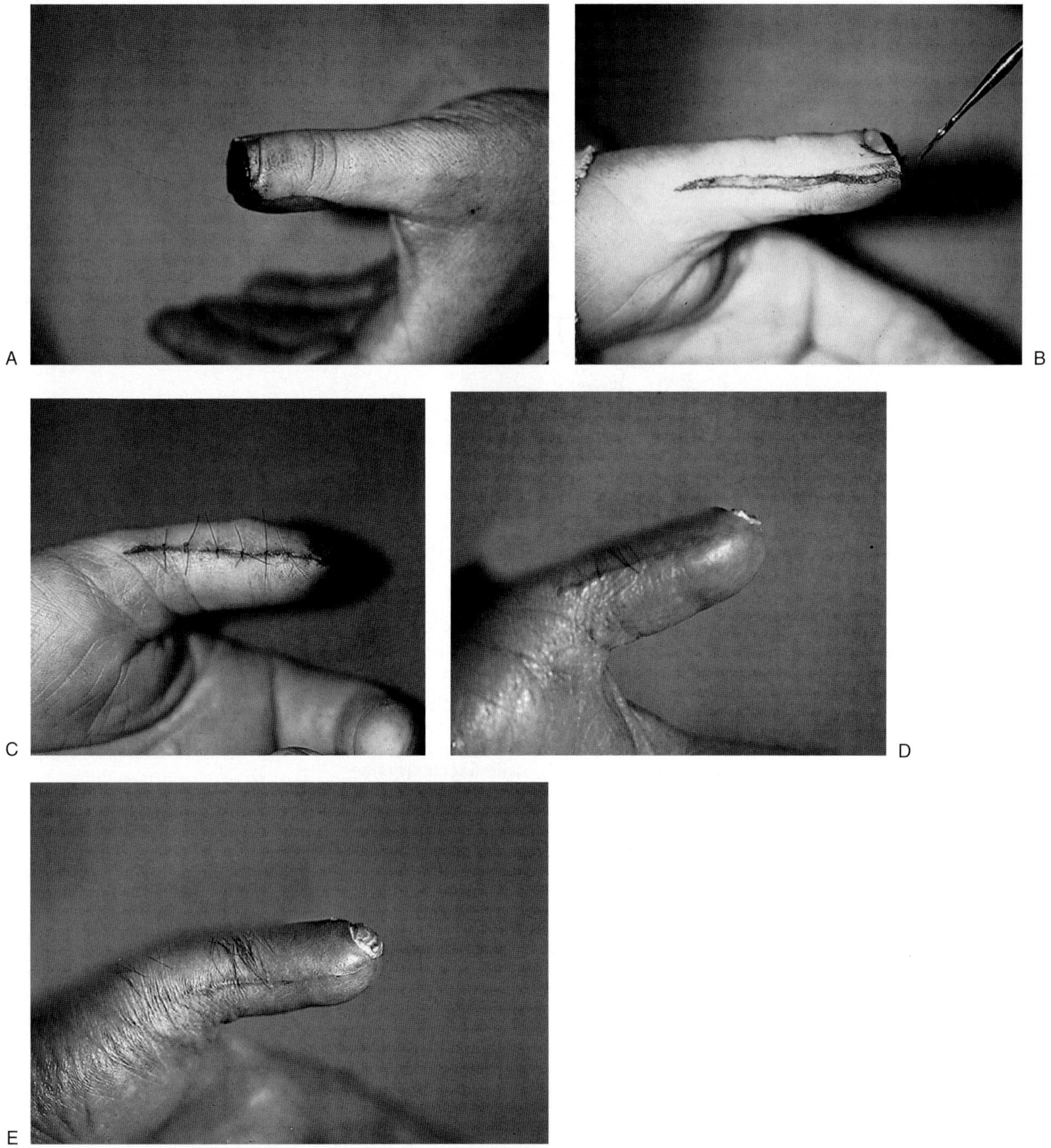

Figure 14-13 The Moberg advancement flap for thumb tip amputations. **A.** Note the transverse amputation through the distal aspect of the left thumb. **B.** A skin hook is used to gently advance the flap that has been incised bilaterally. The flap includes the neurovascular bundles, and is released down to the level of the flexor sheath. **C.** The distal margin of the flap has been advanced to meet the distal edge of the thumbnail, and has been sutured in place with slight flexion of the interphalangeal (IP) joint to facilitate a tension-free closure. **D, E.** Note the excellent pad over the tip of the thumb.

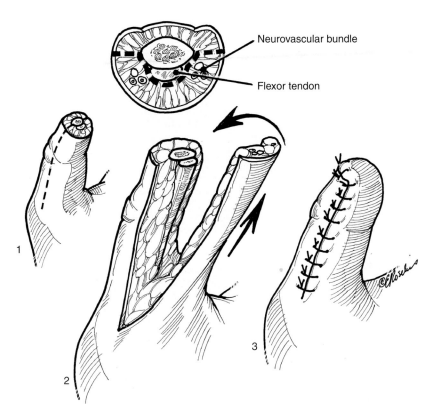

Neurovascular bundle

Flexor tendon

1

2

3

Figure 14-14 Artist's depiction of the Moberg advancement flap. The bilateral midaxial incision is carried to the region of the osseous structures and flexor sheath, and the neurovascular bundle is protected in the flap.

- This can be corrected by removing the nail and trimming the matrix back to the level of the bony support.
- The defect is then closed with an advancement flap without placing any tension on the matrix.

Split and Nonadherent Nail

- Split nails result from a longitudinal scar in the matrix, with an absence of nail-producing cells.
- If the scar is in the dorsal matrix, only a dull streak may appear in the nail plate. If the scar is in the intermediate portion of the germinal matrix, a split or absent nail may occur. If the scar is in the palmar nail or sterile matrix, a split or non-adherence of the nail beyond the scar may occur.
- Nonadherent nails may result from scarring of the germinal matrix, or from a scar in the sterile matrix.
- Treatment involves excising the scar and replacing it with nail matrix.
- Typically, if the defect is large enough to cause a split nail, it cannot be closed primarily and will need a graft.
  - If the defect is in the sterile matrix, it can be treated with a split-thickness graft.
  - The germinal matrix requires a full-thickness graft, which can be taken from the second toe. This will result in a cosmetic defect of a lesser degree than by using the great toe, and still provide adequate matrix for nail regeneration.
- A nonadherent nail typically results from scar in the sterile matrix.
  - This is similarly treated with excision of the scar and placement of a split-thickness matrix graft.
- In severely deformed or bothersome split or loose nails, another option is to remove the entire nail unit and replace it with a split-thickness skin graft.

REPLANTATION

Indications

Indications for replantation have been refined since the first successful limb reattachment was performed in 1962. The current indications for digital replantation are patients with multiple digit amputations, thumb amputations, pediatric patients with amputations, and single digit amputations *distal* to the insertion of the flexor digitorum superficialis tendon. Multilevel amputations offer a greater technical challenge, but may not represent an absolute contraindication to replantation.

Factors such as associated injuries, age, and associated systemic illness all play a role in the decision-making process. Avulsion injuries, and those with massive contamination, may preclude a successful result.

Timing

Muscle tissue is susceptible to irreversible changes after 6 hours of ischemia at room temperature. Digits do not contain muscle, and thus their warm ischemia time is much longer. Successful replantations in digits have occurred after 33 hours of warm ischemia time, and after 94 hours of cold ischemia. These recorded times are at the extreme end of the spectrum of allowable elapsed times prior to replantation; do not take them as an acceptable norm. Thus, transportation of the patient and the amputated part should be as rapid as possible to a center with a replantation capability. When the part has been properly cooled, successful replantation has been achieved in patients after 24 to 30 hours.

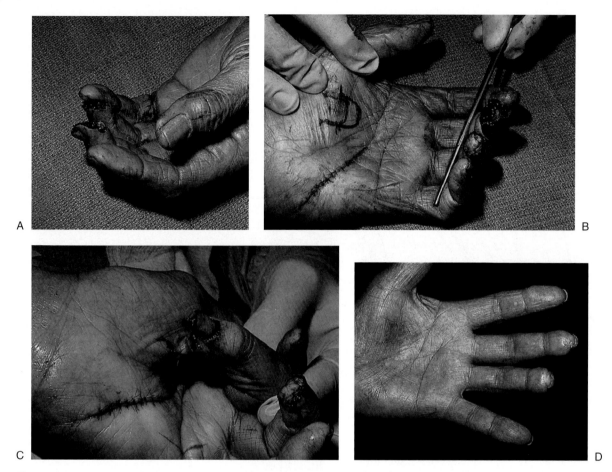

A

B

C

D

Figure 14-15 The thenar flap and color-matched, full-thickness skin graft. **A.** Note the significant loss of pulp in the middle finger, and the loss of skin over the tip of the ring finger. **B.** A full-thickness skin graft was harvested from the hypothenar eminence, the defect closed, and the graft sutured to the ring finger; note the generous length of the thenar flap. **C.** The thenar flap has been elevated and attached to the tip of the middle finger. **D.** Note the excellent functional and cosmetic result.

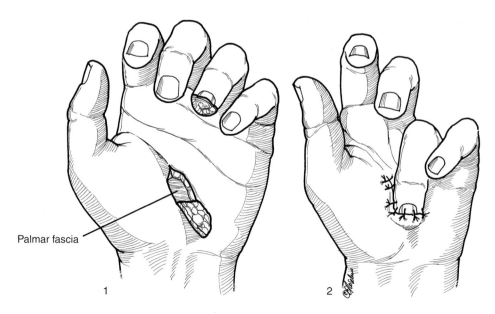

Palmar fascia

1

2

Figure 14-16 Artist's depiction of the technique for the thenar flap.

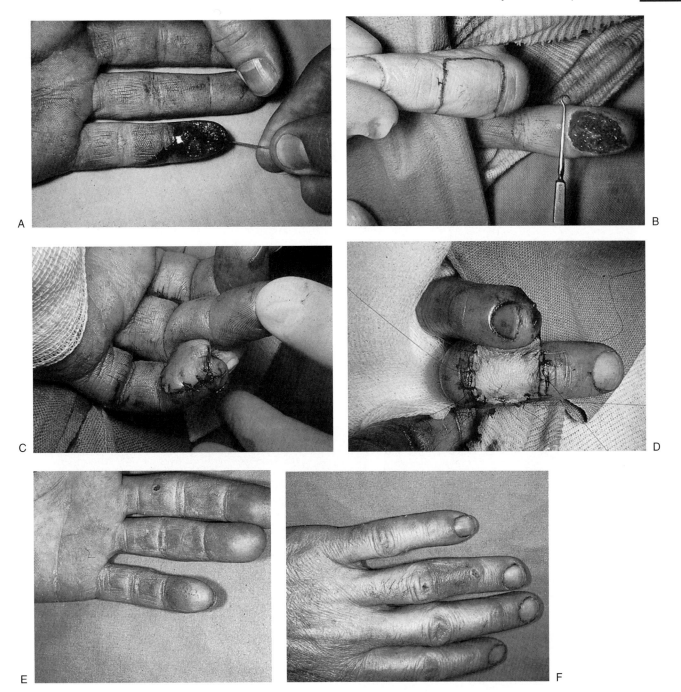

Figure 14-17   The cross-finger pedicle flap.

Steps in Replantation

■ The amputated part must be located and sent with the patient to the most appropriate emergency room. Placing the amputated part in a small plastic bag and laying it on ice is advisable. *The part should not be frozen (no dry ice) or otherwise manipulated.*

■ Ideally, after the patient arrives at the emergency room, an on-call replantation team would divide into two treatment units.

   ■ One team takes the amputated part to the operating room where it is cleaned as needed and kept cool and moist. This team debrides the amputated part as needed and identifies and tags vital structures, including nerves, veins, arteries and tendons.

   ■ The other team should assess the patient with a medical history and physical examination, obtain appropriate laboratory studies, and start general supportive measures as indicated.

■ The details of the replantation procedure is beyond the scope of this text, but they include the shortening and fixation of the bone, repairing flexor and extensor tendons, anastomosis of one or more arteries and two veins, repairing the nerves, and skin coverage.

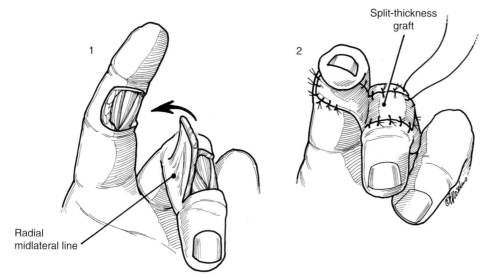

Split-thickness graft

Radial midlateral line

Figure 14-18 Artist's depiction of the cross finger flap.

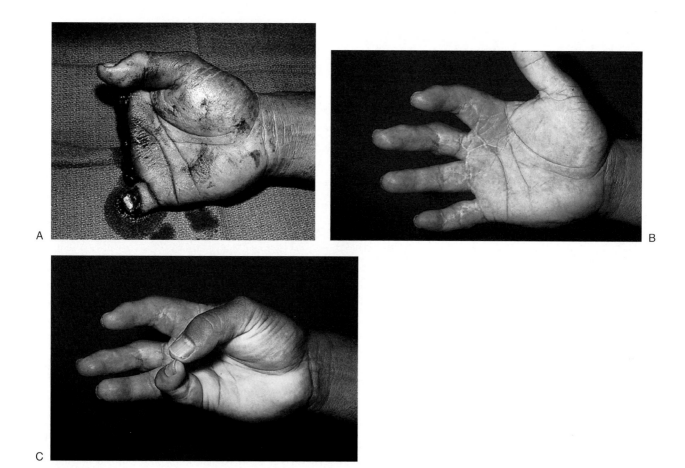

A

B

C

Figure 14-19 Four-finger amputation and successful replantation. **A.** This 34-year-old print shop worker sustained a traumatic amputation of four fingers in a paper cutter. **B.** Successful reattachment was achieved of all four digits. **C.** He regained useful function and sensibility in the hand and returned to work in the print shop.

- Postoperative care includes aspirin for its antiplatelet effect, and some form of anticoagulant therapy of the surgeon's choice. The patient should not be allowed to smoke or drink caffeinated beverages.
- Postoperative monitoring may be accomplished by noting clinical signs such as color, pulp turgor, and capillary refill. However, skin temperature measurements or pulse oximetry may be more reliable.
- Figure 14-19 illustrates a typical replantation patient.

SUGGESTED READING

Atasoy E, Godfrey A, Kalisman M. The antenna procedure for the "hook-nail" deformity. J Hand Surg 1983;8:55–58.

Atasoy E, Ioalimidis, Kasdan ML, Kutz JE. Reconstruction of the amputated fingertip with a triangular volar flap. J Bone Joint Surg 1970;52A:921–926.

Chang J, Jones N. Twelve simple maneuvers to optimize digital replantation and revascularization. Tech in Hand Upper Extremity Surgery 2004;8:161–166.

Chow SP, Ho E. Open treatment of fingertip injuries in adults. J Hand Surg 1982;7:470–476.

Cronin TD. The cross finger flap: a new method of repair. Am Surg 1951;17:419–425.

Das SK, Brown HG. Management of lost finger tips in children. Hand 1978;10:16–27.

Flatt AE. The thenar flap. J Bone Joint Surg 1957;39B:80–85.

Graham B. Major replantation versus revision amputation and prosthetic fitting in the upper extremity: a late functional outcomes study. J Hand Surg 1998;23:783–791.

Kumar VP, Satku K. Treatment and prevention of "hook-nail" deformity with anatomic correlation. J Hand Surg 1993;18A:617–620.

Kutler W. A new method for finger tip amputation. JAMA 1947; 133:29–30.

Moberg E. Aspects of sensation in reconstructive surgery of the upper extremity. J Bone Joint Surg 1964; 46A:817–825.

Yong FC, Teoh LC. Nail bed reconstruction with split-thickness nail bed grafts. J Hand Surg 1992;17B:193–197.

COMPARTMENT SYNDROME

DEFINITIONS

Anatomic Compartments

An *anatomic compartment* is defined as an enclosed space formed by fascia, or a combination of fascia and bone, that contains one or more muscles. An exception to this definition is the carpal tunnel, which contains nine flexor tendons but no muscle—except for those individuals with low-lying muscle fibers from the flexor digitorum superficialis (FDS) that sometimes extend into the carpal canal. The contents of an anatomic compartment are muscles, arteries, veins, and nerves.

Compartment Syndrome

Compartment syndrome is defined as a symptom complex resulting from increased tissue pressure within a limited space that compromises the circulation and function of the contents of that space. This occurs when intramuscular pressure is elevated to a level, and for a period of time, sufficient to reduce capillary perfusion.

The muscle component of the various compartments is the *primary target* of the pathological process; the nerves are the *secondary targets.*

Following sustained vascular compromise, the muscle undergoes necrosis, fibrosis, and contracture; associated nerve injury causes further muscle dysfunction, sensibility deficits, or chronic pain. The end result is a dysfunctional muscle compartment with local and distant manifestations that depend upon the compartment involved and the degree of muscle contracture and nerve dysfunction.

Types

Acute. An acute compartment syndrome results when intramuscular pressure (IMP) exceeds capillary blood pressure for a prolonged period of time. In this circumstance, immediate decompression is required to prevent muscle necrosis.

Chronic or Exertional. This condition occurs when exercise increases IMP enough to cause ischemia, pain, and in some instances, diminished sensibility or neurological dysfunction.

If a particular compartment is hypertrophied or confined by tighter-than-normal fascia, small increases of volume associated with exercise may significantly increase IMP.

Symptoms usually disappear with cessation of the activity but appear again with resumption of the activity. If the activity is continued in spite of pain and neurologic deficit for a sufficient period of time, an acute compartment syndrome may result. This condition is seen most often in the lower extremity, but it also may occur in the upper extremity.

Volkmann's Ischemic Contracture

This condition is defined as the *end result* of irreversible hypoxic damage to muscles, nerves, and vascular endothelium of an anatomic compartment. It may be categorized as mild, moderate, or severe. In its *mild* form, portions of normal muscle are replaced by contractile scar tissue that shortens or contracts the affected muscle. The adjacent nerves are not affected and the resultant deformity may be minimal.

In the *moderate* form the muscle or muscles are more severely involved, and the adjacent nerves may be affected to some degree. The end result is a more significant deformity involving the FDS and flexor pollicis longus (FPL)—and in some instances, portions of the FDS muscles and the median nerve.

In the *severe* type, all of the digital flexors are involved, along with the extrinsic wrist flexors. In some cases, the muscles in the extensor and mobile wad compartment are also involved. The median nerve is severely compromised, and often degenerates into a fibrous tissue thread at its midaspect. Although less likely to be involved, the ulnar nerve may also be compromised. The end result is a severe flexion contracture of the wrist and digits, with significant sensory deficit. Figure 15-1 depicts the clinical and intraoperative appearance of Volkmann's ischemic contracture.

ANATOMIC COMPARTMENTS IN THE UPPER EXTREMITY

There are 13 compartments in the upper extremity from the shoulder to the hand. They are the deltoid, anterior arm, posterior arm, mobile wad of the forearm, flexor forearm, extensor forearm, and pronator quadratus. In the hand they

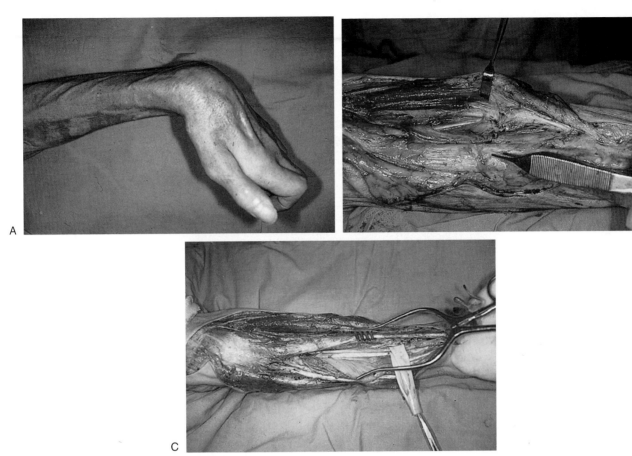

Figure 15-1 Clinical and intraoperative appearance of Volkmann's ischemic contracture in an elderly alcoholic. **A.** Note the fixed and flexed wrist, the adduction contracture of the thumb, and the claw deformity of the fingers. **B.** Note the necrotic muscle at the tip of the forceps. **C.** The median nerve was surrounded by necrotic muscle (Penrose drain).

include the central palmar, adductor, thenar, hypothenar, interosseous, and finger compartments. The central palmar compartment contains the lumbrical muscles, and thus meets the definition of a compartment. The finger or digits, although not a definite compartment, may require release if they are significantly compromised by both internal and external pressure. The *flexor forearm* (Figure 15-2) and the *interosseous* (Figure 15-3) compartments have the greatest clinical significance, since development of a compartment

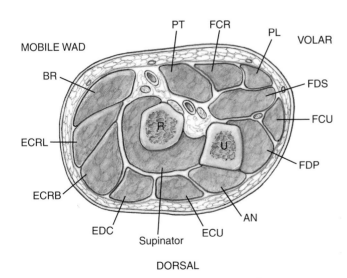

Figure 15-2 The three forearm compartments: the flexor containing the finger, thumb, and wrist flexors; the extensor containing the finger, thumb, and ulnar wrist extensor (ECU); and the mobile wad of three, which is represented by the brachioradialis and the ECRL and ECRB (radial wrist extensors). R, radius; U, ulna.

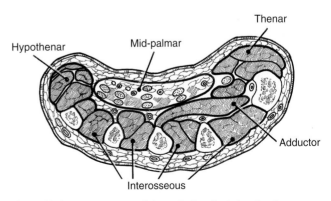

Figure 15-3 Cross section of the midpalm, depicting the thenar, adductor, interosseous, midpalmar, and hypothenar spaces.

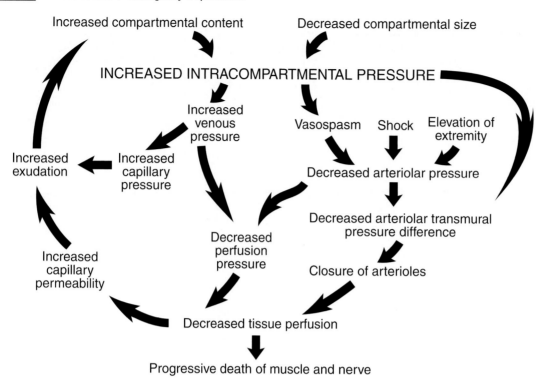

Figure 15-4   Matsen's unified concept of compartment syndrome (see text for details).

syndrome in these two locations probably results in the most significant functional loss and deformity.

ETIOLOGY AND PATHOPHYSIOLOGY

- Compartment syndrome is caused by elevated pressure inside a closed compartment.
- Matsen's unified concept of compartment syndrome is presented in Figure 15-4.
- Increased pressure within a compartment may be caused by either an increased volume within the compartment (such as fracture, hemorrhage, soft-tissue injury, and snake bite) or a decrease in the size of the compartment (such as a tight cast or dressing, burn eschar, or prolonged external limb pressure during anesthesia or during an unconscious state resulting from drugs or alcohol).
- In children, supracondylar fractures of the humerus are a frequent cause because of a cast that fits tightly, or an injury or occlusion of the brachial artery.
- Because of the relatively noncompliant nature of the fascia around the specific anatomic compartments, either of these two situations will result in an increase in pressure.
- Increased pressure within a compartment decreases the blood supply to the soft tissues, resulting in tissue hypoxia and damage.
- The blood flow is determined by several factors, including arterial pressure, venous pressure, resistance within the vessel, and local tissue pressure.
- The difference between the arterial and venous pressures is the arteriovenous gradient.
  - This gradient, and therefore blood flow, will be decreased if venous pressure is increased or if the in-

coming arterial blood pressure is decreased (such as in shock, hemorrhage, or limb elevation).
  - All blood vessels, but particularly the *microcirculation* and veins, are collapsible. Blood flow, therefore, also can be decreased if the surrounding tissue pressure exceeds both the strength of the vessel wall and the pressure within the vessel.
- Tissue pressure affects both the flow through a vessel, and the fluid equilibrium and exchange across the walls of the microcirculation.
- Both the fluid pressure within the capillary and the surrounding tissues, and the respective osmotic pressures within the tissue and plasma, determine fluid exchange.

DIAGNOSIS

The discussion of diagnosis will be focused on the forearm and hand compartments, and will include acute carpal tunnel syndrome.

The six Ps of diagnosis of acute compartment syndrome are given in Box 15-1. Compartment syndrome must be distinguished from arterial injury and nerve injury. Table 15-1, based on five of the six Ps, helps to differentiate compartment syndrome from the ischemia associated with arterial injury or from the findings in nerve injury that might mimic some of the components of compartment syndrome.

Acute Compartment Syndrome of the Forearm

- The diagnosis of forearm compartment syndrome is made by clinical findings, and may be confirmed by measurement of intracompartmental pressure.

BOX 15-1 THE SIX P'S OF DIAGNOSIS OF ACUTE COMPARTMENT SYNDROME

- Pressure (elevated)
- Pain (especially with passive stretch of the involved muscle[s])
- Paresthesia
- Paresis or Paralysis
- Pink skin color
- Pulse (usually intact)

Clinical Findings

- Clinical findings include the following:
  - A swollen, tense, tender compartment with overlying skin that is often pink or red (Figure 15-5).
  - Pain that may seem out of proportion to the injury.
  - Sensory deficits or paresthesias.
  - Paresis or paralysis.
  - Distal pulses are usually intact.
- Pain is usually increased by passive stretch of the muscles in the affected compartment. For pain in the flexor forearm compartment, stretching regimens would include passive extension of the wrist and finger flexors.
  - This finding may not be specific or reliable if there is an associated fracture or blunt trauma.
- Sensory changes usually occur before motor deficits.
  - Radial and ulnar pulses are usually intact, since systolic arterial pressure (+/− 120 mm Hg) exceeds the pressure within the involved compartment.
- If the extremity is swollen, Doppler examination may be useful to determine the status of the pulse.
- Pink or red discoloration of the skin may be absent, and temperature, capillary refill, and compartment turgor may not be reliable signs in many instances.
- *In children, anxiety associated with an increasing analgesic requirement is a very reliable indicator of compartment syndrome.*

TABLE 15-1 DIFFERENTIAL DIAGNOSIS OF COMPARTMENT SYNDROME, ARTERIAL INJURY, AND NERVE INJURY BASED ON FIVE P'S

	Compartment Syndrome	Arterial Injury	Nerve Injury
Pressure in compartment	+	−	−
Pain with stretch	+	+	−
Paresthesia or anesthesia	+	+	+
Paresis or paralysis	+	+	+
Pulses intact	+	−	+

Note: Taken from Hargens AR, Mubarak SJ. Current concepts in pathophysiology, evaluation, and diagnosis of compartment syndrome. Hand Clinics 1998;14:371–384.

Intracompartmental Pressure Measurements

- Although the diagnosis of compartment syndrome may be made clinically, the measurement of the intracompartmental pressure is an additional diagnostic tool that may aid in confirmation of the diagnosis.
- Compartment pressures can be measured by the needle manometer technique, continuous infusion technique, the wick or slit catheter technique, or with transducers that measure pressures digitally.
- Self-contained devices with instructions for use, such as the Stryker and Whitesides pressure monitor, are commercially available.
- It is important to become familiar with at least one of these techniques or devices so that the necessary tools may be readily located in your emergency department, clinic, or hospital, and utilized in a timely fashion.
- The threshold pressures considered consistent with a compartment syndrome range from 45 mm Hg to 20 mm Hg below diastolic pressure.
- Animal studies of compartment syndrome have indicated that clinical signs along with compartment pressures of 30 mm Hg or greater are consistent with compartment syndrome.

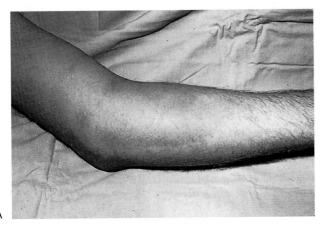
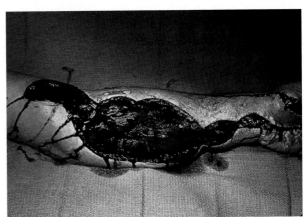

Figure 15-5   Acute compartment syndrome of the forearm. **A.** This patient was obtunded from drugs. He lay on his left arm/forearm for an unknown length of time; note the swelling in the forearm and arm. He complained of severe pain. **B.** He was immediately taken to the operating room, where a comprehensive fasciotomy was performed, which revealed swollen and edematous forearm muscles.

■ Figure 15-6 demonstrates ulnar and dorsal approaches for needle placement in the flexor aspect of the forearm.

Acute Compartment Syndrome of the Hand

Clinical Findings

■ The carpal tunnel, although not a true compartment, may act as a closed space, and the median nerve may be subject to the adverse effects of increased pressure.

■ The hand compartments that may be involved in compartment syndrome are the interosseous (both dorsal and palmar), the thenar and hypothenar, the adductor, and the fingers.

■ The clinical findings in compartment syndrome in the hand are similar to the previously described findings in the forearm, and include pain in the region, pain with passive stretch of the involved muscles, localized swelling, paresthesia in the involved nerve distribution, and muscle paresis.

■ In the hand, all the intrinsic muscles may be evaluated by passively abducting and adducting the digits with the metacarpophalangeal (MCP) joints in extension and the proximal interphalangeal (PIP) joints in flexion.

■ The adductor compartment in the thumb is tested by positioning the thumb in palmar abduction to produce stretching of the adductor.

■ The thenar muscles are stretched by abduction and extension of the thumb, and the hypothenar muscles are stretched by abduction and extension of the little finger.

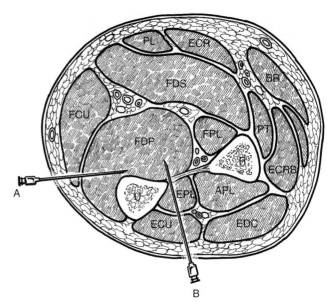

Figure 15-6   Ulnar and dorsal approaches for needle/catheter placement in the flexor forearm to obtain intracompartmental pressure. The starting point for both approaches is at the junction of the proximal and middle third of the *supinated* forearm. **A.** The ulnar approach inserts the needle/catheter into the deep or profundus compartment using the ulna as a guide. **B.** The dorsal approach permits measurement of the dorsal compartment pressures, as well as the deep compartment depending on the depth of insertion. R, radius; U, ulna.

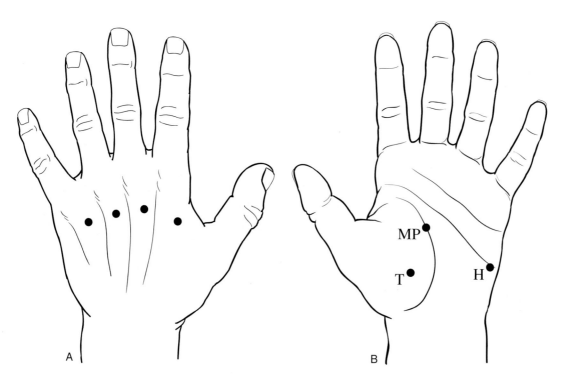

Figure 15-7   Portals for compartment pressure measurements in the hand. **A.** Interosseous compartment pressures may be measured through these four portals on the dorsum of the hand. **B.** The thenar (T), midpalmar (MP), and hypothenar (H) compartments may be measured through these portals.

- Swelling and increased tissue turgor may be noted over the individual involved compartments.
- In the fingers, the amount of swelling and the nature of the injury—as well as the presence of a nonyielding burn eschar—may indicate increased pressure and the need for a fasciotomy.
- Potential compartments are present in the finger due to the presence of fascial bands around the neurovascular bundles, including Grayson's and Cleland's ligaments.

Measurement of Intracompartmental Pressures in the Hand

- Figure 15-7 depicts the sites of needle placement for measurement of compartment pressures in the hand.

TREATMENT OF ACUTE COMPARTMENT SYNDROMES

Forearm Compartment Syndrome

- The goals of treatment are to restore *microcirculation* to the compartment through decompression.

Nonsurgical Treatment

- This includes splitting or removing a tight cast, including the removal of cast padding and tight dressings or bandages of any type *down to the level of the skin.*
- If these maneuvers fail to resolve the problem, then immediate operative decompression is performed.
- Decompression is typically achieved by fasciotomy.

Surgical Treatment

Flexor Forearm Compartment Syndrome

- The forearm compartments (involving the forearm flexor compartment and the mobile wad compartment) are decompressed by a comprehensive incision from the distal arm to the midpalm, as noted in Figure 15-8 and 15-5B.
- The deep fascia is incised from the region of the distal arm to, and including, the carpal canal.
  - The underlying flexor muscles will often bulge dramatically into the wound.
- The median nerve is at risk at four locations: the lacertus fibrosus, the pronator teres, the deep fascial arcade of the flexor digitorum superficialis, and the carpal tunnel.
- If preoperative findings indicate that the ulnar nerve is involved, it is also decompressed as indicated at the cubital tunnel, forearm, and Guyon's canal at the wrist and hand.

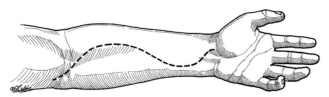

Figure 15-8 Comprehensive incision for release of the volar forearm compartment syndrome. Note that the incision includes the distal arm and should include the carpal tunnel.

- If signs of radial nerve dysfunction are present, decompression of the radial tunnel may also be indicated (see Chapter 7, Entrapment Neuropathies, for details of radial nerve decompression).
- Coexisting forearm fractures are usually stabilized operatively at the time of fasciotomy.
- Skin incisions are left open to accommodate swelling, but are loosely reapproximated to cover the nerves.
- If fractures are open and contaminated, fasciotomy is performed, wounds debrided, and fractures stabilized.
- In contaminated wounds, external fixation or limited internal fixation may be preferable to standard internal fixation methods.
- Skin grafting and limited secondary closure is performed when wounds demonstrate clean granulation tissue.

Release of Extensor Forearm Compartment

- Compartment syndromes involving the forearm extensor compartment are released through a dorsal incision.
- When both the flexor and extensor compartments are involved, it is preferable to release the flexor compartment first; the relaxation afforded by the skin and fascia often decompresses the dorsal compartments.
- Dorsal compartment pressures are used to determine whether or not to release the extensor compartment.
  - If required, it is released through a longitudinal incision 2 cm lateral and distal to the lateral epicondyle. The incision is continued distally to the myotendinous junction of the extensor muscles in the midforearm.
- Fasciotomy is also indicated at the time of limb revascularization if the duration of ischemia has been as much as 4 to 6 hours.
- Post revascularization edema may precipitate compartment syndrome, and prophylactic fasciotomy is indicated.

Hand Compartment Syndrome

- The principles of treatment of hand compartment syndromes are similar to those of the forearm.
- The appropriate incisions for decompression of the various hand compartments are depicted in Figure 15-9.
- The essentials of the deeper dissection for decompression of the hand compartments are given in Figure 15-10.
- Release of swollen fingers may be required based on the amount of swelling and the nature of the skin envelope.
- If a significant burn eschar or swelling is present, digital fasciotomies are performed through midlateral incisions on the nondominant or noncontact side of the digits. The incisions are dorsal to the neurovascular bundles; Cleland's and Grayson's ligaments are incised.
- The dissection usually ends at the flexor sheath.
- The incision is centered over the PIP joint and may extend 2 cm proximal and 2 cm distal to the PIP joint, as described in Figure 15-11.

Prognosis and Caveats for Acute Compartment Syndrome

- The prognosis depends on the *intensity* and *duration* of the elevated compartment pressure.

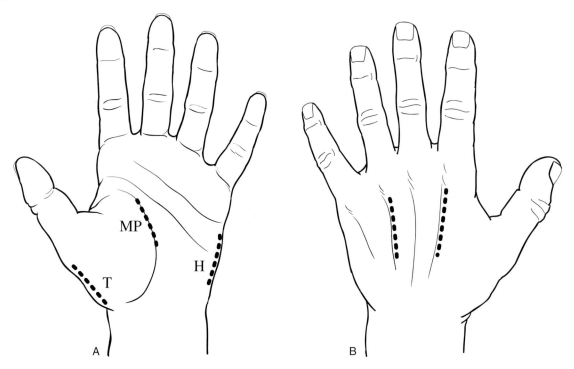

Figure 15-9 Appropriate incisions for release of the hand compartments. **A.** The thenar (T), midpalmar (MP), and hypothenar (H) incisions. **B.** Suitable incisions for release of the interosseous compartments.

■ Therefore, *time is of the essence in the management of compartment syndrome.*

■ If clinical findings and/or pressure readings are suggestive, but not conclusive, remember that the scar from a fasciotomy incision is of relatively minimal consequence compared to an untreated compartment syndrome that results in a Volkmann's ischemic contracture.

TREATMENT OF VOLKMANN'S ISCHEMIC CONTRACTURE

■ Treatment goals are to increase function, decrease associated pain factors if present, and, if possible, restore limb sensibility.

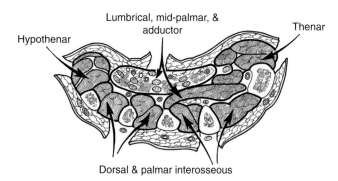

Figure 15-10 Depiction of the details of the deeper dissection for release of the interosseous muscle compartments, the thenar compartment, the midpalmar and adductor compartments (both of which may be released through a midpalmar incision), and the hypothenar compartment.

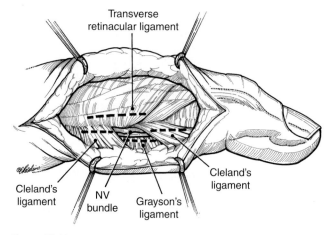

Figure 15-11 Midaxial incision for release of compromised digits in compartment syndrome.

Nonsurgical Treatment

■ Treatment of *mild* contractures depends upon the severity of the deformity and the time interval between injury and initiation of treatment.

■ Contractures of the deep forearm flexors, with normal hand sensibility and preservation of remaining extrinsic muscle strength, are treated by a comprehensive hand rehabilitation program that includes active and passive mobilization, strengthening, and static and dynamic extension splinting. This regimen works to improve thumb web space width, strengthen weak thumb intrinsic muscles, and correct or improve digital flexion contractures.

Surgical Treatment

■ Treatment of *moderate to severe* contractures is based on elimination of contractures, release of secondary nerve compression, and tendon transfers to recover some of the lost function.

■ The surgical procedures employed include excision of the muscle infarct, tendon lengthening, muscles slides, neurolysis (or nerve graft in very severe cases), and various tendon transfers to restore balance and function.

■ Microvascular free tissue transfers of nerve and muscle have been promising in severe cases of Volkmann's contracture.

SUGGESTED READING

Botte MJ, Gelberman RH. Acute compartment syndrome of the forearm. Hand Clinics 1998;14:391–403.

Botte MJ, Keenan MAE, Gelberman RH. Volkmann's ischemic contracture of the upper extremity. Hand Clinics 1998;14:483–497.

Doyle JR. Anatomy of the upper extremity muscle compartments. Hand Clinics 1998;14:343–364.

Hargens AR, Mubarak SJ. Current concepts in the pathophysiology, evaluation and diagnosis of compartment syndrome. Hand Clinics 1998;14:371–383.

Kadiyala RK, Waters PM. Upper extremity pediatric compartment syndromes. Hand Clinics 1998;14:467–475.

Matsen FA III, Clawson DK. Compartment syndromes: a unified concept. Clin Orthop 1975; 113:8–14.

McDougal CG, Johnson GHF. A new technique of catheter placement for measurement of forearm compartment pressure. J Trauma 1991;31:1404–1408.

Mubarak SJ, Hargens AR, Owen CA, et al. The wick-catheter technique for measurement of intramuscular pressure. A new clinical and research tool. J Bone Joint Surg 1976;58A:1016–1020.

Ortiz JA, Berger RA. Compartment syndrome of the hand and wrist. Hand Clinics 1998;14:405–418.

Szabo RM. Acute carpal tunnel syndrome. Hand Clinics 1998;14:419–429.

Tsuge K. Management of established Volkmann's Contracture. In: Green DP, Hotchkiss RN, Pederson WC, eds. Green's operative hand surgery. 4th Ed. New York: Churchill Livingstone, 1999:593–603.

Von Schroeder HP, Botte MJ. Definitions and terminology of compartment syndrome and Volkmann's ischemic contracture of the upper extremity. Hand Clin 1998;14:331–341.

Whitesides TE Jr, Heckman MM. Acute compartment syndrome: update on diagnosis and treatment. J Am Acad Orthop Surg 1996;4:209–218.

INJECTION INJURIES

Injection injuries may occur secondary to penetration of the skin by fluids under high pressure, therapeutic injections (infusions) of chemotherapeutic agents, or self-injection of various narcotic agents in addiction.

HIGH-PRESSURE INJECTION INJURIES

History

These injuries are most often seen in commercial painters, mechanics, heavy equipment operators, and others who work with various fluids under high pressure. The fluids or materials involved may be paint or paint solvents, grease, or hydraulic fluids under high pressure. A common history is that of a painter cleaning his spray gun at the end of the day and checks to see if the gun is clean by spraying the tip of his finger to see if the resultant spray is clear. A similar scenario is that of a heavy equipment operator who notes a leak in a hydraulic line and tries to correct it by holding a rag around the leak. Yet another scenario is the mechanic who wants to know if he still has some grease in his gun, and therefore places the tip of the grease gun on the tip of his finger and pulls the release trigger.

Pathomechanics of Injury

All of the above described scenarios result in the easy penetration of the skin envelope by the various high-pressure fluids. The materials fill the tissue spaces and travel along fascial planes in the line of least resistance. They are very injurious to the tissues, and that—combined with the mechanical factors of increased tissue pressure—produces ischemia and tissue necrosis. Latex or water-based paint is the least noxious of the listed materials, but are still associated with significant soft tissue changes.

Diagnosis and Physical Findings

- The diagnosis is made by the history of what at first may seem a very minimal injury that later develops into a major problem *with pain that may be out of proportion to the physical findings.*

- These patients may be seen in an emergency room setting. The initial findings may not be very striking in terms of appearance of the digit or hand, but as the condition develops they may be associated with severe pain.
- The worker may be hesitant to admit the true mechanism of the injury due to embarrassment.
- The initial physical findings may be negligible, with little or no evidence of penetration except for some swelling in the digit or palm.
- As the chemical irritation develops, there is increased swelling and signs of inflammation. Pain becomes a major factor.

Treatment

- Treatment consists of early decompression through appropriate incisions.
- The aim is to decompress the involved area and to remove as much of the injected material as possible.
- Amputation may be avoided by early treatment that includes wide debridement, open drainage, repeat debridement as indicated, and delayed wound closure (Figure 16-1).

Prognosis

- These injuries result in severe tissue ischemia with necrosis, which may result in amputation.
- Rates of amputation vary from 16% to 48%.
- The outcome from these injuries depends on the type and amount of material injected, the presence of infection, and the interval between injury and removal of the injected material.
- Stiffness is a recognized complication, and the overall prognosis is guarded in these injuries.

THERAPEUTIC INJECTION INJURIES

Injections or infusions are ordinarily safe, but may lead to serious problems because of incorrect placement of needles or catheters, or because of fluid extravasation with tissue necrosis. The latter complication may be seen with

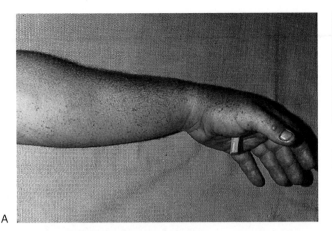

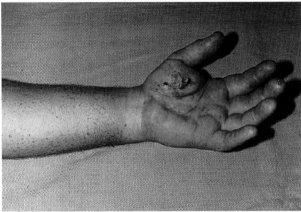

A

B

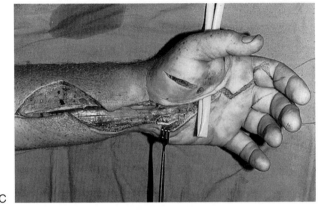

C

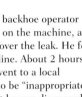

Figure 16-1   **A, B.** This 25-year-old, left-handed backhoe operator detected a small leak in one of the hydraulic lines on the machine, and attempted to stop it by forcibly holding an oil rag over the leak. He felt a stinging sensation in his hand and let go of the line. About 2 hours later he had increasing pain in his left hand and went to a local emergency room, where his pain was considered to be "inappropriate." He was sent home with pain pills. Later that night he was diagnosed with a hydraulic fluid injection injury; the site of entry at the thenar eminence was opened through a small incision, and a small drain inserted. **C.** Further consultation revealed the extensive nature of the injury, and a comprehensive decompression was performed both to remove additional hydraulic fluid and to debride the wound. Delayed wound closure was performed at a later date, and his residuals were those of mild to moderate stiffness in the left thumb.

intravenous chemotherapeutic agents used in cancer therapy, and may result in significant soft tissue loss that requires appropriate soft tissue coverage.

Medications designed for intravenous use mistakenly placed into an artery may result in arterial spasm with muscle ischemia and necrosis. Nerve injuries have been observed in the forearm following extravasation of physiologic intravenous fluids used for rehydration, due to increased hydrostatic pressure rather than any toxicity specific to the fluid. Steroid injection used for treatment of carpal tunnel syndrome, if placed intrafascicularly, may have an adverse effect on nerve function.

SELF-INFLICTED INJECTION INJURIES

These injuries may present in a variety of ways because many different agents may be used. The portal may or may not be

readily evident. Manifestations include infection, edema, and chronic induration of soft tissues. Portals may be intravenous or intra-arterial. If sufficient changes are produced in the arterial lining or wall, ischemia or necrosis may be seen.

SUGGESTED READING

Frederick HA, Carter PR, Littler JW. Injection injuries to the median and ulnar nerves at the wrist. J Hand Surg 1992;17A:645–647.

MacKinnon SE, Hudson AR, Gentili F, et al. Peripheral nerve injection injury with steroid agents. Plastic Reconstr Surg 1982;69:482–489.

Pinto MR, Turkula-Pinto LD, Cooney WP, et al. High-pressure injection injuries of the hand: review of 25 patients managed by open wound technique. J Hand Surg 1993;18A:125–130.

Stanley D, Connolly WB. Iatrogenic injection injuries of the hand and upper limb. J Hand Surg 1992;17B:442–46.

INDEX